BOO~~KS~~

IO856135

MODERN
SKIN THERAPY
with
'GENATOSAN'
MEDICATED CREAMS

A new range of medicated creams prepared with an emulsifying base, characterised by their non-greasy and water-miscible nature and corresponding in formulæ to ointments of recognised value in the treatment of skin diseases. Advantages include rapid absorption and ease of removal from skin or clothing without the aid of soap or friction.

Examples : No. 2, Sulphanilamide 5%; No. 3, Benzyl Benzoate 10%; No. 6, Gentian Violet 0.5%; No. 8, Whitfield's formula; No. 13, Ichthammol 5%; No. 14, Sulphathiazole 5%.

Further information may be obtained from the manufacturers

GENATOSAN LTD.
LOUGHBOROUGH, LEICESTERSHIRE
Telephone: LOUGHBOROUGH 2292

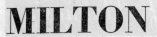

WISE NURSING

In general practice covering the treatment of patients of all ages, it has been found that there is frequent need of alkaline medication for conditions complicated by acidity and irritation of the eliminatory system.

Clinical experience confirms the value of 'Milk of Magnesia' as an antacid for routine use. Composed of a fine suspension of magnesium hydroxide, it is markedly effective in counteracting hyperacidity, while its emollient properties have a soothing effect on the inflamed gastric mucosa.

'Milk of Magnesia' will be found of particular value in relieving colic and vomiting due to digestive upset, while its laxative properties ensure the removal of toxic waste products.

Also 'Milk of Magnesia' Tablets, each equivalent to a teaspoonful of the liquid.

THE CHAS. H. PHILLIPS CHEMICAL CO. LTD.

179 Acton Vale, London, W.3

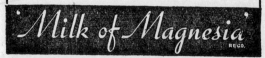
'Milk of Magnesia'
REGD.

'Milk of Magnesia' is the Registered Trade Mark of Phillips' preparation of magnesia.

A SIMPLE CARMINATIVE for

Babies suffering 'WIND=PAIN'

This is usually a temporary discomfort which merely needs a few words of advice to the Mother.

"Gripe Water" made by Woodwards is a simple carminative based on a Doctor's prescription, and used by generations of Mothers for the past 90 years.

A teaspoonful relieves Baby's "Wind-Pain" and sends him back to healthy sleep.

All Babies love "Gripe Water," and it prevents disturbed nights for the Mother.

FROM ALL CHEMISTS

For Delicate Children
THE ANSWER IS
"ROBOLEINE"

Time and time again Nurses are asked: "What is the best food to build him up?"

The answer in one word is "ROBOLEINE," because it is made from Red and Yellow Bone-Marrow, Egg Yolk and Vitamin Concentrate, and each teaspoonful is standardised to contain 190 I.U. of Vitamin A and 140 I.U. of Vitamin D.

This means that, apart from the other good things it contains, **a teaspoonful of "Roboleine" is equivalent in Vitamin D to a tablespoonful of Malt and Oil.**

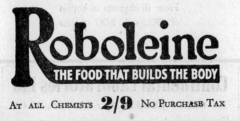

Roboleine
THE FOOD THAT BUILDS THE BODY

AT ALL CHEMISTS **2/9** NO PURCHASE TAX

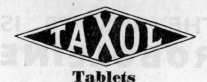
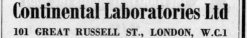

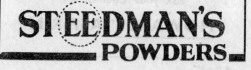

Modern Medical Textbooks

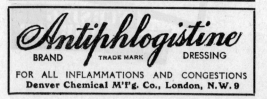

THE

energen

DIETARY SERVICE

The book of detachable Diet
Sheets, as supplied to the medical
profession, and containing diets
for over twenty-six pathological
conditions, can be obtained by
nurses on special request to :—

DIETARY SERVICE DEPARTMENT,
32 BRIDGE ROAD, WILLESDEN,
LONDON, N.W. 10.

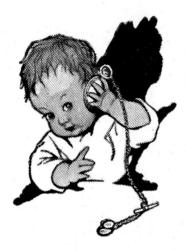

Nestlé's Milk is produced from
England's richest pastures.
It is pure, rich, SAFE Milk.

NESTLÉ'S MILK

PRODUCTS LTD., EASTCHEAP, E.C.3

ANATOMICAL CHART

of the Human Body showing the BONES and ARTERIES

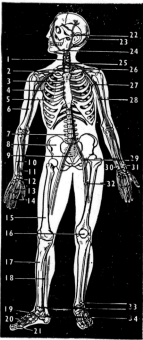

BONES

1 Cervical spine (Neck)
2 Clavicle (Collar bone)
3 Sternum (Breast bone)
4 Scapula (Shoulder blade)
5 Ribs
6 Humerus (Upper arm)
7 Spine (Backbone)
8 Pelvis (Haunch-bone)
9 Sacrum
10 Ulna (Forearm)
11 Radius   ,,
12 Carpus
13 Metacarpus
14 Phalanges
15 Femur (Thigh)
16 Patella (Kneecap)
17 Tibia (Shinbone)
18 Fibula (Brooch-bone)
19 Tarsus
20 Metatarsus
21 Phalanges

ARTERIES

22 Temporal
23 Occipital
24 Facial
25 Carotid
26 Subclavian
27 Axillary
28 Brachial
29 Femoral
30 Ulnar
31 Radial
32 Popliteal
33 Anterior Tibial
34 Posterior Tibial

By courtesy of T. J. SMITH & NEPHEW Ltd., Surgical Dressings Manufacturers, Neptune St., HULL

Facing Title

A NEW
Dictionary for Nurses

COMPILED BY
LOIS OAKES

S.R.N., D.N.(Lond. and Leeds)

*Formerly Sister-Tutor at Stanley Hospital, Brownlow
Hill Infirmary, and Walton Hospital, Liverpool*
Formerly Nursing Editor of " Nursing Illustrated "
Formerly Organizer for the Civil Nursing Reserve, Cambridge
*Nursing Technical Officer to the Ministry of Labour,
Eastern Region*
*Examiner to the General Nursing Council for
England and Wales*

ASSISTED BY
THOS. B. DAVIE

B.A., M.D.(Liverpool), F.R.C.P.(Lond.)

Formerly Pathologist, Walton Hospital
Formerly Professor of Pathology, University of Bristol
George Holt Professor of Pathology, University of Liverpool
*Formerly Examiner to the General Nursing Council for
England and Wales*

NINTH EDITION

EDINBURGH
E. & S. LIVINGSTONE LTD.
16 AND 17 TEVIOT PLACE

1946

First Edition	-	June 1932
Second ,,	-	March 1933
Third ,,	-	April 1934
Fourth ,,	-	April 1936
Fifth ,,	-	January 1938
Sixth ,,	-	January 1940
Seventh ,,	-	June 1941
Reprinted -	-	July 1942
Reprinted -	-	December 1942
Eighth Edition	-	August 1943
Reprinted -	-	April 1944
Ninth Edition	-	January 1946

Made and Printed in Great Britain

PREFACE TO THE NINTH EDITION

THE demand for a Ninth Edition of this dictionary is proof of its continued popularity and usefulness. We desire to acknowledge our thanks to the users of this book for many expressions of appreciation and encouragement. It is our intention to maintain its present standard and to supplement this with new data in order to keep pace with the requirements of modern discoveries and new techniques in medicine, surgery and the practice of nursing.

With this objective, we welcome constructive criticism and suggestions and will endeavour to comply with these without unduly increasing the bulk of the book.

We again wish to record our thanks to the Publishers for their excellent production of this book, which has earned well-merited praise, and for the patience and kindness they have extended to us throughout the trying years of war.

LOIS OAKES.
THOMAS B. DAVIE.

December 1945.

PREFACE TO A PREVIOUS EDITION

IN this, the Eighth Edition of the dictionary, we have completely revised the text and the whole of the section dealing with pronunciation. A new key has been produced and we have avoided the use of all phonetic symbols which might confuse the reader and as far as possible have attempted to reproduce the actual pronunciation with the minimum number of letters distinguished from each other by simple combinations and by simple super-added signs. It is not claimed that all the various sounds utilised in the English language can be represented by the small number of symbols used ; nor do we imagine that the pronunciations given will meet with universal approval. We have, however, attempted to represent by our symbols at least one accepted pronunciation of each word.

We have also added diagrammatic drawings to the first aid section. These deal with a new method of folding blankets round a patient. We trust that these will prove useful and interesting to the users of this book.

We desire to record our grateful thanks to the Publishers for their untiring patience and for the help they have rendered so unstintingly.

LOIS OAKES.
THOMAS B. DAVIE.

August 1943.

CONTENTS

ABBREVIATIONS OF DEGREES, DIPLOMAS, ETC.

A.A.G.B.	American Ambulance (Great Britain).
A.D.M.S.	Assistant Director Medical Services.
A.F.C.	Air Force Cross.
A.H.P.	Assistant House Physician.
A.H.S.	Assistant House Surgeon.
A.M.O.	Assistant Medical Officer.
A.M.S.	Army Medical Staff.
A.R.R.C.	Associate of Royal Red Cross.
A.R.San.I.	Associate Royal Sanitary Institute.
A.T.S.	Auxiliary Territorial Service (Women's).
B.A.O.	Bachelor of Arts.
B.A.O.	Bachelor of Obstetrics.
B.C., B.S., B.Ch.	Bachelor of Surgery.
B.Ch.D., B.D.S.	Bachelor of Dental Surgery.
B.D.A.	British Dental Association.
B.Hy.	Bachelor of Hygiene.
B.M.	Bachelor of Medicine.
B.M.A.	British Medical Association.
B.R.C.	British Red Cross.
B.Sc.	Bachelor of Science.
B.S., B.Ch.	Bachelor of Surgery.
C.B.	Companion Order of the Bath.
C.B.E.	Commander Order of the British Empire.
C.H.	Companion of Honour.
Ch.B.	Bachelor of Surgery.
Ch.M.	Master of Surgery.
C.I.E.	Companion Order Indian Empire.
C.M., Ch.M.	Master in Surgery.
C.M.G.	Companion Order St Michael and St George.
C.N.R.	Civil Nursing Reserve.
C.S.I.	Companion Order Star of India.
C.S.M.M.G.	Chartered Society of Massage and Medical Gymnastics.
C.V.O.	Commander Royal Victorian Order.
D.A.	Diploma in Anæsthetics.
D.A.D.M.S.	Deputy Assistant Director of Medical Services.
D.B.E.	Dame Order of British Empire.
D.C.H.	Diploma in Child Health.

D.C.L.	. .	Doctor of Civil Law.
D.C.M.	. .	Distinguished Conduct Medal.
D.D.M.S.	. .	Deputy Director of Medical Services.
D.D.S.	. .	Doctor of Dental Surgery.
D.F.C.	. .	Distinguished Flying Cross.
D.G.O.	. .	Diploma in Gynæcology and Obstetrics.
D.Hy.	. .	Doctor of Hygiene.
D.M.	. .	Doctor of Medicine.
D.M.D.	. .	Doctor of Dental Medicine.
D.M.R.E.	. .	Diploma of Medical Radiology and Electrology.
D.M.S.	. .	Director of Medical Services.
D.N.	. .	Diplomate in Nursing (*Leeds* and *London*).
D.P.H.	. .	Diploma in Public Health.
D.P.M.	. .	Diploma in Psychological Medicine.
D.R.	. .	Diploma in Radiology.
D.R.C.O.G.	. .	Diploma of the Royal College of Obstetricians and Gynæcologists.
D.S.C.	. .	Distinguished Service Cross.
D.Sc.	. .	Doctor of Science.
D.S.Sc.	. .	Diploma in Sanitary Science.
D.S.O.	. .	Companion Distinguished Service Order.
D.T.H.	. .	Diploma in Tropical Hygiene.
D.T.M.	. .	Diploma in Tropical Medicine.
F.A.N.Y.	. .	First Aid Nursing Yeomanry.
F.C.S.	. .	Fellow of the Chemical Society.
F.E.S.	. .	Fellow of the Entomological Society.
F.G.S.	. .	Fellow of the Geographical Society.
F.I.C.	. .	Fellow of the Institute of Chemistry.
F.L.S.	. .	Fellow of the Linnæan Society.
F.R.A.S.	. .	Fellow of the Royal Astronomical Society.
F.R.C.O.G.	. .	Fellow of the Royal College of Gynæcologists.
F.R.C.P.	. .	Fellow of the Royal College of Physicians.
F.R.C.P.E.	. .	Fellow of the Royal College of Physicians, Edinburgh.
F.R.C.P.I.	. .	Fellow of the Royal College of Physicians of Ireland.
F.R.C.S.	. .	Fellow of the Royal College of Surgeons.
F.R.C.S.E.	. .	Fellow of the Royal College of Surgeons, Edinburgh.
F.R.C.S.I.	. .	Fellow of the Royal College of Surgeons of Ireland.

F.R.F.P.S.	. .	Fellow of the Royal Faculty of Physicians and Surgeons.
F.R.G.S.	. .	Fellow of the Royal Geographical Society.
F.R.M.S.	. .	Fellow of the Royal Microscopical Society.
F.R.S.	. .	Fellow of the Royal Society.
F.R.S.E.	. .	Fellow of the Royal Society of Edinburgh.
F.R.S.L.	. .	Fellow of the Royal Society of Literature.
G.B.E.	. .	Knight Grand Cross Order of the British Empire.
G.C.	. .	George Cross.
G.C.I.E.	. .	Knight Grand Cross Order of the Indian Empire.
G.C.M.G.	. .	Knight Grand Cross Order of St Michael and St George.
G.C.S.I.	. .	Knight Grand Cross Order of the Star of India.
G.C.V.O.	. .	Knight Grand Cross Royal Victorian Order.
G.M.	. .	George Medal.
H.P.	. .	House Physician.
H.S.	. .	House Surgeon.
I.M.S.	. .	Indian Medical Service.
K.B.E.	. .	Knight Commander British Empire.
K.C.B.	. .	Knight Commander Order of the Bath.
K.C.I.E.	. .	Knight Commander Indian Empire.
K.C.M.G.	. .	Knight Commander Order of St Michael and St George.
K.C.S.I.	. .	Knight Commander Order of the Star of India.
K.C.V.O.	. .	Knight Commander Royal Victorian [Order.
L.A.O.	. .	Licentiate in Obstetrics.
L.Ch.	. .	Licentiate in Surgery.
L.D.S.	. .	Licentiate in Dental Surgery.
LL.D.	. .	Doctor of Laws.
LL.M.	. .	Master of Civil and of Canon Law.
L.M.	. .	Licentiate in Midwifery.
L.M.R.C.P.	. .	Licentiate in Midwifery of the Royal College of Physicians.
L.M.S.	. .	Licentiate in Medicine and Surgery.
L.R.C.P.	. .	Licentiate Royal College of Physicians.
L.R.C.S.	. .	Licentiate Royal College of Surgeons.
L.S.A.	. .	Licentiate Society of Apothecaries, London.

M.A.	. .	Master of Arts.
M.A.B.	. .	Metropolitan Asylums Board.
M.A.O.	. .	Master of Obstetrics.
M.B.	. .	Bachelor of Medicine.
M.B.E.	. .	Member Order of British Empire.
M.C., M.S., M.Ch.	. .	Master of Surgery.
M.C.	. .	Military Cross.
M.Ch. (Orth.)	. .	Master of Orthopædic Surgery.
M.D.	. .	Doctor of Medicine.
M.M.	. .	Military Medal.
M.O.H.	. .	Medical Officer of Health.
M.P.A.	. .	Medico-Psychological Association.
M.R.C.O.G.	. .	Member of the Royal College of Obstetricians and Gynæcologists.
M.R.C.P.	.	Member of the Royal College of Physicians.
M.R.C.S.	. .	Member of the Royal College of Surgeons.
M.R.San.I.	. .	Member of the Royal Sanitary Institute.
M.S.	. .	Master of Surgery.
M.S.R.	. .	Member of the Society of Radiologists.
M.V.O.	. .	Member of the Royal Victorian Order.
N.A.	. .	Nursing Auxiliary.
N.H.S.	. .	New Health Society.
O.B.E.	. .	Officer Order of British Empire.
O.M.	. .	Order of Merit.
Ph.D.	. .	Doctor of Philosophy.
P.M.R.A.F.N.S.	.	Princess Mary's Royal Air Force Nursing Service.
P.V.	. .	Public Vaccinator.
Q.A.I.M.N.S.	.	Queen Alexandra's Imperial Military Nursing Service.
Q.A.I.M.N.S.(R.)	.	Queen Alexandra's Imperial Military Nursing Service (Reserve).
Q.A.R.N.N.S.	.	Queen Alexandra's Royal Naval Nursing Service.
Q.I.D.N.	. .	Queen's Institute of District Nursing.
R.A.M.C.	. .	Royal Army Medical Corps.
R.F.N.	. .	Registered Fever Nurse.
R.M.N.	. .	Registered Mental Nurse.
R.M.O.	. .	Resident Medical Officer.
R.M.P.A.	. .	Royal Medico-Psychological Association.
R.N.	. .	Registered Nurse (U.S.A.).
R.N.M.D.	. .	Registered Nurse for Mental Defectives.

R.R.C.	.	Royal Red Cross.
R.S.C.N.	.	Registered Sick Children's Nurse.
Sc.D.	.	Doctor of Science.
S.C.M.	.	State Certified Midwife.
S.I.	.	Sanitary Inspector.
S.M.O.	.	Senior Medical Officer.
S.R.N.	.	State Registered Nurse (England and Wales).
T.A.N.S.	.	Territorial Army Nursing Service.
T.A.N.S.(R.)	.	Territorial Army Nursing Service (Reserve).
T.D.	.	Territorial Army Decoration.
T.F.N.S.	.	Territorial Force Nursing Service.
V.A.D.	.	Voluntary Aid Detachment.
V.C.	.	Victoria Cross.
W.A.A.F.	.	Women's Auxiliary Air Force.
W.R.N.S.	.	Women's Royal Naval Service.
W.V.S.	.	Women's Voluntary Service.

MEDICAL ABBREVIATIONS, ETC.

A	———	argon, anterior, anode.
āā	ana	of each.
abd., abdm.	———	abdomen.
abs. feb.	absente febri	in the absence of fever.
a.c.	ante cibum	before food.
A.C.E.	———	alcohol, 1 part chloroform, 2 parts ether, 3 parts } anaesthetic mixture.
ad.	ad	up to
add.	adde	in addition. Add.
ad effect.	ad effectum	until effectual.
ad grat. acid.	ad gratam aciditatem	to a pleasing acidity.
ad lib.	ad libitum.	as much as is needed.
adv.	adversum	against.
Ag	argentum	silver.

agit.	agitatum	shake.
Al	——	aluminium.
alt. die.	alternis diebus	every other day.
alt. hor.	alternis horis	every other hour.
alt. noct.	alterna nocte	every other night.
amp.	ampere	unit of measurement of strength of an electrical current.
anat.	——	anatomy.
aq.	aqua	water.
aq. bull.	aqua bulliens	boiling water.
aq. cal.	aqua calida	warm water.
aq. dest.	aqua destillata	distilled water.
aq. ferv.	aqua fervens	hot water.
aq. frig.	aqua frigida	cold water.
aq. pur.	aqua pura	pure water.
aq. menth. pip.	aqua menthæ piperitæ	peppermint water.
As	arsenicum	Arsenic.
Au	aurum	gold.
B	——	bowels, Boron.
Ba	——	Barium.
b.b.a.	——	born before arrival.
b.d.	bis die	twice a day.
Bi	——	Bismuth.
b.i.d.	bis in die	twice daily.
biol.	——	biology.
b.o.	——	bowels open.
B.P.	——	1. Blood-pressure. 2. Boiling-point. 3. British Pharmacopœia.
Br	——	Bromine.
bull.	bulliat	let it boil.
C.	——	centigrade, cubic, Carbon.
c.	cum	with.
Ca	——	Calcium.
cap.	capiat	let him take.
cat.	cataplasma	poultice.
c.c.	——	cubic centimetre.
cib.	cibus	food.
Cl	——	Chlorine.
cm	——	centimetre.

c.m.	cras mane	to-morrow morning.
c.m.s.	cras mane sumendus	to be taken to-morrow morning.
c.n.	cras nocte	to-morrow night.
cochl.	cochleare	spoonful.
cochl. ampl.	cochleare amplum	a tablespoonful.
cochl. infant.	cochleare infantis	a teaspoonful.
coch. mag.	cochleare magnum	a tablespoonful.
cochl. med.	cochleare medium	a dessertspoonful.
cochl. parv.	cochleare parvum	a teaspoonful.
co., comp.	compositus	a compound.
cong.	congius	a gallon.
contin.	continuentur	let it be continued.
crast.	crastinus	for to-morrow.
Cu	cuprum	Copper.
cuj.	cujus	of which.
cwt.	———	one hundredweight.
cyath.	cyathus	a glass.
D.	dosis	dose.
d.	da	give.
d.a.h.	———	disorderly action of the heart.
d.d. in d.	de die in diem	from day to day.
decub.	decubitus	lying down.
deg.	———	degree.
destil.	destillatus	distilled.
det.	detur	let it be given.
dieb. alt.	diebus alternis	on alternate days.
dieb. tert.	diebus tertis	every third day.
dil.	dilutus	dilute, diluted.
dim.	dimidius	half.
div.	———	divide.
div. in p. æq.	divide in partes æquales	divide in equal parts.
d.p.	directione propria	with a proper direction.
don.	donec	until.
dr.	———	dram ; also drachm.
dur. dolor.	durante dolore	while the pain lasts.
E.	———	1. Emmetropia. 2. Eye.
e.m.f.	———	electro-motive force.
emp.	emplastrum	a plaster.
en.	———	enema.

exhib.	exhibeatur	let it be exhibited.
ex.	extractum	extract.
ext. liq.	extractum liquidum	liquid extract.
F.		1. Fahrenheit. 2. Fluorine.
F. or ft.	fiat	let it be made.
Fe	ferrum	Iron.
feb. dur.	febri durante	during the fever.
f.h.	fiat haustus	make a draught.
f.m.	fiat mistura	make the mixture.
f. pil.	fiat pilulæ	make the pills.
garg.	gargarisma	a gargle.
g.	——	gram.
gr.	——	grain.
gtt.	guttæ	drops.
guttat.	guttatim	by drops.
H.	——	Hydrogen.
haust.	haustus	a draught.
Hg.	hydrargyrum	Mercury.
hor. decub.	hora decubitus	at bedtime.
h.n.	hac nocte	to-night.
h.s.	hora somni	the hour of sleep, bedtime.
I.	——	Iodine.
id.	idem	the same.
in d.	in die	daily.
inf.	——	infusion.
inj.	injectio	injection.
K.	kalium	Potassium.
kg., kgm.	——	Kilogram.
l.	——	1. Left. 2. Litre.
lat. dol.	lateri dolenti	to the painful side.
lb.	libra	pound.
liq.	——	Liquor.
m.	——	1. Metre. 2. Misce (mix). 3. Mistura (mixture). 4. Mane (m o r n i n g). 5. Minim.
man. pr.	mane primo	first thing in the morning.
m. ft.	mistura fiat	let the mixture be made.

Mg.	——	Magnesium.
ml.	——	millilitre.
mm.	——	millimetre.
Mn	——	Manganese.
M.O.	——	Medical Officer.
MS.	——	manuscript.
mt. or mit.	mitte	send.
N	——	Nitrogen.
n.	nocte	at night.
Na	natrium	Sodium.
ne repetat.	ne repetatur	do not repeat.
No.	——	number.
noct.	nocte	night.
O	——	1. Oxygen. 2. Pint.
ol.	oleum	oil.
o.m.	omni mane	every morning.
omn. bih.	omni bihora	every two hours.
omn. hor.	omni hora	every hour.
o.n.	omni nocte	every night.
oz.	——	ounce.
P	——	1. Pulse. 2. Phosphorus. 3. Pharmacopœia.
Pb	plumbum	Lead.
p.c.	post cibos	after meals.
pil.	pilula	a pill.
p.m.	post mortem	after death, autopsy.
Pot.	——	Potassium.
p.p.h.	——	post-partum hæmorrhage.
p.r.	per rectum	by the rectum.
p.r.n.	pro re nata	as occasion arises.
pt.	——	pint.
pulv.	pulvis	powder.
p.v.	per vaginam	by the vagina.
q.d.	quattuor in die	four times daily.
q.h.	quaque hora	every hour.
q.l.	quantum libet	as much as required.
q.q.h.	quaque quarta hora	every fourth hour; also written 4ts horis.
q.s.	quantum sufficit	a sufficient quantity.
q.v.	quod vide	which see.

R.	——	1. Réaumur. 2. Respiration. 3, Right.
℞	recipe	take.
Ra	——	Radium.
r.d.	——	reaction of degeneration.
rect.	rectificatus	rectified.
rep.	repetatur	let it be repeated.
S	——	Sulphur.
s, ss.	semis, semissis	half.
s.a.	secundum artem	according to rules of the profession (of pharmacy).
Sb	stibium	Antimony.
Si	——	Silicon.
s. or sig.	signetur	let it be labelled, *i.e.* directions.
sing.	singulorum	of each.
s.o.s.	si opus sit	if necessary.
sol	——	solution.
sp. gr.	——	specific gravity.
stat.	statim	immediately.
sum.	sumendus	to be taken.
s.v.	spiritus vini	spirits of wine.
s.v. gall.	spiritus vini gallici	brandy.
s.v.r.	spiritus vini rectificatus	rectified spirit.
syr.	——	syrup.
T.	——	temperature.
tab.	tabella	a tablet.
t.d.	ter die	three times a day.
t.i.d.	ter in die	three times a day.
tinct., tr.	tinctura	tincture.
troch.	——	a troche.
u.	——	unit.
ung.	unguentum	ointment.
ur.	——	urine.
v.	——	volt.
vin.	vinum	wine.
v.m.	——	volt metre.
wt.	——	weight.
Zn	——	Zinc.

COMPARISON OF CENTIGRADE, FAHRENHEIT, AND REAUMAR SCALE

Normal Temperature
=98·4° F.
37° C.
30° R.

CONVERSION OF SCALES

Fahrenheit into Centi-grade—

1. Deduct 32, multiply by 5, and divide by 9.
2. Add 40, multiply by 5, divide by 9, and deduct 40.

Centigrade into Fahren-heit—

1. Multiply by 9, divide by 5, and add 32.
2. Add 40, multiply by 9, divide by 5, and deduct 40.

Reaumur into Fahren-heit—

Multiply by 9, divide by 4, and add 32.

	CENTIGRADE	FAHRENHEIT	REAUMUR
BOILING POINT	100	212	80
	95	203	
	90	194	70
	85	185	
	80	176	
	75	167	60
	70	158	
	65	149	
	60	140	50
	55	131	
	50	122	40
	45	113	
BLOOD HEAT	40	104	
	35	95	30
	30	86	
	25	77	
	20	68	20
	15	59	
	10	50	
	5	41	10
FREEZING POINT	0	32	0
	5		
	10		
	15		10
	18		

Comparison of Thermometric Scales.

WEIGHTS AND MEASURES

APOTHECARIES' WEIGHT.

20 grains =1 scruple.
3 scruples =1 drachm.
60 grains =1   ,,
8 drachms =1 ounce.
12 ounces =1 pound (lb.).

APOTHECARIES' MEASURE.

60 minims =1 drachm.
8 drachms =1 ounce.
20 ounces =1 pint.
2 pints   =1 quart.
4 quarts   =1 gallon.

MÉTRIC WEIGHTS.

1 milligram = ·001 gram.
1 centigram = ·01   ,,
1 decigram   = ·1   ,,
1 gram   =1   ,,
1 Decagram   =10 grams.
1 Hectogram =100   ,,
1 Kilogram   =1,000 ,,
1 Myriogram =10,000 ,,

METRIC LIQUID MEASURE.

1 millilitre = ·001 litre.
1 centilitre = ·01   ,,
1 decilitre   = ·1   ,,
1 litre   =1   ,,
1 Decalitre   =10 litres.
1 Hectolitre =100   ,,
1 Kilolitre   =1,000 ,,
1 Myrialitre =10,000 ,,

AVOIRDUPOIS WEIGHT.

16 drachms =1 ounce.
16 ounces =1 lb.
14 lbs.   =1 stone.
28   ,,   =1 quarter.
4 quarters =1 cwt.
20 cwts.   =1 ton.

LINEAR MEASURE.

12 inches =1 foot.
3 feet   =1 yard.
2 yards   =1 fathom.
5½ ,,   =1 rod, pole, or
                perch.
40 poles =1 furlong.
8 furlongs=1 mile.
1,760 yards=1 mile.

METRIC LINEAR MEASURE.

	Metres.	Inches.
1 millimetre	= ·001 =	·03937.
1 centimetre	= ·01 =	·3937.
1 decimetre	= ·1 =	3·937.
1 metre	=1 =	39·3707.
1 Decametre	=10.	
1 Hectometre	=100.	
1 Kilometre	=1,000.	
1 Myriametre	=10,000.	

GRAINS.

20 grains =1 scruple.
60   ,,   =1 drachm.
480 ,,   =1 ounce.
5,760 ,, =1 lb. (Troy).

APPROXIMATE METRIC AND IMPERIAL EQUIVALENTS

1 cubic centimetre (or 1 millilitre)	=17 minims (16·9) or roughly 15 to 17 minims.
30 millilitres	=1 fluid ounce (or 8 fluid drachms, or 437½ minims).
30 grams	=1 ounce.
1 kilogram	=2¼ lbs. (2·2046 lbs.).
1 litre	=35 ounces, or 1¾ pints (1·7598 pts.).
1 milligram	=0·01543 grains.
1 centimetre	=0·3937 inch.
25 millimetres	=1 inch.
1 kilometre	=⅝ mile.
8 kilometres	=5 miles.
1 minim	=0·059 cubic centimetres.
1 dram (60 grains)	=4 grams.
1 fluid dram (60 minims)	=3½ cubic centimetres (3·552 c.cm.).
1 fluid ounce	=30 millilitres. Also = 437½ grains (28·42 c.cm.).
1 pint (9,600 minims)	=568·4 cubic centimetres (roughly 600 c.cm.) or ½ litre, or 0·57 litre.
1 quart	=1136·8 cubic centimetres, or 1¼ litre.
1 gallon	=4547·2 cubic centimetres, or 4½ litres.
1 ,, of water	=weighs 10 lbs.
1 cubic foot	=6¼ gallons.
1 stone	=6½ kilograms.

DOMESTIC MEASURES

1 teaspoonful	=1 drachm.
2 teaspoonfuls	=2 drachms, or 1 dessertspoonful.
2 dessertspoonfuls	=4 ,, or 1 tablespoonful.
2 tablespoonfuls	=8 ,, or 1 ounce.
1 tumbler	=10 ounces, or ½ pint.

GUIDE TO PRONUNCIATION

Vowels.

a   as in cat (kat).

ā   ,,   tame (tām) ; remain (re-mān′).

å   ,,   father (fàth′-er) ; carcinoma (kår-sin-ō′-má).*

e   ,,   hem ; dead (ded).

ē   ,,   seem (sēm) ; believe (be-lēv′) ; bead (bēd).

é   ,,   bear (bér) ; hair (hér) ; mare (mér) ; there (thér) ; their (thér) ; vary (vé′-ri).

ɪ   ,,   hit ; sitting (sit′-ing) ; story (staw′-ri).

ī   ,,   pike (pīk) ; carditis (kår-dī′-tis).

o   ,,   not ; cough (kof).

ō   ,,   bone (bōn) ; loan (lōn) ; low (lō) ; sew (sō) ; dough (dō).

u   ,,   hut ; butter (but′-er) ; colour (kul′-er).

ū   ,,   mule (mūl) ; dew (dū) ; you (ū).

aw   ,,   awl ; fall (fawl) ; torn (tawn) ; board (bawd) ; taut (tawt) ; caught (kawt).

er   ,,   her ; father (fàth′-er) ; fire (fī′-er).

ïer   ,,   pier ; deer (dïer) ; fear (fïer) ; ampere (am′-pïer).

oi   ,,   poison (poi′-z′n) ; boy (boi).

oo   ,,   moon ; lunar (loon′-à(r)).*

ow   ,,   cow (kow) ; round (rownd) ; bough (bow).

ur   ,,   turn ; worm (wurm).

* *Note.*—When the "à" is terminal it seldom receives its full value, and in rapid speech its pronunciation approaches "er."

xix

Consonants.

ch (=tsh) as in cheese (chēz); search (serch); picture
(pik'-cher).

j (=dzh) ,, judge (juj); rigid (rij'-id).

sh ,, dish; lotion (lō'-shun).

zh ,, vision (vizh'-'n).

ng ,, sing; think (thingk).

g always hard as in good.

r This letter is often left unsounded
or is slurred into the preceding
vowel. In the combination "er"
(see vowels) it is not sounded as a
consonant. Where it receives its
full consonantal value it is usually
placed preceding a vowel; in most
other cases its force is determined
by individual taste and custom.

th No attempt has been made to distinguish between the breathed
sound as in "think" and the voiced
sound as in "them."

Other consonants as in ordinary alphabet.

Accent.—The accented syllable is indicated by a
slanting stroke at its termination, e.g., fibrositis
(fī-brō-sī'-tis).

DICTIONARY
OF MEDICAL TERMS

A.

A. An abbreviation for *accommodation, anode, anterior*. Also a symbol for *Argon*.

A- or An-. A prefix signifying absence of.

āā. Contraction of *ana*, meaning of each; an abbreviation often used in prescription writing.

Ab. A prefix signifying from.

Abactus Venter (ab-ak'-tus ven'ter). An artificial induction of abortion.

Abalienation (ab-āl-i-en-ā'-shun). A term signifying mental deterioration.

Abarticulation (ab-är-tik-ū-lā'-shun). (1) The same as *Dislocation*, (2) *Diarthrosis* (q.v.).

Abasia (ab-ā'-zi-á). Motor inco-ordination resulting in inability to walk.

Abbé's Condenser. A microscope attachment consisting of a mirror and a series of lenses, so arranged as to give a maximum amount of light.

Abdomen (ab-dō'-men). The belly; a cavity immediately below the thorax, from which it is separated by the diaphragm.

Abdominal (ab-dom'-in-al). Pertaining to the abdomen.

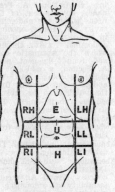

Abdominal Regions

RH, Right hypochondriac region.
LH, Left hypochondriac region.
E, Epigastric region.
RL, Right lumbar region.
LL, Left lumbar region.
U, Umbilical region.
RI, Right iliac fossa.
LI, Left iliac fossa.
H, Hypogastric region.

A

1

A, Aneurysm, aneurysm of the abdominal aorta. **A. Bandage,** one used especially for the abdomen. **A. Breathing,** the use of the diaphragm and abdominal muscles during respiration. **A. Pregnancy,** development of the foetus within the abdominal cavity. **A. Rings,** openings in the lower part of the abdominal wall through which the spermatic cord and round ligament pass. **A. Section,** a mid-line incision opening into the abdomen and reaching from the umbilicus to the pubis.

Abducens (ab-dū'-sens). The sixth pair of cranial nerves.

Abducent. Abducting.

Abduct. To draw away from the median line.

Abduction (ab-duk'-shun). The act of abducting.

Aberration (ab-er-rā'-shun). Deviation from the normal course. **Mental A.,** mental instability not amounting to insanity, *e.g.,* forgetting.

Abiogenesis (ă-bī-ō-jen'-e-sis). Spontaneous generation. The production of animate from inanimate matter.

Abiosis (ă-bī-ō'-sis). Death.

Abiotrophy (ā'-bī-o'-trof-ĭ). Reduced size by reason of failure of development.

Abirritant (ab-ir'-it-ant). Relieving irritation.

Ablactation (ab-lak-tā'-shun).

Cessation of lactation ; weaning.

Ablate (ab-lāt). To take away, especially by excision.

Ablation. Removal of tissue, especially by cutting.

Ablution (ab-loo'-shun). The act of cleansing or purifying by washing.

Abnormal. Deviation from the normal ; unusual.

Abnormality. The state of being abnormal ; malformation.

Aboral (ab'-ōr-al). At a distance from the mouth.

Abort (ab-awrt'). To terminate before full development ; to miscarry.

Abortifacient (ab-awr-ti-fā'-si-ent). An agent which causes abortion.

Abortion (ab-awr'-shun). Expulsion of the foetus from the uterus before it is viable. **Artificial A.,** abortion which is intentionally procured to save the life of the mother. **Criminal A.,** abortion produced when not medically indicated. **Habitual A.,** repeated abortion occurring in several pregnancies. **Induced A.,** same as artificial abortion. **Inevitable A.,** one which cannot be prevented. **Incomplete A.,** that in which parts of the placenta or its membranes are retained. **Missed A.,** non-expulsion of a dead foetus. **Threatened A.,** probable or pending abortion as indicated by signs and symptoms.

2

Tubal A., a rupture of the Fallopian tube when development of the embryo occurs in it, or expulsion of the embryo through the fimbriated end of the tube.

Abrachia (ă-brā'-ki-ȧ). Congenital absence of the arms.

Abrade (ab-rād'). To deface by rubbing off the surface.

Abrasion (ab-rā'-shun). A scraping off of the surface of the skin; excoriation; a superficial wound.

Abreaction (ab-re-ak'-shun). An emotional reaction in which past painful experiences are lived through again, both in speech and action, during the process of psycho-analysis. Also known as *Catharsis.*

Abscess (ab'-ses). The collection of pus in a cavity. **Alveolar A.,** one occurring in the gum or tooth-socket. **Cold A.,** one which develops slowly and without inflammation. **Fæcal A.,** one which contains fæcal matter and which forms in the rectum. **Ischiorectal A.,** occurring in the ischiorectal fossa. **Mammary A.,** breast abscess. **Psoas A.,** a cold abscess from tuberculosis of the lumbar vertebræ; pus burrows down the psoas muscle and locates near its insertion on the lesser trochanter on the inner side of the femur. **Pyæmic A.,** one resulting from pyæmia. **Retropharyn-**

geal A., one formed in the tissues posterior or lateral to the pharynx.

Abscission (ab-sish'-un). Removal of a part by cutting.

Absinthe (ab'-sinth or ab-sant'). The name of a liqueur containing oil of wormwood.

Absinthism (ab-sin'-thizm). Mental hallucinations and deterioration due to excessive drinking of absinthe.

Absorbent (ab-sorb'-ent). Soaking up fluid like a sponge; imbibing or taking up by suction.

Absorptive (ab-sorp'-tiv). Capable of absorption.

Abstinence. Self-denial; voluntary restraint of the appetites, etc.

Abulia (ab-oo'-li-ȧ). Lacking in will-power; indecision of character.

Acacia (ak-ā'-si-ȧ). (1) A genus of trees and shrubs of many varieties. (2) Gum arabic obtained from the **A. Senegal.** It is much used in pharmacy as a vehicle, either in the form of mucilage or syrup. It is a demulcent.

Acapnia (ă-kap'-ni-ȧ). Cessation of respiration due to reduced CO_2 in the blood.

Acardia (ă-kăr'-di-ȧ). Congenital absence of the heart.

Acarus (ak'-ar-us). A parasite of the genus *Arachnoidea,* which includes many varieties of ticks and mites. A well-known example is the itch-

3

mite, or **A. Scabiei**, which is a human parasite. The female, which is twice as large as the male, first becomes impregnated on the surface of the skin, and then starts to burrow beneath the epidermis. The eggs are laid at the end of the burrows, and the female then dies.

Acatalepsy (ă-kat-a-lep′-si). Lack of comprehension ; uncertainty.

Acataphasia (ă-kat-a-fă′-zi-ă). Difficulty or inability to express the thoughts in an orderly sequence.

Acaudal, Acaudate (ă-kaw′ dal). Minus a tail.

Accentuation (ak-sen-tū-ā′-shun). A very marked or increased distinctness.

Accessory (ak-ses′-o-ri). In addition to ; an aid to some more important organ or structure, e.g., the accessory organs of digestion.

Accidental Hæmorrhage. Uterine hæmorrhage resulting from a prematurely detached placenta. It may be either concealed or revealed. In the latter case blood escapes from the vaginal orifice.

Acclimatization (ak-klĭ-mat-i-ză′-shun). Becoming used to new conditions, climate, etc.

Accommodation (ak-kom-mō-dā′-shun). Adjustment, as of the power of the eye to alter the convexity of the lens according to the nearness or distance of objects, to enable the light rays to fall exactly on to the retina.

Accommodative (ak-kom-mō-dā′-tiv). Relating to accommodation.

Accouchement (ak-koosh-mon(g′)). Delivery in childbirth. Confinement.

Accoucheur (ak-koo-sher′). A man skilled in midwifery ; an obstetrician.

Accoucheuse (ak-koo-sherz′). A midwife.

Accretion (ak-krē-shun). An increase of substance or deposit round a central object : an accumulation.

Accumulator. An apparatus for storing electricity.

Acedia (ă-sē′-di-ă). Mental apathy. Lack of interest.

Acephalus (ă-kef-a-lus). A monster without a head.

Acetabulum (as-et-ab′-ŭ-lum). A socket on the external aspect of the innominate bone, into which the head of the femur fits to form the hip joint. Is made by the union of the ilium, ischium, and pubis.

Acetanilide (as-et-an′-il-īd). A colourless crystalline compound derived from aniline and acetic acid, possessing analgesic and antipyretic properties.

Acetate (as′-e-tāt). A salt of acetic acid.

Acetic (as-ē′-tik). Pertaining to vinegar or its acid.

4

Acetonæmia (as-e-tō-nē'-mi-å). The presence of acetone bodies in the blood.

Acetone (as'-e-tōn). A colourless, inflammable liquid. Acetone is sometimes found in the urine under such abnormal conditions as acidosis resulting from starvation, excessive vomiting, and diabetes.

Acetonuria (as-e-tō-nū'-ri-å). The presence of acetone bodies in the urine.

Acetum (as-ē'-tum). Vinegar.

Acet'ylene (C_2H_2). A colourless gas formed by the action of water on calcium carbide, burning with a brilliant illumination.

Achalasia (ak-a-lā'-zi-a). Failure to relax on the part of a sphincter muscle, e.g., the pyloric sphincter.

Achilles Tendon (ak-il'-ēz ten'-don). The large tendinous termination of the soleus and gastrocnemius muscles inserted into the os calcis.

Achillorrhaphy (ak-il-or'-af-i). The operation of stitching the tendo Achillis.

Achlorhydria (å-klor-hid'-ri-å or å-klor-hīd'-ri-å). Absence of hydrochloric acid in the gastric juice.

Acholia (å-kōl'-i-å). Absence of bile secretion.

Acholuria (a-kol-ū'-ri-å). Absence of bile pigment from the urine.

Achondroplasia (å-kon-drō-plā'-zi-å). Arrested growth of the long bones leading to dwarfism. It is sometimes known as fœtal rickets. The intellect is not impaired.

Achromate (å-krō'-māt). Devoid of colour; exhibiting colour blindness.

Achromatic (å'-krō-mat-ik). Without colour; not staining easily.

Achylia (å-kī'-li-å). Absence of chyle.

Acid. The state and also the degree of being acid or sour. An acid when combined with an alkali forms a salt. It will turn blue litmus paper red. **Acetic A.**, a colourless acid. Three kinds are recognized: the *dilute*, 5%; the *strong*, 35%; and the *glacial*, 98·9%. **Amino-acids**, nitrogen containing acids which are the result of the breaking down of proteins. **Boric A.**, **Boracic A.**, (H_3BO_3), a white mildly antiseptic substance existing in powder or crystal form; used for irrigating delicate surfaces, such as the conjunctiva of the eye. **Carbolic A.**, a crystalline compound obtained from the distillation of coal-tar; it is a powerful antiseptic and germicide, and is very poisonous; when employed as an antiseptic for the hands it is used in a strength of 1-40; for instruments, 1-20. **Carbonic A.**, the acid solution of carbon

5

dioxide in water. **Diacetic A.,** the same as **Aceto-acetic A.;** a precursor of **Acetone** in diabetic urine. **Hydrochloric A.** (HCl), a normal constituent of the gastric juice ; it is formed in the oxyntic cells of the stomach. **Hydrocyanic A.,** a deadly poisonous gas liberated by the action of stronger acids on cyanides. **Lactic A.,** formed from milk by the action of ferments. **Nitric A.** (HNO_3), a colourless corrosive liquid ; also used for urine testing. **Oxalic A.,** from wood sorrel, cellulose, etc. **Palmitic A.,** one of the fatty acids. **Picric A.,** a yellow crystalline substance used as an antiseptic and as a dressing for burns. **Acetyl-Salicylic A.,** an antipyretic much used in rheumatism and allied conditions. Synonym, *Aspirin.* **Sulphuric A.** (H_2SO_4), a corrosive poison much used in chemistry. Synonym, *Oil of Vitriol. Concentrated Sulphuric A.* contains 93-98% pure acid. *Dilute Sulphuric A.* contains from 10-15% pure acid. **Tannic A.,** obtained from nutgalls. **Tartaric A.,** a white powder derived from grape-juice and other plants. **Uric A.,** found in urine and in some parts of the body, especially in gouty subjects.

Acidæmia (as-id-ē'-mi-à). Abnormal acidity of the blood. An increase in the hydrogen-ion content of the blood.

Acid-fast. A term applied to bacilli which, when stained, do not become decolorized when subjected to dilute acids, *e.g.,* tubercle bacilli.

Acidimetry (as-id-im'-et-ri). The process of finding out the amount of free acid in a solution.

Acidity (as-id'-it-i). The state of being acid or sour.

Acidosis (as-id-ō'-sis). A condition associated with an abnormal formation of acid or an abnormal loss of alkali ; seen in diabetes, terminal stages of chronic nephritis, shock, burns, poisoning, and fasting. The commonest form is associated with an abnormal production of di-acetic acid and β-hydroxybutyric acids (" Ketone bodies "), brought about by a disturbance of metabolism of fats, following a deprivation of carbohydrates (as in fasting), or an inability of the body to oxidize carbohydrates (as seen in diabetes due to lack of formation of insulin). This condition is known as " Ketosis," which is only one form of acidosis.

Acidum. Latin for *Acid.*

Acme (ak'-mē). The turning-point or crisis of an illness.

Acne (ak′-nē). A general term denoting inflammation of the sebaceous glands of the skin. *Papules, pustules,* and blackheads form on the face, chest, and back of adolescents. **A. Rosa′cea,** a chronic inflammation of the face and nose often, but not always, due to alcoholism. **A. Vulgaris,** the common form of acne.

Aconite (ak′-o-nīt). *Monkshood.* A poisonous drug obtained from the root of the Aconitum Napellus. Is sedative, diaphoretic, and diuretic.

Aconitine (ak-on′-it-ēn). The very poisonous chief alkaloid of *Aconite.*

Aconuresis (ak-on-ū-rē′-sis). Involuntary emptying of the bladder.

Acos′ta′s Disease. Mountain sickness.

Acoumeter (ak-ow′-mē-ter). An instrument for measuring the acuteness of hearing.

Acousmatamnesia (ak-oos-matam-nē′-si-à). Inability to call up mental images of sound.

Acoustic (ak-oos′-tik). Relating to the sense of hearing.

Acoustics (ak-oos′-tiks). The science of sound.

Acrid (ak′-rid). Burning ; pungent.

Acriflavine (ak-ri-flā′-vin). Same as *Flavin.* A powerful antiseptic and germicide.

Acrocyanosis (ak-rō-sī-an-ō′-sis). Coldness and blueness of the extremities, associated with chilblains and due to loss of vasomotor tone.

Acrodynia (ak-rō-din′-i-à). Epidemic erythema. Reddening of the extremities. Closely related to ergotism.

Acromegaly (ak-rō-meg′-a-li). A disease state due to a tumour of the eosinophil cells of the anterior lobe of the pituitary and characterized by enlargements of the extremities—of hands, feet, and lower jaw. Also known as *Marie′s Disease.*

Acromion (ak-rō′-mi-on). The extreme outer end of the spine of the scapula.

Acronyx (ak′-rō-niks). An ingrowing toe-nail.

Acrophobia (ak-rō-fō′-bi-à). Morbid fear of being at a height.

Acrotic (ā-krot′-ik). Absence of the pulse.

Actinic (ak-tin′-ik). Ultraviolet. Pertaining to the rays beyond the visible violet end of the spectrum.

Actinium (ak-tin′-i-um). A chemical element found in the ore of uranium, and possessing radio-active properties.

Actinocutitis (ak-tīn-ō-kū-tī′-tis). Dermatitis resulting from continued exposure to X-rays.

Actinogram (ak-tin′-ō-gram). *See* Skiagram.

7

Actinomyces (ak-tīn-ō-mī'-sēz). A genus of parasitic fungus having a radiating mycelium. The ray fungus.

Actinomycosis (ak-tīn-ō-mī-kō'-sis). A disease caused by the ray fungus. It commonly attacks the jaw, lungs, or intestines.

Actinoscopy (ak-tīn-os'-ko-pi). Examination by means of X-ray.

Actino-therapy (ak-tīn-ō-the'-rap-i). A method of treating disease by means of the use of the actinic light rays. Often known as "sunlight" treatment, ultra-violet ray treatment, etc.

Action. The activity or function of any part of the body. Reflex A., a specific involuntary motor response to a sensory impulse.

Activate. To render active.

Activator. A substance which renders some other substance active. A term often used in connection with enzymes and hormones, *e.g.*, *Secretin*, an intestinal hormone, activates the *pancreas*; *Enterokinase* activates *trypsinogen*, etc.

Active (ak'-tiv). Energetic; mobile; not passive.

Actual (ak-tū-al). Real.

Acuity (ak-ū'-it-i). Sharpness and clearness, as of vision.

Acuminate (ak-ū'-min-āt). Tapering to a point.

Acupressure (ak-ū-presh'-ur). Compression of a bleeding artery by passing needles beneath it.

Acupuncture (ak-ū-pungk'-tūr). The introduction of needles into the tissues for the purpose of withdrawing fluid or of producing counter-irritation.

Acute (a-kūt'). Short and severe; not long drawn out or chronic.

Acute Yellow Atrophy. A necrosis of the liver which may result from poisoning with phosphorus, T.N.T., or other chemicals or as a manifestation of toxæmia of pregnancy.

Acyesis (ā-sī-ē'-sis). Absence of pregnancy.

Acystia (a-sis'-ti-ā). Absence of the bladder.

Adam's Apple. A prominence in front of the neck, especially in the adult male, due to the thyroid cartilage.

Adaptation (ad-ap-tā'-shun). (1) The power of the eye to adjust itself to alterations in the intensity of light. (2) The ability of an organism to adapt itself to its environment.

Add. An abbreviation for the Latin, *adde* or *addetur*, meaning "add to."

Addict (ad'-ikt). A person who is unable to resist indulgence in some habit, such as the drug habit.

Addiction (ad-ik'-shun). The

8

state of being given up to a habit.

Addison's Disease. A disease of the *suprarenal cortex* (often tuberculosis), accompanied by marked bronzing of the skin, asthenia, pigmentation of the mucous membranes, glossitis, and other gastric disturbances. The untreated disease terminates fatally in from one to three years.

Adducens Oculi (ad-ū'-sens ŏk'-ū-lē). The *internal rectus* muscle of the eye.

Adducent (ad-ū'-sent). Drawing towards the centre, as to the median line of the body.

Aden (ā'-den). A gland.

Adenectomy (ad-en-ek'-to-mi). Surgical removal of a gland.

Adenitis (ad-en-ī'-tis). Inflammation of a gland.

Adenocarcinoma (ad-en-ō-kǎ(r)-sin-ō'-mǎ). A malignant cancerous growth of glandular tissue.

Adenoid (ad'-en-oid). (1) Resembling a gland. (2) An overgrowth of the glandular tissue of the posterior nares.

Adenoidectomy (ad-e-noid-ek'-to-mi). Surgical removal of adenoid tissue.

Adenoma (ad-en-ō'-mǎ). A non-malignant swelling or tumour consisting of glandular tissue.

Adenomatome (ad-en-ō'-mǎ-tōm). An instrument used for excising adenoid growths.

Adeps. Lard. **A. Lanæ,** wool fat or lanoline.

Adherent. Closely approximated ; sticking firmly.

Adhesion (ad-hē'-zhun). An abnormal connection between parts : the act of sticking to. Membranous bands which tend to form when two inflamed surfaces are in contact with each other : (1) **Primary A.,** healing by first intention ; (2) **Secondary A.,** healing by the formation of granulations.

Adiaphoresis (ā-dī-ā-for-ē'-sis). Absence or lack of perspiration.

Adipic (ad'-ip-ic or ǎ'-dip-ik). Pertaining to fat.

Adipocele (ad'-ip-ō-sēl). A hernia containing fat or fatty tissue.

Adipocere (ad'-ip-ō-sēer). A waxy substance from animal decomposition in moist soils.

Adipose (ad'-ip-ōz). Fat ; of a fatty nature.

Adiposity (ad-i-pos'-it-i). The state of being fat.

Aditus (ad'-it-us). An entrance or opening.

Adjustment. The mechanism by which the tube of a microscope is raised or lowered.

Adjuvant (ad-joo'-vant). A substance included in a prescription which aids the action of other drugs.

Adnexa (ad-neks'-ǎ). Structures which are in close proximity to a part. **A. Oculi,** the lachrymal apparatus. **A. Uteri,** the ovaries and Fallopian tubes.

Adolescence (ad-ō-les'-sens). The age between puberty and full maturity ; youth.

Adoral (ad-awr'-al). Near the mouth.

Adrenal (ad-rē'-nal). Near the kidney. The same as *Suprarenal.*

Adrenalin (ad-ren'-a-lin). The internal secretion of the medulla of the *suprarenal gland.* It raises the blood-pressure ; is a cardiac stimulant and a styptic ; is commonly used in a strength of 1-1,000 solution. The same as *Epinephrin.*

Adsorption (ad-sawrp'-shun). The act of sucking up or attracting fluids or gases. Not the same as capillary attraction.

Advancement (ad-vans'-ment). A surgical operation for the cure of strabismus.

Adventitia (ad-ven-tish'-i-à). The external coat of an artery or vein.

A d y n a m i c (ā-dī-nam'-ĭk). Lacking vital activity and power ; asthenic.

Ægophony (ē-gof'-o-ni). A goat-like bleating sound heard on auscultation of the chest.

Aerate (ēr'-āt). (1) To impregnate or charge with air. (2) To charge a liquid with CO_2.

Aerobia (ēr-ō'-bi-à). The con-

dition of life which requires oxygen for its maintenance.

Aerobic (ēr-ō'-bik). Pertaining to aerobia ; needing air.

Aerophagy (ēr-of'-a-ji). Air-swallowing.

Aerotropism (ēr-ō-trō'-pizm). The growth of organisms either toward or away from air. *See* **Tropistic Action.**

Æsculapius (ēs-kū-lā'-pi-us). The God of Medicine. Also *Asclepios.*

Æther. The same as *Ether.*

Ætiology (ē-ti-ol'-o-ji). A science dealing specially with the causation of disease. Also spelt *Etiology.*

Afebrile (ā-feb'-rīl). Without symptoms of fever.

Affect. A psychological term denoting the emotional part of an instinct.

Afferent (af'-er-rent). Conveying to ; from the periphery to the centre.

Affinity (af-in'-i-ti). (1) Common relationship ; attraction. (2) A chemical attraction between two substances, as, for example, oxygen and hæmoglobin.

A f f u s i o n (af-ū-zhun). A method of reducing temperature by pouring water on the body.

After-birth. The placenta, cord, and membranes which are expelled from the uterus shortly after the birth of the child.

After-image. A visual im-

10

pression of an object which persists after the object has been removed. Such an impression may be either *positive* or *negative*. In the former case the image is seen in its natural bright colours without any alteration; but in the latter case the bright parts become dark, while the dark parts are light.

After-pains. The uterine pains which are felt after the birth of the child, due to contraction and retraction of the muscle fibres.

Agalactia (ă-gal-ak'-ti-ă). Absence of secretion of milk.

Agar (ā'-gàr). A gelatinous substance prepared from Ceylon moss and similar sea-weeds. It is used very extensively in the preparation of solid media for bacterial culture. It has no nutritive value; it merely serves to solidify or stiffen the media.

AgCl. Silver chloride.

Age (Mental). The age of a person with regard to his mental development; this is determined by a series of mental tests as devised by Binet. Thus if a woman of thirty can only pass the tests of a child of twelve, she is said to have a mental age of twelve.

Agglomerate (ag-lom'-er-āt). To congregate; to form into clumps or masses.

Agglutina'tion. The clumping

of bacteria as effected by the specific immunity antibodies, called agglutinins, developed in the blood serum of a previously infected person.

Agony (ag'-o-ni). Severe or excruciating pain.

Agoraphobia (ag-or-ō-fō'-bi-ă). Fear of being at a height.

Agranulocytosis (ă-gran-ū-lō-sī-tō'-sis). A condition of the blood characterized by an absence of, or marked reduction in, the number of granulocytes or polymorphonuclear leucocytes. (*See also* Angina.)

A g r a p h i a (a-grăf'-i-ă). Inability to express the thoughts in writing.

Ague (ā-gū). Malaria. A condition characterized by intermittent paroxysms of fever and rigors. The disease is conveyed by mosquitoes, and there are two or three different varieties. Thus if the rigors occur every 24 hours it is known as *quotidian malaria*; if every 48 hours, *tertian malaria*; if every 72 hours, *quartan malaria*.

Air. The gaseous mixture which makes up the atmosphere. It consists of *oxygen*, 20·94%; *nitrogen*, 78·09%; CO_2, 0·03%; *argon*, 0·94%, and traces of *ozone*, *neon*, *helium*; also *water vapour* in varying amounts. **A.-Bed**, a rubber bed filled with air. **Complemental A.**, the extra air that can be drawn

11

into the lungs by deep inspiration. **A.-Hunger**, a condition resulting from extreme shock, such as may result from hæmorrhage ; the breathing is sighing and gasping, on account of the shortage of oxygen in the blood. **Residual A.**, that which still remains in the alveoli of the lung after forced expiration. **Supplemental A.**, the extra amount of air expired when breathing out with great effort. **Tidal A.**, that which passes in and out of the lungs without special effort, *i.e.*, during quiet breathing.

Akinesia (ă-kĭn-ē-zĭ-á). Loss of the power of motion.

Ala (ā-lá). Any wing-like process. **A. Magna**, the greater wing of the sphenoid. **Alæ Nasi**, the nostrils. *Adj.* **Alar.**

Alalia (ă′-lā-lĭ-á). Defective speech due to a local lesion of the vocal cords.

Alastrim (al-as′-trĭm). Milk-pox ; a mild form of smallpox chiefly found among the black races of South Africa. Also known as *Amaas.*

Alba (al′-bá). White. **Mist. A.**, white mixture.

Albino (al-bē′-nō). An individual who lacks pigment. The hair is white, the skin very fair, and the eyes are pink, with very weak vision.

Albumin (or Albumen) (al-bū′-min). A variety of protein ; the white of egg is pure albumin. Its chemical composition is not fully determined, but is known to contain *carbon, hydrogen, nitrogen, oxygen, sulphur.* **A. Water**, after removing the specks from 2 eggs, separate the white from the yolk, and then cut the whites across several times, but do not beat. Add ½ pint of cold boiled water. Stir lightly and add a pinch of salt or a few drops of lemon. For infants the lemon is omitted, and the albumin water must be strained through gauze.

Albuminuria (al-bū-min-ŭ′-rĭ-á). An abnormal condition characterized by the presence of albumin in the urine.

Albumose (al′-bū-mōz). A substance formed during the early digestion of protein. It is an intermediate stage between albumin and peptones.

Albumosuria (al-bū-mōz-ŭ′-rĭ-á). The presence of albumose in the urine.

Alcohol (al′-kō-hol) ($C_2H_5.OH$). A colourless volatile liquid, which is stimulant in small amounts, but in large quantities acts as a narcotic. It boils at 78° C., and freezes at −139° C. ; is distilled from fermented wines or spirits, repeated distillations producing a stronger alcohol. Various strengths are recognized, *e.g.*, 20-95%. **Absolute A.,** alcohol containing no water.

Alembroth (al-em'-broth). A crystalline salt, a compound of mercuric chloride and ammonium chloride. It is used as an antiseptic. Wool, gauze, and lint are impregnated with the salt, and these dressings are usually coloured blue as a distinguishing mark.

Aleukæmia (ā-lū-kē'-mi-ā). A deficiency of leucocytes in the blood.

Alexander-Adams' Operation. An operation used in the repair of backward displacements of the uterus by a method of shortening the round ligaments. Named after *William Alexander*, of Liverpool, and *James Adams*, of Glasgow.

Alexia (ă-leks'-i-ā). Word blindness; loss of the ability to interpret the significance of the printed or written word, but without loss of visual power. Due to a brain lesion.

Algesia (al-jē'-zi-ā). Excessive sensitiveness to pain; hyperæsthesia.

Algesimeter (al-jes-im'-et-er). An instrument which registers the degree of sensitivity of the skin.

Alienation (ā-li-en-ā'-shun). Mental derangement; insanity.

Alienist (ā'-li-en-ist). *See* **Psychiatrist.**

Alimentary. Pertaining to food. **A. Canal,** the canal down which the food passes during digestion; it commences at the mouth and ends at the anus; the structures forming it are the *mouth, pharynx, œsophagus, stomach, small intestine, colon, and rectum.* **A. Duct,** same as the *thoracic duct.*

Alimentation (al-i-men-tā'-shun). The method or process of introducing food into the body. **Artificial A.,** the nourishment of persons who are too weak and ill to take food in the ordinary way. **Forced A.,** forcible feeding. **Rectal A.,** the passing of food into the rectum. **Subcutaneous A.,** the introduction of nourishment by means of subcutaneous injections.

Alkalæmia (al-kal-ē'-mi-ā). An excessive alkalinity of the blood due to a decrease in the *hydrogen-ion* concentration of the blood. Also referred to as *Alkalosis.*

Alkali (al'-kal-ī). A series of soluble, corrosive bases analogous to, and including soda, potash, and ammonia which neutralize acids forming salts and combine with fats to form soaps. Alkaline solutions turn red litmus blue.

Alkaline (al'-kal-īn). Possessing the properties of an

alkali. Alkaline solutions contain an excess of hydroxyl over hydrogen ions ; neutral solutions contain them in equal numbers, and acid solutions contain an excess of hydrogen ions.

Alkalinuria (al-kal-in-ūr′-i-à). Alkalinity of urine.

Alkaloid (al′-kal-oid). Resembling an alkali. A name often applied to a large group of organic bases found in plants, and which possess important physiological actions. Morphine, quinine, caffeine, atropine, and strychnine are well-known examples of alkaloids.

Alkalosis (al-kal-ō′-sis). *See* **Alkalæmia.**

Alkapton (al-kap′-ton). A decomposition product of proteins found in the urine and cerebrospinal fluid under certain pathological conditions.

Alkaptonuria (al-kap-ton-ūr′-i-à). The presence of alkapton in the urine which causes it to turn dark on standing.

Allantois (al-an′-toiz). A sac which is developed from the hind-gut of the early embryo. Later it curves round to envelop the embryo completely.

Allergy (al′-er-ji). An altered or exaggerated susceptibility to various foreign substances or physical agents which are harmless to the great majority of individuals.

Alloy (al′-oi). The combination of two or more metals by fusion.

Aloes (al′-ōz). The dark, bitter, inspissated juice of several species of aloe ; laxative. Decoction aloes co., ½-2 fl. oz.

Aloin (al′-ō-in). A bitter, active principle of aloes. By varying the dose it is both laxative and purgative.

Alopecia (al-ō-pē′-si-à). Loss of hair from any part of the body, but more particularly from the scalp ; baldness. **A. Areata,** sharply defined, rounded patches of baldness, due to nervous disturbances.

Alterative (ol′-ter-a-tiv). A medicine which favourably changes bodily nutrition and excretion by some method or process not known.

Alternating Current. An electrical current which rapidly and periodically alters its direction.

Alternation of Generation. A type of reproduction found in some of the lower forms of life, in which one generation reproduces sexually and the next asexually.

Alum. Aluminium and potassium sulphate ; is astringent and styptic, and is soluble in water but not in alcohol.

Aluminium (al-ū-min′-i-um). A metallic white element with an atomic weight of 27 and a specific gravity of 2·58. Used for surgical instruments and splints. Symbol, Al.

14

Alveolar (al-vē'-ō-lår). Pertaining to the alveoli. **A. Processes,** the teeth sockets.

Alveolus (al-vē'-ō-lus). (1) An air-vesicle of the lung. (2) A tooth-socket. (3) A gland follicle.

Amalgam (a-mal'-gam). An alloy containing mercury.

Amastia (ă-mas-ti-å). Congenital absence of the breasts.

Amaurosis (ă-mor-ō'-sis). Partial or complete blindness due to causes other than ophthalmic changes in the eye. May be caused by such diseases as nephritis, brain lesions, and diabetes.

Am'ber. A yellow fossil resin from extinct trees.

Ambergris (am-ber-grēs). A rare and valuable substance excreted from the intestines of the sperm whale. It is sometimes found floating in greyish masses on the surface of the sea. Is used chiefly as a perfume.

Ambidextrous (am-bi-deks'-trus). Able to use both hands equally well.

Amblyopia (am-bli-ō'-pi-å). Defective vision approaching blindness.

Amboceptor (am'-bō-sep'-ter). An intermediary substance found in blood serum which has the specific power of binding the *complement* to the cell. One of the antibodies. *See* **Ehrlich's Side-chain Theory.**

Ambrine (am'-brēn). A proprietary preparation used for the treatment of burns. A good substitute consists of betanaphthol, eucalyptus and olive oils, hard and soft paraffin wax.

Ambulatory (am-bū-lā'-tor-l). Mobile; able to walk; not confining the patient to bed.

Amelia (ă-mē'-li-å). Absence of the limbs.

Amelioration (ă-mē-li-or-ā'-shun). Cessation of the severity of symptoms. Improvement in the general condition.

Amenorrhœa (a-men-o-rē'-å). Absence of the menses. **Primary A.,** when menstruation has not been established at the time when it should first appear. **Secondary A.,** absence of the menses after they have once commenced.

Amentia (ă-men'-shi-å). Absence of intellect; idiocy.

Ametria (ă-mēt'-ri-å). Congenital absence of the uterus.

Ametropia (ă-met-rō'-pi-å). Defective sight due to imperfect refractive power of the eye.

Amidopyrine (am-i-dō-pī'-rin). A colourless crystalline compound or white powder used medicinally as an antipyretic and analgesic; is tasteless, odourless, and soluble in water and alcohol. Synonym, *Pyramidon.*

Amino-acids (am-ēn'-ō-as-ĭdz).

15

Organic acids in which one or more of the hydrogen atoms are replaced by the amino group (NH_2). The amino-acids may be likened to the building stones of which a protein is formed. There are many different amino-acids. Among the more important are *tryptophane, lysine, glycine, phenylalanine, tyrosine, leucine, histidine* and *cystine*.

Amitosis (ā-mī-tō′-sis). Multiplication of a cell by the method of direct fission.

Ammonia (am-ō′-ni-ȧ). A colourless gas (NH_3) soluble in water. In solution it is a volatile alkali with a penetrating odour. Medicinally it is antacid and stimulating.

Amnesia (am-nē′-zi-ȧ). Temporary loss of memory, especially for words.

Amnion (am′-ni-on). The inner membrane forming the sac which directly encloses the embryo and forms a sheath for the umbilical cord.

Amniotic (am-ni-ot′-ik). Pertaining to the amnion. **A. Fluid,** the fluid contained in the amniotic sac. *See* **Liquor Amnii**

Amœba (am-ē′-bȧ). A minute, unicellular, animal organism. It exists in shallow ponds or pools, and is found in great numbers in the green slime on the top of the water. They are also found in the

16

mud at the bottom. They possess an outer translucent substance called the *ectosarc*, and an inner denser substance, the *endosarc*, which contains the nucleus. It feeds by surrounding its victim and enclosing it in the so-called

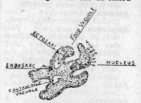

The Amœba.

food-vacuole. Oxygen is absorbed from the surrounding water, and CO_2 is eliminated through the *contractile vacuole*. The organism moves by pushing out parts of the cell protoplasm. These projections are called *pseudopodia,* or false legs. Reproduction occurs either by *direct fission,* or, more rarely, by a method of *encystment.* There are various types of amœbœ, but one type is especially well known as being parasitic to man, the *Entamœba histolytica,* which causes amœbic dysentery.

Amœbic (am-ē′-bik). Of the nature of an amœba.

Amœbiasis (am-ō-bī'-a-sis). Infection with pathogenic amœbæ.

Amœboid (am-ē'-boid). Resembling an amœba in shape or movement.

Amorphous (am-awr'-fus). Having no regular shape.

Ampere (am'-pier). The unit of measurement of the strength of an electric current.

Amphibia (am-fib'-i-å). A class of vertebrates capable of living both on land and in water. A good example is the frog.

Amphoric (am-for'-ik). Relating to a bottle. A breath sound, sound heard on auscultation resembling that produced by blowing across the mouth of a bottle.

Ampoule (am'-pool). A small glass phial containing a drug ready sterilized and in the correct dosage for immediate use. The same as *Ampule*.

Ampulla (am-pul'-å). Any flask-like dilatation. **A. of Vater,** the enlargement formed by the union of the common bile duct with the pancreatic duct where they enter the duodenum.

Amputation (am-pū-tā'-shun). The removal of a part of the body. **Accidental A.,** loss of the whole or part of a limb through an accident. **Bloodless A.,** amputation without loss of blood. **Circular A.,** a circular cut at right angles to the long axis of a limb; the raw edge is covered by a single flap; a method of amputation much used during the Great War. **Syme's A.,** amputation at the ankle joint.

Amyasthenia (ā-mī-as-thēn'-i-å). Great muscular weakness, especially of the limbs.

Amyl Nitrite. A yellow volatile liquid. Acts as a vasodilator, and is much used in *angina pectoris.* Dose 2-5 minims by inhalation.

Amylase (am'-i-lāz). An enzyme which converts starches into sugar.

Amyloid Disease (am'-i-loid). A fatty disease which sometimes affects the liver, spleen, and kidneys. These organs become wax-like in appearance. Also known as *Lardaceous Disease.*

Amyotonia (ā-mī-ō-tōn'-i-å). Great muscular weakness, often congenital. Same as *Myatonia.*

Amyotrophia (ā-mi-ō-trō'-fi-å). Muscular wasting.

Anabolism (an-ab'-ol-izm). Constructive metabolism. A form of metabolism in which a comparatively simple substance is built up into one which is more complex. The opposite is katabolism.

Anacidity (an-as-id'-it-i). Lacking in acid. Often used in connection with gastric juice when hydrochloric acid is deficient. Achlorhydria.

17

Anacrotic (an-a-krot′-ik). Relating to anacrotism.

Anacrotism (an-a-krot′-izm). An oscillation in the ascending curve of a sphygmographic pulse tracing.

Anadicrotic (an-a-dī-krot′-ik). A variety of pulse in which the sphygmographic record shows a double wave in the ascending curve.

Anæmia (an-ē′-mi-à). A deficiency of the hæmoglobin content of the blood. **Addison's A.**, a very grave form of anæmia often ending fatally. The same as *Pernicious A.*, *Primary*, *Idiopathic*, or *Essential A.* A form of anæmia arising without obvious cause. **Secondary A.**, a form of anæmia which follows some other disease or abnormal condition, *e.g.*, cancer, sepsis, and hæmorrhage.

Anaerobe (an′-ĕr-ōb). A microorganism which does not need oxygen or air for its existence.

Anæsthesia (an-es-thēz′-i-à). Loss of sensation. **Local A.**, insensibility of one part of the body only. **General A.**, insensibility of the whole body. **Spinal A.**, anæsthesia caused by the injection of an anæsthetic into the spinal subarachnoid space. Same as *Intrathecal Anæsthesia*.

Anæsthetic (an-es-thet′-ik). A drug which produces anæsthesia.

Anæsthetist (an-ēs′-the-tist). One who administers anæsthesia.

Anal (ā-nal). Pertaining to the anus.

Analgesia (an-al-jē′-zi-à). Loss of painful impressions without loss of tactile sense.

Analysis (an-al′-i-sis). A term used in chemistry to denote the determination of the composition of a compound substance. *See* **Psycho-analysis**.

Analyst (an′-a-list). One who conducts an analysis.

Anaphase (an′-a-fāz). A stage in mitosis when the newly divided chromosomes move towards the opposite poles of the chromatic spindle to form the *diaster*. *See* **Karyokinesis**.

Anaphrodisiac. *See* **Antaphrodisiac**.

Anaphylaxis (an-a-fil-aks′-is). A hypersensitive state of the body to a foreign protein, so that the injection of a second dose brings about an acute reaction ; known also as *protein sensitization* and *serum sickness*. The reaction does not occur if the initial dose has been administered not more than ten days previously. To prevent anaphylaxis the second dose of serum should be given gradually, *i.e.*, it must be divided into small doses, with a short interval between. Some doctors prefer to give half

18

the dose, and the remainder after half-an-hour's interval.

Anasarca (an-a-sàrk'-à). The infiltration of the subcutaneous cellular tissue with serous fluid ; dropsy.

Anastomosis (an-as-to-mō'-sis). (1) A term denoting the inter-communication of the branches of two or more arteries or veins. (2) In surgery the word indicates an artificial union of two structures, *e.g.*, *End-to-end A.*, of two parts of the intestine.

Anatomic (an-a-tom'-ik). Relating to anatomy.

Anatomist (a-nat'-o-mist). One who studies anatomy or who performs dissections.

Anatomy (a-nat'-o-mi). The science which deals with the structure of the body through dissection. **Applied A.**, especially applied to the diagnosis of disease and its treatment. **Comparative A.**, comparing the bodily structures and anatomical relations between the lower animals and man. **Descriptive A.**, that which describes distinct and separate parts of the body with reference to their relation to other parts. **Gross A.**, naked-eye structure of the body ; not needing a microscope. **Microscopic A.**, histology ; the study of minute structures requiring the use of a microscope. **Regional A.**, a detailed description of some particular region or part.

Anatoxin (an-a-toks'-in). Bacterial toxin modified by formalin so as to reduce its harmful effects without reducing its antigenic powers.

Andria (an'-dri-à). A pseudo-male hermaphrodite.

Andro (an'-drō). A prefix signifying man.

Androgyna (an-drō-jī'-nà). A pseudo-female hermaphrodite, *i.e.*, one in whom the female characteristics are predominant.

Androphobia (an-drō-fō'-bi-à). A morbid dislike or fear of men.

Anencephalous (an-en-kef'-a-lus). Without a brain. A term used in connection with fœtal monsters. The condition is incompatible with life.

Anergia (an-er'-ji-à). Inactivity.

Aneroid (an'-er-roid). Without liquid. A term used in connection with barometers and sphygmomanometers.

Aneuria (an-ū-rī-à). Deficiency or lack of nervous energy.

A n e u r y s m (an'-ūr-izm). A local dilatation in the course of an artery ; may occur in any artery, but is most common in the arch of the aorta, thoracic aorta, femoral artery, popliteal artery, and abdominal aorta (the latter more rarely). Such tumours

19

are recognized by the presence of pulsations which correspond to each systole of the heart. A *bruit* is also heard on auscultation. **Arterio-venous A.,** an aneurysmal communication between an artery and a vein. **Arterial A.** are of three main varieties : (1) *Dissecting A.,* in which the blood forces its way between the fibres of the muscular coat so that the inner half is pushed towards the intima and the outer half to the adventitia; (2) *Fusiform A.,* in which the coats are all equally expanded throughout the circumference of the vessel ; (3) *Sacculated A.,* when the arterial wall only bulges on one side of the vessel. **A. Needle,** a large blunt needle fixed to a metal handle and with the eye-end turned up.

Angina (an-jī'-nâ). Spasmodic attacks of pain accompanied by a sensation of suffocation and impending death. There are several different types of this condition. **Agranulocytic A.,** inflammation and ulceration of the pharynx associated with marked reduction or even complete absence of the polymorphonuclear leucocytes of the blood. **A. Ludovici or Ludwig's A.,** an acute inflammation of the struc-

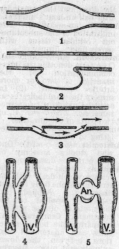

Types of Aneurysms.

Arterial—
1, Fusiform.
2, Saccular.
3, Dissecting.
Arterio-venous—
4, Aneurysmal varix.
5, Varicose aneurysm (the aneurysm is false).

A., Artery.   V., Vein.
An., Aneurysm.

tures of the floor of the mouth and submaxillary region. **A. Pectoris**, a condition characterized by agonizing pain directly behind the sternum, due to temporary ischæmia of the heart muscle. The pain, which often radiates down the left arm, is so acute that the sufferer is unable, or afraid, to move, and retains the position assumed when the attack commenced. The face is pale, and the skin cold and clammy. A capsule of amyl nitrite, broken in a clean handkerchief, is held beneath the nose of the patient, so that the fumes are inhaled. This immediately relieves the heart by dilating the peripheral arterioles. **Vincent's A.**, an inflammatory condition of the throat, due to infection with spirilla and fusiform bacilli.

Angioma (an-ji-ō'-må). A tumour formed of blood-vessels. **A. Telangiectatic**, one consisting of dilated capillaries. See **Nævus**.

Angiomyoma (an-ji-ō-mī-ō'-må). A tumour containing both vascular and muscular structures.

Angioneurotic (an-ji-ō-nū-rot'-ik). Pertaining to *angioneurosis*; a defect or abnormality of the vasomotor nerves, *e.g.*, **A. Œdema**, a neurosis characterized by localized non-inflammatory dropsical swellings.

Angle (ang'-gl). The space between two lines which converge towards a given point.

Anhidrosis (an-hi-drō'-sis). A diminution of sweat.

Anhydrous (an-hī'-drus). Entirely without water; dry.

Aniline (an'-il-ēn). An oily compound obtained from the dry distillation of coal and much used in the preparation of dyes.

Animalcule (an-im-al'-kūl). A minute animal organism which is invisible to the naked eye.

Anion (an'-I-on). See **Ion**.

Anisocytosis (an-I-sō-sī-tō'-sis). Inequality in the size of the red blood corpuscles.

Ankle (ang'-kl). The joint between the leg and the foot; the tarsus. **A. Clonus**, a series of rapid muscular contractions of the calf muscle when the foot is suddenly flexed by pressure upon the sole.

Ankyloblepharon (ang-ki-lō-blef'-a-ron). Adhesion of the edges of the eyelids.

Ankylosed (ang'-ki-lōzd). Rigid; immovable; fixed by ankylosis.

Ankylosis (ang-ki-lō'-sis). The fusion or union of the bones forming the joint, resulting from inflammation or injury. Fixation of the joint.

Ankylostoma (ang-ki-lō-stō'-

21

má). The hook-worm. A minute parasite which infests the intestines, and known as the *A. duodenale*. The disease is also known as *hook-worm disease* and *ankylostomiasis*.

Ankyroid (ang'-ki-roid). Hook-shaped.

Annular (an'-ū-lår). Ring-shaped. **A. Ligament**, the ligament round the ankle and wrist.

Anoci Association (an-ō'-si as-sō-si-ā'-shun). Criles' method of preventing post-operative shock by a method of nerve-blocking, *i.e.*, the injection of a local anæsthetic such as novocain into the sensory nerves leading from the field of operation. Quinine - urea - hydrochloride is also used for this purpose.

Anodal (an-ō'-dal). Pertaining to the anode.

Anode (an'-ōd). The positive pole of a galvanic battery.

Anodyne (an'-ō-dīn). A remedy which relieves pain, such as opium, morphine, codeine, etc.

Anoesia (an-ō'-zi-å). Lack of understanding; idiocy.

Anomaly (an-om'-a-li). That which is unusual or differs from the normal.

Anonymous (an-on'-i-mus). Without a name; nameless; innominate.

Anopheles (an-of'-i-lēz). A genus of mosquitoes. The females are the host of the malarial parasite, and their bite is the means of transmitting the disease to man.

Anorchus (an-awr'-kus). Without testicles. A male without testicles in the scrotum, either through absence or failure of descent.

Anorexia (an-o-reks'-i-å). Loss or deficiency of appetite for food.

Anosmia (an-oz'-mi-å). Absence of the sense of smell.

Anoxæmia (an-oks-ē'-mi-å). Insufficient oxygenation of the blood.

Antacid (ant'-as-id). A substance which corrects acidity; that which neutralizes or counteracts acidity.

Antagonism (an-tag'-on-izm). Having an opposite effect; working in opposition, as said of drugs, muscles, and organisms.

Antaphrodisiac (ant-af-rō-diz'-i-ak). An agent that diminishes sexual desire; absence of sexual impulse. Also **Anaph'rodisiac**.

Anteflexion (an'-tē-flek'-shun). The bending forward of an organ. Commonly applied to the position of the uterus.

Antemortem (an'-tē-mawr'-tem). Before death.

Antenatal (an-tē-nā'-tal). Before birth.

Antepartum (an'-tē-pår'-tum). Before birth. More generally confined to the period im-

22

mediately preceding delivery. **A. Hæmorrhage,** bleeding from the uterus before delivery; may be either concealed or revealed, and accidental or inevitable.

Anterior. The front surface of anything; situated in front of.

Antero (an'-te-rō). Prefix signifying before.

Anteroposterior. Passing from before backwards.

Anteversion (an'-tē-ver'-shun). The forward displacement or tilting of the whole organ.

Anthelmintic (an-thel-min'-tĭk). A remedy or cure for intestinal worms. *See* **Enema, Anthelmintic.**

Anthracosis (an-thra-kō'-sis). A pigmentation of the lungs, especially of coal miners, from the inhalation of coal dust or smoke.

Anthrax (an'-thraks). A malignant disease caused by the *Bacillus anthracis.* Workers in wools, hides, and brushes are commonly affected. The disease may attack the lungs, *Woolsorters' disease,* or the alimentary tract, the *gastrointestinal* type, or the loose cellular tissues giving rise to *anthrax œdema,* or more commonly it occurs in the form of a pustule known as an *anthrax boil* or *malignant pustule.* The disease often proves fatal. It is treated with Sclavo's serum. *See* **Bacteria.**

Anthropoid (an'-thrō-poid). Relating to man; a term often used in connection with the man-like apes.

Antibodies. Substances existing in blood which are antagonistic to the growth and harmful action of bacteria. They are reaction substances similar to those under the influence of which they were formed. Examples of such are *antitoxins, bacteriolysins, agglutinins, precipitins,* etc.

Anticus (an'-tē-kus or an-tī'-kus). Latin for anterior.

Antidote (an-ti-dōt). A remedy which counteracts or neutralizes the action of a poison.

Antienzyme (an-ti-en'-zīm). Any substance which neutralizes an enzyme.

Antifebrile (an'-ti-feb-rīl). Efficacious in reducing or allaying fever.

Antigen (an-ti-jen). A substance which under favourable conditions can produce the formation of antibodies.

Antikamnia (an-ti-kam-ni-á). A proprietary medicine having an antipyretic and analgesic action.

Antiluetic (an-ti-loo-et'-ik). An agent which prevents or cures syphilis.

Antimonium, Antimony (an'-tim-o-ni). A metallic element, bluish in colour.

23

Symbol, Sb. Atomic weight, 120·2. Often used medicinally. A constituent of tartar emetic, etc.

Antipathy (an-tip'-a-thi). Dislike; a revulsion of feeling; repulsion of feeling.

Antiperiodic (an-ti-pier-ri-od'-ik). An agent which prevents the periodic return of a disease, *e.g.*, the use of quinine in malaria.

Antiperistalsis (an-ti-pe-ri-stal'-sis). A reversal of the normal peristaltic action, *i.e.*, occurring from below upwards.

Antiphlogistin (an-ti-flō-jis'-tin). A proprietary preparation. It is much used for poultices, acting as an antiseptic, analgesic, and counter-irritant in cases of deep-seated inflammation. It has largely superseded the linseed poultice, being lighter and retaining the heat longer. It is renewed every 6-24 hours.

Antipyretic (an-ti-pī-ret'-ik). An agent which allays or reduces fever.

Antipyrin (an-ti-pī'-rin). A derivative of coal-tar products. It is antipyretic, antirheumatic and analgesic in action. Dose 5-10 gr. *See* Phenazone.

Antirachitic (an-ti-rak-it'-ik). Preventing or curing rickets. *See* Rachitis.

Antiscorbutic (an-ti-skawr-bū'-tik). An agent which prevents or cures scurvy.

Antisepsis (an-ti-sep'-sis). The prevention of sepsis; introduced into surgery in 1880 by Lord Lister, who used carbolic acid.

Antiseptic (an-ti-sep'-tik). A substance which counteracts putrefaction by preventing the growth of bacteria. The following are some common antiseptics and the strengths in which they are generally used:—

> Boracic acid, a saturated solution, or 1-25.
> Biniodide solution, 1-500. Commonly 1-1000.
> Carbolic solution, 1-20 for instruments; 1-40 for hands; 1-60 for gargle.
> Creosote, 3Ĭ to water OĬ for inhalation.
> Corrosive sublimate, 1-1000.
> Iodine, 22% solution for painting on the skin. For baths, etc., 3Ĭ to water OĬ
> Izal, 3Ĭ to water OĬ.

Antispasmodic (an-ti-spaz-mod'-ik). A substance which allays or relieves spasms, *e.g.*, *valerian.*

Antisyphilitic (an-ti-sif-il-it-ik). A remedy for syphilis.

Antisyphonage (an-ti-sī'-fon-āj). Preventing syphonage. A. Pipe, a 2-in. pipe placed beyond the trap of a water-closet pedestal. It passes through the wall, and continues upwards through the roof, with a wire cage at the top like a soil-pipe. Air passes down and into the trap, and by acting as a buffer, prevents the water-seal from being syphoned out by the rush of excreta down the soil-pipe.

Antitoxin (an-ti-toks'-ĭn). A substance formed in blood plasma by the injection into the body of the toxins produced by certain bacteria, such as the *B. tetani*. It acts by combining with the haptophore group of the molecules of the toxin, thus rendering it inert. *See* **Ehrlich's Theory of Immunity.**

Antivenine (an-ti-vě'-nin). A serum prepared from animals injected with the venom of snakes, and used as an antidote in cases of poisoning by snake-bite.

Antrum (an'-trum). A cavity, especially in a bone, such as the **A. of Highmore** in the *superior maxillary* bone.

Anuria (an-ū'-ri-ă). Absence of the secretion of urine by the kidneys. *See* **Suppression of Urine.**

Anus (ā'-nus). The extreme termination of the rectum. It is formed of a sphincter muscle which relaxes to allow fæcal matter to pass through. **Artificial A.,** one

produced surgically in some higher part of the bowel in cases of obstruction through any cause. **Imperforate A.,** one which has no opening; may be acquired or congenital.

Aorta (ā-awr'-tă). The large artery of the body which leaves the left ventricle of the heart; the main arterial trunk. **Abdominal A.,** the part which passes through the diaphragm into the abdomen. **Arch of the A.,** the curved part of the aorta after it leaves the heart. **Thoracic A.,** that which continues from the arch down through the thoracic cavity.

Aortic (ā-awr'-tik). Pertaining to the aorta. **A. Valve,** the semilunar cusps guarding the entrance to the aorta.

Aortitis (ā-awr-tī'-tis). Inflammation of the aorta.

Apathy (ap'-ath-i). Indifference; lack of interest.

Apepsia (ă-pep'-si-ă). Imperfect gastric secretion resulting in impairment of the digestive function.

Apepsinia (ă-pep-sin'-i-ă). Complete absence of pepsin or pepsinogen in the gastric juice.

Aperient (a-pier'-ri-ent). A mild laxative drug causing an evacuation of the bowels.

Aperture. An opening or orifice.

25

Apex (ā'-peks). The summit or top of anything which is cone-shaped. **A. Beat**, the beat of the apex of the heart against the chest wall, normally felt in the fifth intercostal space. **A. Pulmonis**, the apex of the lung.

Aphagia (ă-fā'-ji-ă). Inability to swallow.

Aphasia (ă-fā'-zi-ă). Loss of speech due to a brain lesion. **Motor A.**, loss of ability to articulate. **Sensory A.**, loss of power to recognize the written or spoken word.

Aphonia (ă-fō'-ni-ă). Loss of voice not brought about by a lesion of the brain. **A. Clericorum**, clergyman's sore throat. **Hysterical A.**, loss of speech due to hysteria.

Aphrodisiac (af-rō-diz'-i-ak). An agent which stimulates sexual excitement.

Aphthæ (af'-thē). Same as *Thrush*; small whitish spots occurring inside the mouth.

Aphthous (af'-thus). Relating to or infected with aphthæ.

Apical (ā'-pik-al). Pertaining to the apex.

Aplasia (ă-plā'-zi-ă). Incomplete development of tissue; absence of growth.

Apnœa (ap'-nē-ă). A transitory cessation of breathing.

Apodia (ă-pō'-di-ă). Congenital absence of the feet.

Apomor'phine Hydrochlor'ide. An alkaloid derived from morphine; is a strong and prompt emetic. Dose: expectorant, 1/64-1/32 gr.; hypnotic and emetic, 1/32-1/8 gr.

Aponeurosis (ap-on-ū-rō'-sis). A broad glistening sheet of tendon-like tissue which serves to invest and attach muscles to each other, and also to the parts that they move.

Aponeurositis (ap-on-ū-rō-si'tis). Inflammation of an aponeurosis.

Aponia (ă-pō'-ni-ă). Freedom from pain.

Apophysis (ap-of'-is-is). A projection, protuberance, or outgrowth. Usually used in connection with bone, *e.g.*, the **Basilar A.**, the Basilar process.

Apoplexy (ap-ō-pleks'-ĭ). Sudden unconsciousness caused by rupture of an artery in the brain resulting in extravasation of blood into the cerebral substance.

Appendicectomy (ap-pen-disek'-to-mi). Excision of the vermiform appendix. Also *Appendec'tomy.*

Appendices Epiploicæ (ap-pen'di-sēs ep-i-plō'-i-sē). Pouches of peritoneum, filled with fat and attached to the colon.

Appendicitis (ap-pen-di-sī'-tis). Inflammation of the appendix.

Appendicostomy (ap-pen-dikos'-to-mi). An operation in which the appendix is brought to the surface through an abdominal incision, and an opening made in it.

Appendix Vermiformis (appen-'diks ver-mi-fawr'-mis). A worm-like appendage of the cæcum about the thickness of a pencil and measuring from 1 to 6 in. in length. It is apparently functionless.

Apperception (ap-per-sep'-shun). The mental process whereby new knowledge is organized and interpreted in the light of past knowledge and experiences.

Appetite (ap'-pe-tīt). The desire for food ; hunger ; a great longing.

Applicator (ap'-li-kā-tor). An instrument for applying local remedies.

Apposition (ap-ō-zish'-un). The approximation or bringing together of two surfaces or edges.

Aqua (ak'-wà). The Latin for water. **A. Bulliens,** boiling water. **A. Callida,** warm water. **A. Destillata,** distilled water. **A. Fortis,** nitric acid (*q.v.*). **A. Frigida,** cold water. **A. Menthæ Piperitæ,** peppermint water. **A. Pura,** pure water.

Aqueduct (ak'-wi-dukt). A canal. **A. of Sylvius,** the canal connecting the third and fourth ventricles of the brain.

Aqueous (ā'-kwi-us). Watery. **A. Humor,** the fluid contained in the anterior chamber of the eye.

Arachnida (ar-ak'-nid-à). A group of arthropoda to which belong spiders and scorpions.

Arachnoid (ar-ak-noid). Resembling a spider's web. **A. Membrane,** the middle serous membrane of the cranial meninges.

Arantius (ar-ant'-i-us). An Italian anatomist and physician of Bologna (1530-89). **Corpus Arantii,** minute round bodies situated at the edge of the semilunar valves of the heart. **Duct of A.,** the ductus venosus.

Arbor (àr'-bor). Latin, a tree. **A. Vitæ,** the tree-like appearance of the cerebellar cortex as seen in a median section.

Arch. A curve or loop. **A. of Aorta,** the curved part between the ascending and descending aorta. **Palmar A.,** the arch formed by the union of the *radial* and *ulna* arteries in the palm. **Plantar A.,** the arch formed by the union of the *plantar* and *dorsalis pedis* arteries in the foot. **Pubic A.,** the arch formed by the ascending rami of the ischia ; it is immediately below the *symphysis pubis. See* **Pelvis.**

Area (èr'-i-à). A circumscribed space ; one having definite boundaries. **Association A.,** areas in the cerebrum which link up and

27

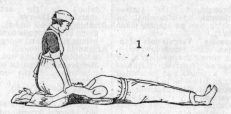

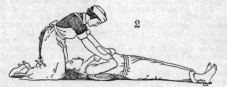

Artificial Respiration (Sylvester's Method).

correlate the various nerve centres.

Areola (ar-ē'-ŏ-là). The pigmented area round the nipple of the breast. **Secondary A.,** a dark circle of pigmentation which surrounds the primary areola in pregnancy. **Areolar Tissue,** a fine, delicate connective tissue.

Argenti Nitras (ar-jen'-ti nI'-tras). Silver nitrate ; argentum (ar-jen-tum) silver.

Argon (ar'-gon). One of the chemical inert gases of the atmosphere ; only exists in small quantities, 0·94%.

Argyll-Robertson Pupil. A pupil which reacts to accommodation but not to light.

Argyrol (ar-jI'-rol). An organic silver compound with a brown coloration in solution. It is much used for conjunctivitis, 5-10%, and cystitis, strength 10-40%.

Arithmomania (ar-ith-mŏ-mā'-ni-à). An anxiety neurosis

28

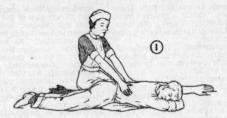

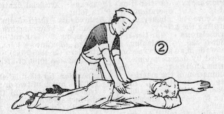

Artificial Respiration (Schafer's Method).

characterized by counting objects and repeating numbers.

Arnica (àrn'-ik-à). A herb, the tincture of which is used as a local sedative for bruises.

Arrhythmia (à-rith'-mi-à). Any deviation from the normal rhythm of the heart-beat.

Arsenic (àr'-sen-ik). A heavy lustrous solid, compounds of which are much used medicinally. In solution these are useful for many skin complaints and as a tonic. Symptoms of *A. poisoning*

29

must be watched for. These are chiefly gastric pain, vomiting, and diarrhœa. Liquor arsenicalis, 1%, 2-8 minims.

Arsenobenzol (ár-sen-ō-benz'-zol). An arsenical preparation used in the treatment of syphilis.

Artefact (árt'-i-fakt). Any artificially produced alteration in a structure ; an unnatural change.

Arteriole (ár-tier'-ri-ōl). A small artery.

Arteriorrhaphy (ár-tier-ri-or'-raf-i). An operation for the cure of aneurysm by suturing the artery.

Arteriosclerosis (ár-tier-ri-ō-skler-ō'-sis). Hardening of the walls of an artery, accompanied by degeneration.

Arteritis (ár-te-rī'-tis). Inflammation of the arteries.

Artery (ár'-te-ri). A blood vessel which carries blood from the heart to the various tissues.

Arthralgia (árth-ral'-ji-á). Articular neuralgia. Pain in the joints.

Arthrectomy (árth-rek'-to-mi). (1) The operation of opening into a joint cavity with the object of removing dead or diseased tissue. (2) Excision of a joint.

Arthritis (árth-rī'-tis). Inflammation of a joint. It may arise from many different causes, *e.g.*, **A. Deformans**, a

chronic condition characterized by atrophy of the bone and soft tissues, resulting in pain and marked deformity and stiffening. **A. Nodosa**, arthritis accompanied by chalky deposits around the joints. **Gonorrhœal** (or **Gonococcal**) **A.**, that resulting from infection with the gonococcus. **Gouty A.**, occurring in persons suffering with gout.

Arthrodesis (árth-rō-dē'-sis). Ankylosis induced by surgical means. Artificial fixation of a joint.

Arthrodynia (árth-rō-din'-i-á). Pain in a joint ; arthritis.

Arthrotomy (árth-rot'-o-mi). An opening into a joint.

Articular (ár-tik'-ū-lár). Pertaining to a joint or articulation.

Articulation (ár-tik-ū-lā'-shun). (1) The union of two or more bones ; a joint. (2) Clear, distinct speech.

Artificial (árt-i-fish'-al). Not natural ; made or invented by man. **A. Respiration**, a method of restoring suspended animation by causing air to enter and leave the lungs ; the best known methods are those of *Sylvester, Howard, Laborde, Schultze, Schafer,* and *Marshall-Hall.* **A. Ventilation**, the air is filtered, washed, and warmed before it is propelled into the various rooms ; the air

30

inlets are situated near the ceiling and the outlets low down; the chief systems are (1) the plenum, (2) the vacuum, (3) the balance.

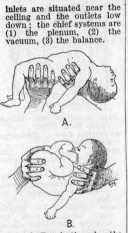

A.

B.

Artificial Respiration in the New-born (Byrd's Method).

Arytenoid (ar-ĭ-tēn′-oid). Funnel or pitcher shaped. **A. Cartilage**, the cartilages forming the posterior wall of the upper rim of the larynx.

Asafetida (as-a-fet′-i-dà). A gum-resin of fœtid odour; antispasmodic.

Asbestos (as-bes′-tos). A fibrous mineral substance which is an excellent heat resistant, non-conductor of heat, and therefore is used for covering steam-pipes.

Asbestosis (as-bes-tō′-sis). Fibrosis of the lungs resulting from the inhalation of fine asbestos dust and fibrils.

Ascariasis (as-kar-ī′-a-sis). The condition of being infected with the *ascarides*.

Ascaris (as′-kar-is). A nematode worm belonging to the family Ascaridæ, and commonly infesting the intestinal canal. **A. Lumbricoides**, the round-worm. **A. Vermicularis**, the thread-worm.

Aschheim-Zondek Test. A test for pregnancy which depends upon the presence of a hormone in the urine. Injections are made of the early morning urine of a woman suspected of pregnancy, into female immature mice. If the woman is pregnant, postmortem examination of the mouse will show congestion and hæmorrhage of the ovaries with maturation of the follicles. The test is 98-99% accurate.

Ascites (as-sī′-tēz). Dropsy of, and free fluid in, the abdominal cavity.

Asclepiads (as-klē-pi′-adz). An order of physicians and priests of Asclepios.

Asclepios, Æsculapius (as-

31

klĕp'-i-os,   ās-kū-lā'-pi-us).
The Greek god of medicine.

Asepsis (ă-sep-sis). A condition of being free from bacteria, obtained by sterilization by heat or by the use of strong antiseptics like lysol.

Aseptic (ă-sep-tik). Pertaining to asepsis.

Asexual (ă-seks'-ū-al). Not sexual. **A. Reproduction,** a method of reproduction not involving the mating of the two sexes.

Asphyxia (as-fĭks'-i-ă). A state of suspended animation caused by obstructed breathing due to gas inhalation, submersion in water, smothering, or strangulation. **A. Livida,** suspended respiration in the new-born; the face is blue or livid. **A. Pallida,** a similar condition in which the skin surface is cold and pallid.

Aspiration (as-pi-rā'-shun). (1) The act of drawing in the breath; inspiration. (2) The withdrawal of fluids from a body cavity by means of a suction or syphonage apparatus.

Aspirator (as'-pi-rā'-tor). An instrument used for aspirating fluids from cavities.

Assimilation (as-sim-l-lā'-shun). The same as **Anabolism.** The process whereby the already digested food-stuffs

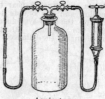

Aspirator.

are absorbed and utilized by the tissue cells.

Association Centre. Co-ordinating centre.

Astasia (as-tā'-zi-ă). Inability to stand due to motor ineo-ordination.

Asteatosis (ă-sti-a-tŏ'-sis). Insufficient sebaceous secretion resulting in dryness of the skin.

Aster (as'-ter). The stellate rays forming round the dividing centrosome during mitosis. *See* Mitosis.

Astereognosis (ă-ste-ri-og-nŏ'-sis). Loss of power to recognize the shape and consistency of objects.

Asthenia (as-thĕ'-ni-ă). Weakness; debility.

Asthenic. Pertaining to asthenia.

Asthenopia (as-thĕ-nŏ'-pi-ă). Weak-sightedness.

Asthma (asth'-mă). A respiratory disease characterized by paroxysms of acute dyspnœa associated with a sense of suffocation; the definite cause is unknown, but may be due to increased sensitiveness to certain proteins. **Cardiac A.**, a type occurring in persons suffering with advanced heart disease.

Asthmatic (asth-mat′-ik). Pertaining to asthma; one who suffers with asthma.

Astigmatism (as-tig′-mat-izm). Defective vision caused by inequality in the curvature of the cornea and lens so that the light rays do not converge to a point on the retina.

Astragalus (as-trag′-a-lus). The ankle bone; the second largest bone of the ankle. *See* Tarsus.

Astraphobia (ast-ra-fō′-bi-á). A morbid fear of thunder and lightning.

Astringent (as-trin′-jent). A substance which dries up a discharge or over-secretion from a mucous membrane by causing contraction of the small blood-vessels, *e.g.*, iron, tannin, alum, and adrenalin.

Astrocytoma (as-trō-sī-tō′-má). A slowly growing tumour of the glial tissue of brain or cord.

Asylum (as-ī′-lum). A place of refuge; a place where special care and treatment is given to those in need of it. **Lunatic A.**, a hospital for the care of the mentally sick.

Asymmetry (ă-sim′-et-ri). Lacking in proportion; unevenness.

Asynclitism (ă-sin′-klit-izm). A lateral oblique presentation of the fœtal head in the brim of the pelvis; a parietal presentation.

Atactic (ă-tak′-tik). Incoordinated; irregular.

Atavism (at′-a-vizm). The reappearance of an hereditary trait which has skipped one or more generations; a reversion to ancestral type.

Ataxia, ataxy (ă-taks′-i-á, ă-taks′-i). Defective muscular control resulting in irregular and jerky movements.

Atelectasis (at-el-ek′-ta-sis). Imperfect expansion of the lungs of a new-born child. Collapse of lung tissue.

Atelia, Ateliosis (at-ē′-li-á, at-ē-li-ō′-sis). The retention of childish characteristics in the adult.

Atheroma (ath-e-rō′-má). Degenerative changes in the walls of an artery.

Athetosis (ath-e-tō′-sis). A condition marked by purposeless movements of the hands and feet; is generally due to a brain lesion.

Atlas (at′-las). The first cervical vertebra. (*v.* p. 34.)

Atmosphere (at′-mŏs-fier). The air surrounding the earth. It exerts a pressure of 14·7 lbs. per sq. in. at sea-level, which is measured by means

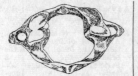

The Atlas.

of a barometer. The composition of the atmosphere is—

Oxygen	.	20·94%
Nitrogen	.	78·09%
CO_2	.	0·03%
Argon	.	0·94%
		100·00

Also there is a varying amount of water vapour and traces of *helium, neon, ozone, iodine.*

Atom (at'-om). A minute particle or unit, two or more of which form a chemical compound. Modern science formulates the theory that an atom is formed of still smaller units, known as electrons (*q.v.*). **Atomic Theory,** formulated by Dalton, who taught that all matter is composed ultimately of atoms. **Atomic Weight,** the weight of different atoms as compared with that of *hydrogen,* which is the lightest, and is represented as 1; the heaviest known is that of *uranium. Oxygen* is 16.

34

Atomizer (at'-om-ī-zer). An instrument producing a spray.

Atonic (ā'-ton-ĭk). Lacking in tone; weak; slack.

Atophan (at'-ō-fan). A drug sometimes used in gout and rheumatism.

Atremia (ā-trē'-mi-à). Inability to walk, caused by hysteria.

Atresia (ā-trē'-zi-à). The closure of a normal opening.

Atrium (ā'-tri-um). An auricle of the heart. One of the two upper chambers of the heart.

Atrophy (at'-ro-fĭ). Wasting of a part from lack of nutrition or use. **Progressive Muscular A.,** a very chronic disease, marked by general weakness and wasting of the muscles, with loss of their function.

Atropine (at'-ro-pēn). An alkaloid obtained from the plant, Atropa Belladonna. Used to check the secretions. and for this reason is often given hypodermically prior to the administration of an anæsthetic; is also much used as drops, which, when instilled into the eyes, cause dilatation of the pupils. Dosage: Atropine sulphate, 1/240-1/60 grain.

Attenuated (at-ten'-ū-ā-ted). Wasted; thin; weakened.

Attraction (at-rak'-shun). That which tends to draw one particle to another. The affinity existing between one chemical substance and another.

Atypic (ă-tip'-ik). Not typical; unusual; irregular.

Audiometer (aw-di-om'-et-er). An instrument for testing the sense of hearing.

Audition (aw-dish'-un). The act of hearing; listening.

Auditory (aw'-dit-o-ri). Pertaining to the sense of hearing. **A. Area**, the part of the brain concerned with hearing. **A. Meatus**, the entrance into the ear. **A. Nerves**, the eighth pair of cranial nerves. **A. Ossicles**, the small bones of the middle ear, viz., (1) *malleus*, (2) *incus*, (3) *stapes*.

Auerbach's Plexus (ow'-er-bak). A plexus of sympathetic nerve fibres situated between the longitudinal and circular fibres of the muscular coat of the stomach and intestines. Also called the *Myenteric Plexus*.

Aura (aw'-ră). A premonition; a peculiar sensation or warning of an oncoming attack, such as occurs in epilepsy.

Auricle (aw'-rik-l). One of the upper chambers of the heart.

Auricular (aw-rik'-ū-lá(r)). Pertaining to the cardiac auricle. **A. Ventricular Tract**, a neuromuscular bundle of nerve fibres which pass, as the bundle of His, from the right auricle into the ventricle. *See* **Pulse** and **Heart-Block**.

A. Fibrillation, irregular and rapid contractions of the auricles which work independently of the ventricles.

Auriscope (aw'-ris-kŏp). An instrument for examining the ear.

Auriscope.

Aurum (aw'-rum). The Latin for gold.

Auscultation (aws-kul-tā'-shun). A method of listening to the body sounds for diagnostic purposes, particularly the heart, lungs, and fœtal circulation. It may be (1) *immediate*, by placing the ear directly to the skin of the patient; (2) *mediate*, by the use of a stethoscope.

Autoclave (aw'-tŏ-klāv). An apparatus for high-pressure steam sterilization.

Autodestruction (aw-tŏ-de-struk'-shun). Self-destruction.

Auto-eroticism (aw-tŏ-e-rot'-is-izm). A perverted sex instinct in which self-gratification is obtained. *See* **Masturbation**.

Autogenous (aw-toj'-e-nus). Self-produced. **A. vaccine**, one prepared from bacteria obtained from the patient's own infection.

Auto-infection (aw-tŏ-in-fek'-shun). Re-infection.

Automatism (aw-tom'-at-izm). The performance of unconscious acts, *i.e.*, non-volitional acts.

Autonomic (aw-tŏ-nom'-ik). Independent. **A. Nervous System**, the distinct system of nerve cells and fibres constituting the sympathetic and para-sympathetic nerves.

Autopsy (aw-top'-si). A post-mortem examination. The examination of a dead body after death, performed for diagnostic purposes.

Auto-suggestion (aw-tŏ-su-jest'-yun). Self-suggestion.

Auto-transfusion (aw-tŏ-transfū'-zhun). A method of treating internal hæmorrhage by returning the patient's own extravasated blood to the circulation. The apparatus required is a beaker, glass rod, two cups or small bowls, a funnel, and 250 c.cm. ampules of 2% sodium citrate; the quantity being used is 10 c.cm. for each 90 c.cm. of blood. The apparatus for giving intravenous saline is also prepared, together with some physiological salt solution (0·9 %). After opening the abdomen the blood is allowed to run into the cup, which is then emptied into the beaker

containing the sodium citrate. The mixture is continually stirred by the nurse. After discovering and arresting the cause of the hæmorrhage, the rest of the blood is baled out, and the citrated blood now filtered through several layers of gauze (15-20) over the glass funnel into the saline flask, so that it enters the blood-vessel with the saline. *Contra-indications* are : (1) obviously infected blood ; (2) stale blood, *i.e.*, when bleeding has been going on for several days.

Avertin (a-ver'-tin). A tribromethanol ; a white crystalline substance with a melting-point of 79°-80° C. (174°-176° F.), and which is 3½% soluble in water at a temperature of 40° C. It vaporizes at the temperature of steam, and should be protected from light and air.

Avitaminosis (ā-vi-tam-in-ō'-sis). Any disease resulting from a deficiency of vitamins in the diet.

Axilla (aks-il'-á). The arm-pit.

Axillary Artery (aks-il'-a-ri art'-e-ri). The artery passing through the axilla. That section of the main artery which lies between the *sub-clavian* and *brachial* arteries.

Axis (aks'-is). (1) The second cervical vertebra. (2) A medial line. **A. Traction Forceps**, special forceps which are applied to the presenting head during child-

The Axis.

birth and which exert force along the normal axis of the pelvis. *See* Forceps. A. Cylinder, *see* Axon.

Axon (aks'-on). The same as *Axis Cylinder*. The core of a nerve fibre formed from an elongation of a dendrite from the nerve cell.

Azoospermia (ā-zō-ŏ-sperm'-i-ă). Sterility of the male through non-production of spermatozoa.

Azotæmia (a-zō-tē'-mi-ă). The presence of (an excess of) nitrogenous substances in the blood: usually seen in uræmia due to nephritis, but may be due to non-renal causes. (From *azote*, a synonym for *nitrogen*.)

Azygos (az'-i-gos). Occurring singly; not paired. A. veins, three unpaired veins of the abdomen and thorax which empty into the *inferior vena cava*.

B.

Babin'ski's Reflex. A test performed on patients suffering with nerve diseases. When the sole of the foot is gently stroked with the thumb, there is extension instead of flexion of the toes. It is normally present in infants at birth.

Baciliform (bas-il'-i-form). Shaped like a bacillus; rod-shaped.

Bacilluria (bas-il-ū'-ri-ă). The presence of bacilli in the urine.

Bacillus (bas-il'-us). A rod-shaped micro-organism belonging to the genus *Schizomycetes*. Pl. *Bacilli*. *See* Bacteria.

Back-pressure. Pressure caused by the damming back or by the actual backward flow of blood in a vein or in one of the chambers of the heart.

Bacteria (bak-tier-ri-ă). Minute unicellular organisms, containing no chlorophyll although belonging to the vegetable kingdom; they divide by direct fission. Acid-fast B., bacteria which are not decolorized by exposure to strong mineral acids; examples are the *Tubercle B.*, the *Smegma B.*, and the *B. Lepræ*. Aerobic B., bacteria requiring oxygen for their development. Anaerobic B., those

37

which thrive best without the presence of oxygen. **Chromogenic B.**, bacteria which produce a pigment. There are three great groups of bacteria. (1) *Cocci*, which are rounded in shape: these may occur singly; in pairs, *diplococci*; in chain formation, *streptococci*; or in clusters, *staphylococci*. (2) *Bacilli*, or rod-like organisms, *e.g.*, *B. Tuberculosis*, *B. Anthracis*, *B. Tetani*. (3) *Spirilla*, these are curved or spiralled, and cause such diseases as Asiatic cholera and syphilis. Bacteria may possess *motility* or movement, may produce poisons or *toxins*, and sometimes develop *flagellæ* and *spores*, the latter being an element of encystment. Bacteria are best destroyed by prolonged heat, and also by the use of chemicals in gaseous or liquid form.

Bacteriæmia (bak-te-rēm'-i-à). The presence of bacteria in the blood. Also called *Bacillæmia*.

Bacterial (bak-tier'-ri-al). Pertaining to bacteria.

Bactericide (bak'-ter-i-sīd). Any agent capable of destroying bacteria, *e.g.*, antiseptic lotions, great heat or cold.

Bacteriological (bak-tier'-ri-ō-loj'-ik-al). Pertaining to bacteriology

Bacteriologist (bak-tier'-ri-ol'-o-

jist). One who studies or is skilled in bacteriology.

Bacteriology (bak-tier'-ri-ol'-o-jē). The science which deals with the study of bacteria.

Bacteriolysin (bak-tier'-ri-ō-li'-sin). An antibody formed in the blood as the result of infection, and capable of destroying the organism causing the infection by lysis or solution.

Bacteriolytic (bak-tier'-ri-ō-lit'-ik). Pertaining to the destruction of bacteria.

Bacteriophage (bak-tier'-ri-ō-fāj). Ultra-microscopic organisms which are parasitic to bacteria, and normally exist in the intestinal tract.

Bacteriostatic (bak-tier'-ri-ō-stat'-ik). Preventing the growth or development of bacteria.

Bag. Any sac-like structure. **Barnes B.**, a bag used for dilating the cervix uteri; another used for the same purpose is **Champetier de Ribes B. Ice B.**, a bag filled with ice for applying cold to the body. **Politzer's B.**, a rubber bag for inflating the middle ear. **B. of Waters**, the fœtal sac enclosing the liquor amnii.

Baker's Itch. A form of eczema occurring on the hands of bakers from continual contact with flour.

Balanitis (bal-an-ī'-tis). Inflammation of the glans penis.

BACTERIA

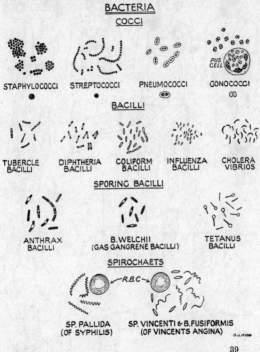

COCCI

STAPHYLOCOCCI   STREPTOCOCCI   PNEUMOCOCCI   GONOCOCCI

PUS CELL

BACILLI

TUBERCLE BACILLI   DIPHTHERIA BACILLI   COLIFORM BACILLI   INFLUENZA BACILLI   CHOLERA VIBRIOS

SPORING BACILLI

ANTHRAX BACILLI   B.WELCHII (GAS GANGRENE BACILLI)   TETANUS BACILLI

SPIROCHAETS

R.B.C

SP. PALLIDA (OF SYPHILIS)   SP. VINCENTI & B.FUSIFORMIS (OF VINCENTS ANGINA)

39

ROLLER BANDAGING

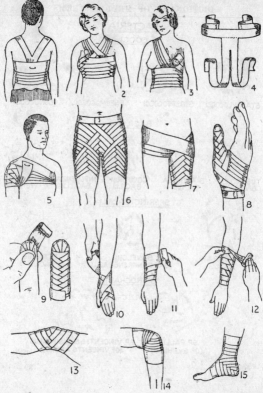

See foot of next page

Ballottement (bal-lot'-mon(g)). A method of diagnosing pregnancy by inserting a finger into the vagina and pushing the uterus, causing the embryo to rise and fall again like a heavy body in water.

Balneology (bal-nē-ol'-o-ji). The science of baths, especially with relation to their medical uses.

Balneum (bal'-ni-um). A bath.

Balsam (bawl'-sam). A resinous, fragrant, vegetable fluid. **Canada B.**, often used in preparing microscope slides. **Friars' B.**, compound tincture of benzoin. **B. of Peru**, an expectorant and sedative. **B. of Tolu**, a stimulant, expectorant, and stomachic.

Bandage (band'-āj). A strip of gauze, muslin, cotton, or flannel used for keeping dressings and splints in position, or for the support of some part of the body. **Abdominal B.**, same as *Many-tail*. **Capeline B.**, one which is applied to the head like a cap; it may be done with one 6-yd. bandage, but more generally two are used. **Many-tailed B.**, an abdominal bandage with four to six bands at each side; is used after an operation. **Roller B.**, a 6-yd. bandage, varying from 1-6 in. in width, according to the part of the body to which it is to be applied. **Spica B.**, a bandage taken once round the body and once round the limb. **Spiral B.**, one wound spirally round a limb. **Suspensory B.**, a bandage used for supporting the scrotum. **T. Bandage**, one shaped like the letter T used for keeping perineal dressings in position. **Triangular B.**, especially used for first aid purposes and for arm-slings.

Banti's Disease. A form of anæmia accompanied by enlargement of the spleen, hæmorrhages, and cirrhosis of the liver.

Banting's Diet. A method of dieting in which farinaceous

Roller Bandaging.

1, Many-tail bandage for chest.
2, Double-breast bandage.
3, Single-breast bandage.
4, T-bandage.
5, Ascending shoulder spica.
6, Double-groin spica.
7, Single-groin spica.
8, Thumb spica.
9, Finger bandage, figure-of-eight.
10, Hand bandage.
11, Spiral bandage for forearm.
12, Reverse bandage for forearm.
13, Knee bandage, half flexed.
14, Knee bandage, full flexed.
15, Heel bandage.

B *

TRIANGULAR BANDAGING

1

2

3

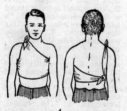

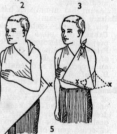

4

5

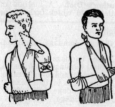

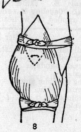

6

7

8

9

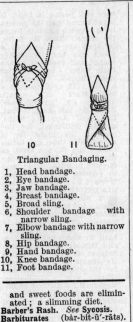

10 11

Triangular Bandaging.

1, Head bandage.
2, Eye bandage.
3, Jaw bandage.
4, Breast bandage.
5, Broad sling.
6, Shoulder bandage with narrow sling.
7, Elbow bandage with narrow sling.
8, Hip bandage.
9, Hand bandage.
10, Knee bandage.
11, Foot bandage.

and sweet foods are eliminated ; a slimming diet.

Barber's Rash. *See* Sycosis.

Barbiturates (bàr-bĭt-ū´-rāts). A group of widely used non-habit forming, hypnotic drugs. Some of the commoner examples are evipan, dial, nembutal, luminal, and sodium pentothal.

Barium (bér-i-um). Ba. A metallic element, the salts of which are opaque to X-rays, and the pure barium sulphate is therefore valuable for the examination of the alimentary tract, being used as an alternative to bismuth compounds.

Barograph (bar´-ō-graf). An apparatus by which the movements of a barometer are recorded on a revolving drum.

Barren (bar´-ren). Unable to reproduce ; sterile.

Bartholin's Glands (bàr´-tō-linz). Two small glands situated at the sides of the lower part of the vagina. Their ducts open just outside the hymen.

Barton's Fracture (bàr´-ton). Fracture of the distal end of the radius.

Basal (bā´-zal). Pertaining to the base ; fundamental.

Basal Metabolism (me-tab´-o-lizm). The energy output of a body at complete rest, *i.e.*, the energy necessary just to maintain body warmth and the necessary cardiac and respiratory activity required for life.

Basal Narcosis (nàr-kō-sis). The pre-anæsthetic administration of narcotic drugs which reduce fear and anxiety,

43

induce sleep, and thereby minimize post-operative shock.

Base (bās). (1) The lowest part of anything. (2) The main part of a compound. (3) In chemistry the substance which combines with an acid to form a salt.

Basedow's Disease (bas'-id-of). Exophthalmic goitre. Hyperthyroidism (*q.v.*).

Basement Membrane. A delicate transparent layer underlying the epithelium of mucous membranes and glands.

Basilar (baz-il'-ár). Relating to the base.

Basilic (bas-il'-ik). Prominent. An important vein, the **Median B.**, at the bend of the elbow. This vein is generally chosen for introducing fluids, such as saline or blood, into the body, or for withdrawing blood from the body.

Basophilic (băz-ŏ-fĭl'-ĭk). Having an affinity for basic stains—used in the study of histology.

Bath. To immerse in water or sand for cleansing purposes. A **Hot B.**, 100°-110° F. **Warm B.**, 85°-95° F. **Tepid B.**, 70°-85° F. **Cold B.**, 60°-70° F. **Acid B.**, one to which acid has been added to the water. **Alkaline B.**, one containing washing soda or other alkali. **Blanket B.**, a method of bathing a very sick person in bed; it is performed with the patient lying between blankets, hence the name. **Bran B.**, 3 lbs. of bran are enclosed in a gauze bag and thoroughly soaked and squeezed in the bath water; emollient for skin diseases. **Brand B.**, a cold bath used to reduce temperature in certain diseases, *e.g.*, *typhoid fever*. **Brine B.**, salt bath. **Foot, Leg, and Arm B.**, baths, usually medicated, for immersing the limbs for a considerable time, *e.g.*, *iodine baths*. **Hip B.**, the same as the *Sitz Bath*. **Mud B.**, immersion in warm mud; said to possess medicinal value. **Mustard B.**, mustard is mixed to a smooth paste and added to a warm, *not hot*, bath, 1 oz. to every gallon of water; useful in chill, rheumatism, and convulsions in children. **Sitz B.**, a shallow bath, in which only the hips and buttocks are immersed. **Sulphur B.**, one containing ℥iv potassa sulphurata; used for the cure of scabies and other skin complaints. **Vapour B.**, a method of immersing the body in steam.

Battery (bat'-er-ri). A series of Leyden jars or galvanic cells which generate electricity.

Battledore Placenta (bat'-el-dawr pla-sen'-tá). *See* Placenta.

Baudelocque's Diameter (bŏd'-lok). The external conjugate measurement of the pelvis. **B. Method**, a method of converting a face presentation into that of a vertex.

B.C.G. Abbreviation for Bacillus of Calmette and Guerin. A vaccine of attenuated tubercle bacilli used for the inoculation of infants to render them immune against tuberculosis. This method is still in the experimental stage.

Bead-test. A method of testing the activity of the digestive process in different parts of the alimentary tract. Beads covered with different types of food are attached by a thread and enclosed in a capsule which the patient swallows after a meal. The time taken for elimination of the beads per rectum is noted, and the remaining food on the beads is carefully examined.

Bearing-down. A feeling of pressure in the pelvis, due to expulsive efforts to deliver the child.

Beat (bēt). Pulsation of the blood in the heart and blood-vessels.

Bed-sore. A sore skin caused by lack of circulation in the part. Inanition, damp, and creases in the sheet are also causative. A bed-sore may be *threatened* if the skin is merely red, or *actual* if the skin is broken. In the latter case the wound may vary from a broken skin to a large, deep, septic wound, such as are liable to arise in conditions of paralysis, spine injuries, and other nerve diseases. They are also a complication of fractures. The parts most liable to be affected are bony prominences, such as the *shoulders*, *sacrum*, and *buttocks*, *knees*, *elbows*, and *heels*. Treatment is both *preventive* and *curative*.

Belladonna (bel-à-don'-à). *Atropa belladonna*, a poisonous plant, the deadly nightshade. It is used *internally* to check secretion, and *externally* is sometimes combined with glycerine for application to the skin. Atropine is an alkaloid of belladonna, B. Radix, ½-2 grs.

Bellini's Ducts (bel-ē'-nēz). The straight tubules of the kidneys, into which the collecting tubules open and which carry the urine to the calyces of the renal pelvis.

Bellocq's Sound (bel'-oks). An instrument used for plugging the posterior nares.

Bence-Jones' Albumose. Protein bodies appearing in the urine of persons suffering from disease of the bone-marrow. On heating the urine a precipitate forms at about 60° C. ; this disappears on further heating to boiling point, and reappears on cooling to 60° C.

Bendien's Test. A precipitation test carried out in varying concentrations of blood serum and colloidal vanadic acid, reputed to be of diagnostic value in cancer.

Benedict's Reagent. A solution used in testing for glucose. It is formed of 173 grs. of sodium or potassium citrate, 200 grs. of crystallized sodium carbonate dissolved in 800 cc. of boiling water. After cooling and filtering, 17·3 grs. of copper sulphate are added and the whole diluted to 1 litre with water.

Benign (be-nīn'). A term applied to tumours which are not malignant ; innocent.

Benzene (ben'-zēn). A colourless inflammable liquid obtained from coal-tar. It is a solvent of iodine, sulphur, phosphorus, fats, and resinous bodies.

Benzoin (ben'-zō-in). A resinous balsam obtained from a tree in Sumatra, the *Styrax benzoin*. It is antiseptic, expectorant, and healing ; is greatly used as an inhalation in pulmonary diseases. One drachm of the compound tincture is put into a Savar's inhaler, and 1 pint of boiling water added, and the vapour is inhaled.

46

Benzol. Same as *Benzene*.

Beriberi (ber'-ē-ber'-ē). A tropical disease resulting from lack of vitamin B_1 ; it is met with in persons who live on polished rice. The symptoms are mainly those of neuritis, weakness, muscular wasting, and œdema.

Bernard's Canal (ber'-nård'). *See* **Santorini's Duct.** **B. Center,** the "sugar-controlling" centre in the floor of the fourth ventricle.

Beta-naphthol (bē-tá-naf'-thol). A parasiticide and intestinal disinfectant. Derived from naphthalin.

Bicellular (bī-sel'-ū-lár). Having two cells.

Bicephalic (bī-kef'-al-ik). A double-headed monster.

Biceps (bī'-seps). A muscle possessing two heads or points of origin, *e.g.*, the flexor biceps in front of the humerus.

Biconcave (bī-kon'-kāv). Concave or hollow on both sides.

Biconvex (bī-kon'-veks). Convex on both sides.

Bicornuate (bī-kåwn'-ū-āt). Having two horns, generally applied to a double uterus or a single uterus possessing two horns. Pregnancy may occur in either or both, although the latter is very unusual.

Bicuspid (bī-kus'-pid). Having two cusps or points. **B. Teeth,** the two teeth situated next to the canine on either side of the jaw. **B. Valve**, the cardiac valve between the left auricle and ventricle. Also known as the *Mitral Valve*.

Biennial (bī-en′-i-al). Lasting for two years, or occurring every two years. Used in connection with certain plants which complete a life-cycle every second year.

Bier's Hyperæmia (Bierz). A method of treating acute inflammation by inducing artificial hyperæmia in the part by means of an air-pump, suction glasses, or by means of an elastic bandage placed above the diseased area.

Bifurcate (bī′-fur-kāt). Forked; having two prongs or branches; divided into two.

Bilateral (bī-lat′-e-ral). Having two sides.

Bile (bīl). A viscid, orange-greenish coloured fluid secreted by the hepatic cells and stored in the gall-bladder; has a disagreeable bitter taste, and is alkaline in reaction. Its constituents are—

Water .	. Biliverdin.*
Sodium glyco-cholate	Bilirubin.*
Sodium tauro-cholate	Lecithin.
Mucin .	. Cholesterin.

* Pigments.

Bile Ducts. These are the *hepatic ducts* which join the *cystic duct* coming from the gall-bladder. Together these form the **Common Bile D.** The latter unites with the *pancreatic duct* to form the ampulla of Vater which opens into the duodenum, thus allowing pancreatic juice and bile to enter the intestine together. *See Diagram of Liver.*

Bilharzia (bil-hárt′-si-à). A species of parasitic flukes which infest the liver. They are also found in the portal vein, mesenteric veins, and the urinary tract, and may be discharged in the urine. The main symptoms are severe anæmia, hæmaturia, and diarrhœa.

Biliary (bil-i-ar-i). Pertaining to bile. **B. Fistula**, an un-natural communication of the bile ducts either with the surface of the body or with one of the internal organs.

Biliousness. A disturbance of the digestive system associated with an excess of bile. The symptoms are sickness, severe headache, and severe prostration. The condition is often associated with constipation.

Bilirubin (bī-li-roo′-bin). The pigment which gives bile its orange colour; is derived from hæmoglobin.

Biliuria (bĭ-li-ū'-rĭ-à). The presence of bile in the urine.

Biliverdin (bĭ-li-ver'-din). The green pigment of bile formed from bilirubin through oxidation.

Bimanual (bĭ-man'-ū-al). Performed with both hands. A method used in gynæcology, when the fingers of one hand are inserted in the vagina, while the other hand is placed on the abdomen just above the symphysis pubis.

Binary (bĭn'-a-rĭ). Consisting of only two elements or parts.

Binder. A broad belt for passing round the abdomen.

Biniodide of Mercury (bin-I'-ŏ-dĭd). A powerful and efficient antiseptic; is closely allied to *perchloride of mercury*, but is less irritating; is coloured pink as a distinguishing mark. One biniodide tablet containing 3·75 grs. added to 1 pint of water makes 1-1,000 solution.

Binocular (bin-ok'-ū-lár). The use of both eyes in vision. An optical instrument requiring both eyes for its use.

Bio. Pertaining to life.

Biochemistry (bĭ-ŏ-kem'-ĭs-trĭ). The chemistry of living tissues and of vital processes occurring in the body.

Biodynamics (bĭ-ŏ-dĭ-nam'-ĭks). The science which deals with the vital forces.

Biogenesis (bĭ-ŏ-jen'-e-sĭs). The production of life from living matter as opposed to *abiogenesis*.

Biogenetic (bĭ-ŏ-jen-et'-ĭk). Relating to biogenesis.

Biologist. A person who makes a special study of biology.

Biology (bĭ-ol'-o-jĭ). The science that deals with life and all living things. Some of its many branches are anatomy, histology, zoology, botany, and both animal and plant physiology.

Bioplasm (bĭ-ŏ-plazm). The substance of which a living cell is formed; protoplasm.

Biot's Breathing. Rapid short respirations interrupted by pauses up to half a minute; often seen in meningitis when it is a bad prognostic sign.

Bipalatinoid (bĭ-pal-at'-in-oid). A gelatin capsule containing two compartments.

Biparietal (bĭ-par-I'-et-al). Pertaining to both parietal bones.

Biparous (bip'-a-rus). Bearing two offspring at a time.

Biped (bĭ'-ped). Having two feet.

Bipolar (bĭ-pō-lár). Having two poles.

B.I.P.P. A paste which came into prominence during the Great War. It is used for deep septic cavities. The wound is first thoroughly irrigated to clear it of pus, and then the cavity is swabbed out quite dry

48

(this last is an important point). The paste is spread on ribbon gauze and packed, not too tightly, into the cavity until it is filled up. Outer dressings of sterile gauze and wool are applied, and these are not removed for two or three days. The letters stand for Bismuth, Iodoform, Paraffin Paste.

Birth (burth). The act of expelling the young from the uterus ; delivery ; being born.

Bisexual (bī'-seks-ū-al). Having the characteristics of both sexes ; hermaphrodite.

Bismuth (biz'-muth). A crystalline metal, the salts of which are much used medicinally. They are astringent and sedative, and opaque to X-rays. When given for this purpose, carbonate of bismuth is added to a bowl of bread and milk, and this is known as a B. Meal.

Bistoury (bis'-tū-ri). A small knife used in surgery ; may be straight or curved.

Bitumen (bit'-ū-men). Mineral pitch ; asphalt.

Biuret (bī'-ū-ret). A substance obtained from urea. B. Reaction, when a few drops of Fehling's solution are added to protein, a violet colour results. B. Reaction for urea, when a few drops of solution of copper sulphate and an excess of caustic soda

are added to biuret a reddish or deep violet colour results.

Bivalve (bī'-valv). Having two valves.

Black Draught. Mist. Sennæ Co. B.P. Purgative.

Black Wash. Lotio Hydrargyri Nigra. Particularly useful for syphilitic sores. Synonym, *Lotio Nigra.*

Blackwater Fever. A malignant form of malaria occurring in the tropics, especially Africa. There is great destruction of red blood cells, and this causes a very dark-coloured urine, due to the presence in it of hæmoglobin products.

Bladder (blad'-er). A sac-like structure. Gall-B., a pear-shaped bag, on the under surface of the liver, measuring about 4 in. by 1 in. ; its function is to store and concentrate the bile. Urinary B., a muscular bag situated in the pelvis ; it acts as a reservoir for the urine.

Bland. Mild ; non-irritating ; soothing.

Blast. Usually a suffix indicating a primitive cell type, *e.g.,* erythroblast, myeloblast. Also the destructive wave of high pressure emanating from an explosion.

Blastoderm (blast'-ō-derm). A delicate membranous lining of the zona pellucida of the fertilized ovum. The rudimentary structure from which the embryo is formed.

Blastoma (blast-ō′-ma). A granulomatous mass caused by a micro-organism.

Blastomycetes (blas-tō-mī-sē′-tēz). *See* **Saccharomyces**.

Blastomycosis (blas-tō-mī-kō′-sis). An infectious skin disease caused by the *Blastomycetes*.

Bleaching Powder. Chlorinated lime ; used for bleaching clothes, and also for cleansing the pans of water-closets, etc.

Bleb. A watery blister forming on the skin ; a bulla.

Bleeder. *See* **Hæmophilia**.

Blennophthalmia (blen-of-thal′-mi-à). Catarrh of the conjunctiva caused by inflammation.

Blennorrhagia (blen-o-rāj′-i-à). A copious vaginal discharge, especially when due to gonorrhœa. Same as *Blennorrhœa*.

Blennorrhœa (blen-or-ē′-à). (1) A copious discharge of mucus from the urethra or vagina. (2) Gonorrhœa.

Blennorrhœal (blen-or-ē′-al). Pertaining to blennorrhœa.

Blepharitis (Blef-a-rī′-tis). Inflammation of the edges of the eyelids.

Blepharospasm (blef-a-rō-spazm). A spasmodic closure of the eyelids, as when a foreign body suddenly enters the eye.

Blind. Without sight ; absence of vision. **Colour B.**, unable to distinguish colours ; may be partial or complete ; probably due to a defect in the rods and cones layer of the retina. *See* **Daltonism**. **Day Blindness**, defective vision by day, but normal at night. **Mind B.**, inability to recognize an object seen. **Night B.**, normal vision by day, but subnormal at night. **Psychic B.**, same as *Mental* or *Mind Blindness*. **Snow B.**, loss of sight due to the glare of the sunlight upon the snow. **Word B.**, inability to understand the written or printed word due to a brain lesion.

Blinking. Involuntary winking.

Blister. A vesicle filled with fluid. Also a vesicant or irritant fluid or plaster for producing a skin blister. **Flying B.**, a series of blisters, each one being applied to a fresh skin surface. **Water B.**, one filled with a watery fluid.

Blood. The red viscid fluid filling the heart and blood-vessels. *Reaction*, alkaline, sp. gr. 1,060. *Weight*, 1/12-1/14 of the body-weight.

Blood-clotting *See* **Coagulation**.

Blood-count. The count of the number of red and white blood cells in an accurately measured quantity of blood. Normally there are 5,000,000 red cells per c.mm., and 7,000-10,000 white cells.

Blood Crisis. The appearance of large numbers of nucleated red blood cells or erythroblasts in the blood-stream.

Blood-letting. *See* Venesection.

Blood-pressure. The pressure exerted by the blood on the walls of the arteries. It is estimated by using an instrument known as a *sphygmomanometer*, which consists mainly of an inflatable armlet or cuff attached to a mercury column or other indicator of pressure. The normal systolic pressure is about 120 mm. of mercury. The factors controlling the blood-pressure are : (1) the condition of the heart muscle ; (2) the elasticity of the arterial walls ; (3) arteriolar resistance ; (4) the volume and viscosity of the blood.

Blood Sugar. The amount of sugar normally existing in blood. It varies between 0·1 and 0·18 gms. per cent. If it rises above this figure the sugar *threshold* is said to have been reached, and the excess sugar commences to leak through into the urine.

Blood Transfusion. The passing

BLOOD FILMS.

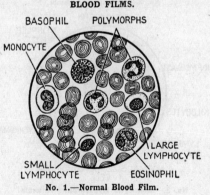

BASOPHIL   POLYMORPHS

MONOCYTE

LARGE LYMPHOCYTE

SMALL LYMPHOCYTE   EOSINOPHIL

No. 1.—Normal Blood Film.

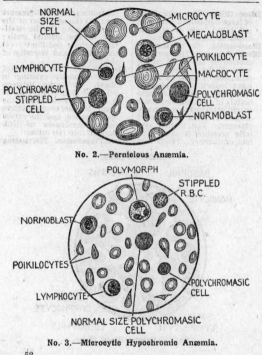

No. 2.—Pernicious Anæmia.

No. 3.—Microcytic Hypochromic Anæmia.

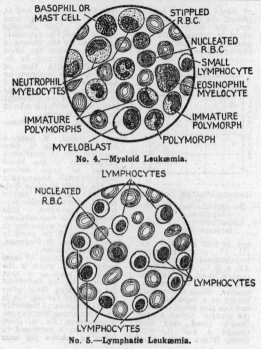

BASOPHIL OR MAST CELL

STIPPLED R.B.C.

NUCLEATED R.B.C.

SMALL LYMPHOCYTE

NEUTROPHIL MYELOCYTES

EOSINOPHIL MYELOCYTE

IMMATURE POLYMORPH

IMMATURE POLYMORPHS

POLYMORPH

MYELOBLAST

No. 4.—Myeloid Leukæmia.

LYMPHOCYTES

NUCLEATED R.B.C.

LYMPHOCYTES

LYMPHOCYTES

No. 5.—Lymphatic Leukæmia.

53

of blood from a healthy person, the donor, to someone, the recipient, whose blood is deficient either in quantity or quality. The blood of all persons falls into

DONOR CORPUSCLES				
GROUP GROUP	AB	A	B	O
AB	−	−	−	−
A	+	−	+	−
B	+	+	−	−
O	+	+	+	−

Hæmagglutination Reactions.

−, No agglutination, therefore compatible.

+, Agglutination, therefore incompatible.

one of four groups, I., II., III., IV., or under the new international nomenclature AB, A, B, O. Group AB may receive blood from anyone, and is known as a *universal receiver*. Group O is similarly known as a *universal donor*, and can give blood to any of the groups. Group A must receive blood only from Groups A and O, while Group B can receive blood only from Groups B and O. Group O receives only from Group O. This grouping of the blood is extremely important for the success of transfusion, since the blood of one person may be incompatible with that of another. This is shown by agglutination or clumping of the corpuscles when the blood serum of one is brought into contact with the cells of an unsuitable group.

Bloody Sweat. Same as *Hæmidrosis*.

Blue. A colour. **B. Baby,** a baby whose skin is very cyanosed due to insufficient oxygenation of the blood caused by some serious developmental abnormality of the heart such as pulmonary stenosis and/or patent inter-ventricular septum. Synonyms, *Blue Disease* and *Morbus cœruleus*. **B. Line,** a line appearing at the margins of the gums in lead poisoning. **B. Ointment,** mercurial ointment.

B.M.R. Abbreviation for *basal metabolic rate*, which is the minimum amount of heat produced by an individual in the resting state after twelve hours' fasting. It is generally measured indirectly by determining the oxygen consumption for a short period, and is expressed in terms of calories per hour per square metre of body surface.

Boil.—An acute inflammatory swelling occurring round a hair follicle. A *furuncle*. *See* **Furunculosis.**

Bolus (bō'-lus). A round soft mass. A name given to the soft pulpy mass of food in the mouth after mastication is completed. The bolus is formed by the tongue, which then conveys it to the throat ready for swallowing.

Bone (bōn). The material which forms the skeleton of vertebrate animals.

Bone Cell. Small cells included in the minute porosities of bone. They were originally osteoblasts which have become included within the bone they have laid down.

Bone Graft. The transplantation of a piece of bone from one part of the body to another, or from one person to another, in order to repair a defective bone.

Boracic Acid. *See under* **Acid.**

Borax (bor'-aks). The combination of boric acid with sodium.

Borborygmus (bawr-baw-rig'-mus). A rumbling noise caused by the movement of flatus in the intestines.

Boric Acid. Same as *Boracic Acid.*

Boron (bawr'-on). Symbol, B. A non-metallic element in the form of crystals or powder; is the base in boric acid.

Botallo's Foramen. Same as the *foramen ovale* between the auricles in the cardiac septum. (Leonardo Botallo, Italian physician of sixteenth century.)

Botany (bot'-an-i). The science which deals with plants and the whole of the vegetable kingdom. One of the branches of *biology.*

Bothriocephalus Latus (both-ri-ō-kef'-a-lus). A genus of tape-worm.

Botulism (bot'-ū-lizm). A form of poisoning resulting from eating canned or preserved foods which are infected by the *Clostridium botulinum.*

Bougie (boo-zhē). A cylindrical instrument made of gum-elastic or metal. Used in varying sizes for dilating orifices such as the urethra and rectum.

Bouillon (boo'-yong). A culture media much used in the laboratory for growing bacteria. A clear, sterile broth made of 3 grms. of beef, 5 grms. of sodium chloride, 10 grms. of pure peptone, and 1 litre of water, dissolved by boiling and then filtered.

Bovine (bō'-vīn). Pertaining to the cow or ox. **B. Tuberculosis,** the form of tuberculosis found in cattle; is transmissible to man through the milk.

Bowel (bow'-el). The intestine; gut. **Small B.,** the first

20 ft. of intestine, the first 12 in. of which is the *duodenum* ; the next 2/5 is the *jejunum*, and the remaining 3/5 the *ileum*. Large B. measures 6 ft. in length, but is larger in diameter than the small intestine, and has other distinguishing features.

Bowman (bō'-man). Sir William Bowman, an English physician of the nineteenth century. B.'s Capsule, the spherical capsule which surrounds the renal glomerulus. *See* Malpighian Bodies.

Boyle's Law. At any stated temperature a given mass of gas varies in volume inversely as the pressure. B. Mica Flap, a ventilator used for the outlet of vitiated air. It is placed in the part of the wall which opens into the chimney. On the posterior side of it are flaps made of mica which automatically shut down, preventing a reflux of foul air from the chimney, while allowing used air to pass freely from the room.

Bozeman's Catheter (bōz'-e-manz). An intra-uterine irrigating catheter. It is grooved in such a way that the fluid introduced can return freely.

B.P. Abbreviation for *British Pharmacopœia*, *Blood Pressure*, or *Boiling Point*.

Brachia (brā-ki-a). The arms, or any arm-like appendage. Singular = brachium.

Brachial (brā'-ki-al). Pertaining to the brachium.

Brachiocephalic (brāk-i-ō-kef-al'-ik). Pertaining to the arm and head.

Bradycardia (brā-di-kàr'-di-à). An abnormally slow pulse-rate.

Braidism (brād'-izm). A synonym for *Hypnotism*, named after James Braid, an English surgeon.

Brain (brān). An organ situated in the cranial cavity. It is composed entirely of nervous matter, and is covered and protected by the *meninges*. It consists essentially of five divisions : (1) the cerebrum ; (2) cerebellum ; (3) pons varolii ; (4) mid-brain ; (5) medulla oblongata. There are twelve pairs of cranial nerves. Abdominal B., an old term for the solar plexus. Mid-B., the mesencephalon. B. Sand, the gritty substance sometimes found in the pineal and pituitary bodies and in some meningeal tumours known as psammomas. B. Stem, the parts of the brain not included in the cerebrum and cerebellum.

Bran. The husk of grain. The coarse outer part of cereals, especially wheat. B. Bath, *see* Bath.

Branchial (brang'-ki-al). Pertaining to the fissures or gills, which occur on each side of the neck of the human embryo, and which enter into the development of the nose, ears, and mouth.

Brand's Bath. *See* Bath.

Brandy (bran'-di). An alcoholic liquor obtained from wine by means of distillation. It varies in flavour and colour, these depending upon its age and the wood of which the cask is made. Also called *Spiritus Vini Gallici*.

Braun's Blunt Hook (brawnz). A hook used for decapitating a fœtus which cannot be delivered.

Braxy (braks'-i). The anthrax of sheep.

Bread (bred). Cereals ground to flour, and after being mixed with yeast and water left to rise, and then baked in a hot oven. **Brown B.,** bread made from flour in which the outer husk is retained, thus ensuring the presence of vitamin. **Diabetic B.,** bread in which the carbohydrate is reduced to a minimum; generally of almond flour.

Breast (brest). The anterior upper part of the thorax. The mammary gland. **B. Bone,** the sternum.

Breath (breth). The air inhaled and exhaled by the lungs.

Breech. The buttocks; the rounded prominence at the lower posterior part of the trunk formed by the gluteal muscles; the rump. **B. Presentation,** presentation of the fœtus with the buttocks descending first.

Bregma (breg'-ma). The anterior fontanelle (*q.v.*).

Bright's Disease. A term used to include acute and chronic nephritis and other diffuse chronic sclerosing affections of the kidney. Usually associated with œdema of the tissues and with albuminuria and casts. Named after Richard Bright, an English physician.

Brilliant Green. An antiseptic dye of a brilliant green colour; sometimes used in pre-operative skin preparation.

Brim. An edge or rim. The edge between the true and false pelvis. The iliopectineal line.

British Thermal Unit. The amount of heat required to raise 1 lb. of water through 1° F. Often abbreviated *B.Th.U.*

Broadbent's Sign. Visible retraction of the left side and back, synchronous with each heart beat and due to adherent pericardium.

Broca's Area (brŏk'-à). The motor centre for speech. Situated at the commencement of the Sylvian fissure in the left hemisphere of the cerebrum. Injury to this centre results in inability to articulate.

Brodie's Abscess (brō'-dē). Chronic abscess of bone, most frequently in the head of the tibia.

Bromide (brō'-mīd). A salt formed by the combination of bromine with a base such as potassium. Is sedative in action and useful in hysteria, epilepsy, and allied conditions.

Bromidrosis (brōm-i-drō-sis). A profuse fœtid perspiration, especially when it occurs in the feet.

Bromine (brō'-mēn). A non-metallic liquid element. A dark brownish-red volatile fluid, sp. gr. 2·99; symbol Br. Gives off obnoxious fumes. Obtained from sea-water and saline springs.

Brominism (brō'-min-izm). Poisoning produced by bromine or one of its compounds.

Bronchi (brong'-kī). The two tubes into which the trachea divides at its lower end. The plural of bronchus.

Bronchial Tubes. Subdivisions of the bronchi after they enter the lungs.

Bronchiectasis (brong-ki-ek'-tas-is). Dilatation of the bronchial tubes associated with a profuse, fœtid, purulent expectoration.

Bronchiole (brong'-ki-ōl). One of the minute subdivisions of the bronchi which terminate in the alveoli or air sacs of the lungs.

Bronchitis (brong-kī'-tis). Inflammation of the bronchial tubes.

Bronchocele (brong'-kō-sēl). Swelling of the thyroid gland due to cystic goitre; a cyst of the bronchus.

Bronchophony (brong-kof'-o-ni). Vocal resonance heard over the bronchi during auscultation.

Broncho - pneumonia (brong-kō-nū-mō-ni-à). The same as *lobular pneumonia*. Patchy inflammation of the lobules of the lung; often commences in the bronchi and usually follows some other disease. *See* Pneumonia.

Bronchorrhœa (brong-kō-rē'-à). An excessive discharge of mucus from the respiratory tract.

Bronchoscope (brong'-kō-skōp). An instrument used for examining the interior of the bronchi.

Bronchospasm (brong'-kō-spazm). Sudden constriction of the bronchial tubes.

Brow. The region of the supra-orbital ridge.

Brownian Movement (brow'-ni-an). A rhythmic rapid movement observed microscopically in minute particles suspended in fluid.

Brucellosis (broo-sel-ō'-sis).

Disease due to infection with organisms of the Brucella group, *e.g.*, Malta fever.

Bruise (brooz). A discoloration of the skin due to an extravasation of blood in the underlying tissues ; there is no abrasion of the skin.

Bruit (broo′-ē). A murmur heard on auscultation. **Aneurysmal B.**, a blowing sound heard over an aneurysm. **B. de Diable,** a peculiar hum heard over the large veins in anæmic persons; a humming noise ; from the Fr. *diable*, a humming-top. **Systolic B.**, an abnormal sound heard in the heart during its systole or contraction.

Brunner's Glands. Small glands situated in the submucous lining of the duodenum ; also called *Duodenal Glands.*

Bubo (bū′-bō). A lymphatic glandular swelling, especially of the axilla and groin.

Bubonic (bū-bon′-ik). Pertaining to buboes. **B. Plague,** Oriental plague.

Bubonocele (bū-bon′-ō-sēl). Incomplete inguinal hernia.

Buccal (buk′-al). Relating to the mouth.

Buccinator (buk′-sin-ā-tor). One of the cheek muscles.

Buccula (buk′-ū-lā). The fleshy fold known as double chin.

Buchu (boo′-koo). The name of a drug derived from the dried leaves of *Barosma betulina* ;

is mainly diuretic in its action. Dose, infusion, 1-2 fl. oz.

Budding (bud′-ing). A form of reproduction in the lower forms of life. Also in plant life the method by which new leaves are produced.

Bulb. A rounded globular part of a structure.

Bulbar (bul′-bár). Pertaining to a bulb or to the medulla.

Bulimia (bū-lim-i-á). Excessive hunger. Great increase in the appetite.

Bulla (bool′-á) . A large watery blister.

Bunion (bun′-yan). Inflammation and swelling of the bursa of the large toe joint.

Bunsen Burner. A special gas burner fitted with air-holes which are capable of adjustment, thus excluding or admitting air in such a way as to produce a luminous or non-luminous flame. The mixture of air with gas generates great heat instead of light, and the flame burns with a bluish colour, due to the complete oxidation of the hydrocarbons, etc., of the gas.

Burette (bū-ret′). A graduated glass tube ending in a tap ; used for the accurate measurement of fluids.

Burn. A lesion of the skin or deeper tissues caused by dry or moist heat. Many authorities recognize six degrees of burns, but these are now

59

often reduced to only three, viz.: (1) burns involving the skin and superficial tissues; (2) those affecting the muscles and deeper layers; (3) charring of the bones.

Bursa (bur'-sä). A membranous sac lined with synovial membrane and containing a small quantity of synovial fluid. Bursæ are found between (a) tendon and bone (b) skin and bone, (c) muscle and muscle. Their function is to facilitate without friction movement between these surfaces.

Bursal (bur'-sal). Pertaining to a bursa.

Bursitis (bur-sī'-tis). Inflammation of a bursa.

Buttermilk. The fluid remaining over after making butter; a refreshing drink.

Buttocks (but'-oks). See Breech.

Butyl (bū'-til). A hydrocarbon radicle.

Butyrate (bū'-tir-āt). A salt of butyric acid.

Butyric (bū-tir'-ik). Derived from butter. B. Acid, one of the volatile acids of butter.

C.

Cacao (ka-kā'-o). See **Theobroma.** C. Butter, oil of theobroma; is a soft, yellowish substance with an odour like chocolate, and of the consistency of tallow; does not become rancid, and melts at body temperature; is largely used as a base for suppositories.

Cachet (kash'-ā). A flat capsule formed of rice-paper enclosing a drug which is to be taken internally.

Cachexia (ka-keks'-i-ä). A term denoting a state of constitutional disorder, malnutrition, and general ill-health. The chief signs of this condition are bodily emaciation, sallow, unhealthy skin, and heavy, lustreless eyes.

Cachinnation (kak-in-ā'-shun). A paroxysm of hysterical laughter.

Cacidrosis (kak-id-rō'-sis). Fœtid perspiration.

Cacodyl (kak'-ō-dil). A colourless liquid derived from arsenic; has a very nauseous smell, and is inflammable in air.

Cacodylate (kak-ō-dī'-lāt). A salt of cacodylic acid; is prescribed medicinally for skin diseases, malaria, tuberculosis, etc.

Cadaver (kad-ā'-ver). A dead body; a human corpse.

Cadaveric Rigidity (kad-a-ver'-ik). Rigor mortis.

Cadaverous (kad-av'-e-rus). Resembling a human corpse.

Cadmium (kad'-mi-um). A bluish-white metal found in several zinc ores. Symbol, Cd.

Cæcum (sē'-kum). The blind

pouch which forms the commencement of the colon; is separated from the ileum by the ileocæcal valve.

Cæsarean Section (sĕ-zĕr-i-an sek'-shun). An operation by which the fœtus is delivered through a median abdominal and uterine incision. The operation is used when natural labour is impossible or inadvisable, thereby saving the lives of mother and infant. It is said to be named after Cæsar, who is supposed to have been born in this way.

Caffeine (kaf'-ēn or kaf'-ān). An alkaloid present in coffee and tea. At first it exerts a stimulative effect on the cerebral cortex, but later has a depressant and narcotic action. It is also a powerful diuretic, and for this reason is useful in cardiac dropsy. Dose, caffeine citrate, 2-10 gr.

Caffeinism (kaf'-ēn-izm). An abnormal state arising from an excessive use of caffeine. The main symptoms are nervousness, insomnia, and tachycardia.

Caisson Disease (kā'-son). A condition which may affect persons who are subjected to an increased atmospheric pressure, such as deep-sea divers and men who work in caissons, diving-bells, etc.

Cajuput (kaj'-u-put). An East Indian tree, the leaves of which yield a volatile oil used as a stimulant, carminative, and antispasmodic. Dose, oil of cajuput, 1-3 minims.

Cal. Abbreviation for large calorie (q.v.).

cal. Abbreviation for small calorie (q.v.).

Calabar Bean (kal'-a-bár bēn). The dried seed of the West African plant, the Physostigma venenosum. The chief alkaloid is known as physostigmine or eserine. Is a spinal sedative and depressant, and is much used in conditions associated with disease or irritation of the spinal cord, e.g., tetanus. It is also much used in diseases of the eye.

Calamine (kal'-a-min or kal'-a-mēn). Native zinc carbonate. C. Lotion, a watery suspension of the powdered calamine from which the coarser particles have been strained. The powder and lotion are much used in eczema and other skin diseases.

Calcaneum (kal-kā'-nē-um). The heel bone; the os calcis.

Calcaneus (kal-kā'-nē-us). The same as Calcaneum. Also a form of club-foot in which only the heel touches the ground.

Calcareous (kal-kā'-ri-us). Pertaining to or containing lime or calcium; of a chalky nature.

Calcarine (kal'-kå-rīn). Spur-shaped.

Calciferol (kal-sif'-e-rol). A substance obtained by irradiation of ergosterol. It is almost pure vitamin D.

Calcification (kal-sif-i-kā'-shun). The hardening of an organic substance by a deposit of calcium salts within it.

Calcination (kal-sin-ā'-shun). The withdrawal of moisture from a substance by heat, *e.g.*, roasting. Pulverization or drying up by heat.

Calcium (kal'-si-um). One of the metallic elements, symbol Ca; is found in nearly all tissues, particularly bone and teeth. The salts are one of the essential factors in producing the coagulation of blood. *See* **Coagulation.**

Calculus (kal'-kū-lus). A concretion formed within certain of the body cavities, especially the kidneys, ureter, urinary bladder, gall-bladder, and bile ducts. More rarely they may be found in salivary, pancreatic, or prostatic glands, etc. **Biliary C.**, a gall-stone in the bile ducts or gall-bladder; it is composed chiefly of cholesterin, inorganic salts, and bile pigment; often multiple and faceted through contact with each other. **Urinary C.,**

a stone formed in any part of the urinary tract; in the kidney it is termed a *Renal C.*, and in the bladder it is known as a *Vesical C.*

Calf. Pl. *calves.* The muscular portion at the back of the leg, formed principally by the bellies of the soleus and gastrocnemius muscles.

Calf-bone. The fibula.

Calibrator (kal'-i-brā-tor). An instrument for measuring the diameter of an opening.

Caliper (kal'-ip-er). Sometimes also spelt **Calliper.** A surgical appliance for measuring the diameter of a round body. Usually in the form of a compass with curved legs, used chiefly in pelvimetry. *See* **Pelvimeter.** Also a two-pronged instrument with sharp points used for insertion into the lower end of a long bone, such as the femur, when it is fractured. A weight is attached to the caliper, thus ensuring a steady pull on the distal end of the bone. **Ice C.,** tongs used in handling large blocks of ice. **Walking C.,** a form of splint in which the two struts are attached to the heel of the boot. Used in the later or ambulant stage of treatment of fractures of the lower limbs.

Callosity (kal-os'-it-i). A local hardening of the skin caused by pressure or friction. The epidermis becomes hypertrophied. Most commonly seen on the feet and palms of the hands.

Callous (kal'-us). Hard; like callus.

Callus (kal'-us). The partly calcified tissue which forms about the ends of a broken bone; is the agent by means of which a fracture unites.

Calmative (kăm'-a-tiv). Sedative.

Calmette's Reaction (kal'-met). An inflammatory reaction of the conjunctiva after instillation of a drop of tuberculin into the eye. The reaction is much more severe in sufferers from tuberculosis than in normal persons.

Calomel (kal'-ō-mel). Subchloride of mercury (HgCl). A white, heavy, almost tasteless insoluble powder used as an antisyphilitic and purgative. Dose, ½-3 gr. Is sometimes given 1 gr. hourly until the 3 gr. are given. Should be followed in a few hours by a dose of salts. This increases the purgative action of calomel and prevents its retention in the intestine.

Calor (kal'-or). Latin for heat. Natural or moderate heat.

Cal. Fervens, boiling-point, 100° C. (212° F.). **C. Lenis**, gentle heat.

Calorie (kal'-or-ē). A unit of heat, being the amount of heat required to raise 1,000 g. of water 1° C. This is known as a **Large C.**, and is the one used in the study of metabolism. A **Small C.** is the amount of heat required to raise 1 g. of water through 1° C.

Calorific (kal-or-if'-ik). Pertaining to heat. Heat producing. **C. Value**, the number of calories produced by a given amount of any food substance. Thus 1 g. of protein = 4·1 calories; carbohydrate = 4·1 calories; fat = 9·3 calories.

Calorimeter (kal-or-im'-e-ter). An apparatus for determining the amount of heat yielded or produced by any substance. In physiology the apparatus can be used to estimate the heat production of an animal within a given time. In the study of metabolism a **Bomb C.** is used in which a known quantity of a food-substance is burnt with a view to estimating its calorific value.

Calvarium (kal-vē'-ri-um). The vault of the skull; also the skull itself.

Calx (kalks). 1. Lime or chalk; calcium oxide. There are many preparations, of which chlorinated lime is one. 2. The heel.

Calyx (kāl'-iks). A cup-like sheath.

Calyces (kăl'-i-sēz). Plural of calyx. **C. of Kidney.** The cup-like extensions of the renal pelvis which surround the apices of the pyramids.

Camphor (kam'-for), $C_{10}H_{16}O$. A solid volatile oil obtained from the wood of *Cinnamomum camphora*; is translucent and crystalline with a bitter, pungent taste. Will float on water, and is only slightly soluble in it, but is very soluble in spirit, ether, or chloroform. Its action is chiefly antispasmodic, antaphrodisiac, carminative, and cardiac stimulant.

Camphoraceous (kam-for-ā'-si-us). Resembling camphor.

Camphorated (kam'-for-ā-ted). Impregnated with camphor.

Canal (kan-al'). A narrow tube or duct; a passage. **Alimentary C.,** the passage made up of the mouth, pharynx, œsophagus, stomach, large and small intestines. **C. of Arantius,** the ductus venosus. **Auditory C. (external),** the passage leading from the external auditory meatus to the membrana tympani; **(internal),** the channel for the auditory and facial nerves through the petrous bone. **Digestive C.,** *see* Alimentary C. **Haversian C.,** the network of minute canals in the compact tissue of bone; they serve to convey arteries, veins, and lymph vessels through the bone. **Inguinal C.,** a passage leading from the internal to the external abdominal ring; it contains the spermatic cord in the male and the round ligament in the female. **Lachrymal C.,** the opening in the lachrymal bone through which the lachrymal duct passes. **Medullary C.,** the central cavity of a long bone; it contains the *medulla* or marrow. **Semicircular C.'s,** three bony semicircular canals opening into the vestibule of the internal ear; they are concerned with equilibrium. **Santorini's C.,** *see* Santorini's Duct.

Canaliculus (kan-a-lik'-ū-lus). A minute capillary passage. Any small canal, such as the passage leading from the edge of the eyelid to the lachrymal sac, or one of the numerous small canals leading from the Haversian canal, and terminating in the lacunæ of bone. Pl. *canaliculi.*

Cancellous (kan-sel'-us). Resembling lattice-work; light and spongy; like a honeycomb. **C. Bone,** that which underlies the compact tissue of bone; the interstices of bone cancellous tissue are filled with red bone marrow.

Cancer (kan'-ser). A malignant tumour.

Cancerophobia (kan-se-rō-fō'-bi-à). Extreme fear of cancer.

Cancerous (kan'-se-rus). Pertaining to or resembling cancer.

Caneroid (kang'-kroid). A cutaneous lesion showing a mild degree of malignancy.

Cancrum Oris (kang'-krum or'-is). Acute gangrenous stomatitis attacking the inner side of the cheek. It results in sloughing of the tissues, causing great disfigurement. Death occurs from exhaustion and from absorption of toxins. May follow as a complication of measles and typhoid fever, but is to be guarded against in any septic or foul condition of the mouth.

Canine (kān'-īn). Resembling a dog. C. Teeth, the *eye teeth*, situated between the incisors and the bicuspids. They correspond to the fangs of animals. *See* Teeth.

Canker (kang'-ker). An old term signifying ulceration of the mouth.

Cannabis Indica (kan'-ab-is in'-dik-à). Indian hemp; also known as *Bang* and *Hashish*. Prepared from the flowering resinous tops of the *C. sativa* grown in India. Medicinally it is hypnotic and anodyne. In large doses produces disordered consciousness, hallucinations, and feelings of great exaltation with grandiose delusions. The chief preparations are the *extract*, dose ¼-1 gr., and the *tincture*, dose 5-15 minims.

Cannula (kan'-ū-là). A hollow tube for introduction into some body cavity with the object of either withdrawing or introducing fluid. A sharp-pointed trocar may be inserted into the lumen of the tube before inserting the cannula. When the latter is *in situ*, the trocar is withdrawn. Commonly used for giving intravenous saline or blood transfusion.

Cantharides (kan-thar'-i-dēz). A blistering substance prepared from the dried Spanish beetle, the bodies of which form a greyish-white powder. The main preparations of cantharides are in the form of *tincture, plaster, ointment,* and *liquor epispasticus, i.e.,* blistering fluid. *See* Blister.

Cantharis (kan'-thar-is). The singular of *cantharides.*

Canthus (kan'-thus). The angle at either end of the opening between the eyelids. The inner is known as the **Nasal C.**, and the outer as the **Temporal C.**

Caoutchouc (koo'-chook). Indiarubber.

Capacity (kap-as'-it-i). The ability and power to hold or contain. **Vital C.**, the volume of air that can be expelled after a full inspiration. **Stomach C.,** the amount of fluid or food capable of being retained in the stomach. **Thermal C.,** the amount of heat absorbed by a body when raised 1° C. in temperature.

Capeline (kap´-e-līn). A bandage applied to the head. Consists of two 6-yd. bandages sewn together so that a double-headed roller bandage is made, the head of

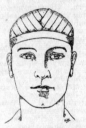

Capeline Bandage.

one bandage being rolled till it is larger than the other.

Capillarity (kap-il-lar´-it-i). The name given to certain phenomena which appear when open tubes of narrow bore are placed into liquids, with reference to the differ-

ence of level of the liquid inside and outside the tube.

Capillary (kap-il´-a-ri). Resembling hair; microscopic blood-vessels which act as a connecting link between the arterioles and venules.

Capitellum (kap-it-el´-um). A small, smooth, rounded protuberance on the lower outer end of the humerus. It articulates with the head of the radius.

Capsicum (kap´-si-kum). Cayenne pepper; stimulant, counter-irritant, and carminative.

Capsule (kap´-sūl). (1) The ligaments which surround any joint. (2) A gelatinous or rice-paper container for noxious drugs. (3) The outer membranous covering of certain organs, such as the kidney, liver, spleen, suprarenals. **Bowman's C.,** the globular enlargement forming the commencement of a uriniferous tubule.

Caput Succedaneum (ka´-put suk-si-dā´-ni-um). A swelling which forms on the presenting part of the fœtus during labour, due to congestion and œdema following pressure by the dilated os uteri. It is not harmful, and disappears in the course of a few days.

Caramel (kar´-à-mel). Burnt sugar; used as a browning

agent. Also useful for flavouring.

Carbohydrate (kär-bō-hī′-drät). Organic compounds, including starches, sugars, and cellulose, composed of carbon, hydrogen, and oxygen, the two latter elements being in the proportion to form water. *Monosaccharids* ($C_6H_{12}O_6$) *e.g.*, glucose, dextrose, levulose, and galactose. *Disaccharids* ($C_{12}H_{22}O_{11}$), *e.g.*, cane sugar, lactose, and maltose. *Polysaccharids* ($C_6H_{10}O_5$)n, including starch, glycogen, cellulose, and dextrin. Each of these contains the so-called carbohydrate group ($C_6H_{10}O_5$) either singly or in multiplication. Thus monosaccharids $= C_6H_{10}O_5 + H_2O = C_6H_{12}O_6$, disaccharids contain two, and polysaccharids many of these groups, plus water.

Carbolfuchsin (kär-bol-fook′-sin). A brilliant red stain used in histology and bacteriology. It consists of a solution of fuchsin in weak carbolic acid.

Carbolic Acid. *See Acid.*

Carbolize (kär′-bol-īz). To disinfect with solution of carbolic acid.

Carboluria (kär-bol-ū-ri-à). The presence of carbolic acid in the urine. This gives the urine an olive-green colour.

Carbon. Symbol, C.; atomic weight, 12. A non-metallic element existing widely in nature. It is found almost in the pure state in the diamond, charcoal, and graphite. **C. Dioxide** (CO_2) is formed in the body through the oxidation of carbon. **C. Monoxide** (CO), a very poisonous gas sometimes formed in coal mines; present also in coal gas; has a great affinity for hæmoglobin of the red blood cells, forming the stable compound, carboxyhæmoglobin.

Carbonate (kär′-bon-āt). A salt of carbonic acid.

Carbuncle (kär′-bung-kl). Inflammation of a localized area of subcutaneous tissue, commencing as a tense reddened swelling, but later the skin becomes thinned, and bursts at several points, discharging pus. This suppurating mass finally sloughs away, leaving an ulcer cavity. Constitutional symptoms are usually severe, and the local condition is exceedingly painful.

Carcinogenesis (kär-sin-ō-jen′-e-sis). The production of cancers. *Carcinogenic compounds*, chemical substances capable of inducing cancerous growths when applied to or injected into tissues.

Carcinoma (kär-sin-ō′-mà). Cancer; a malignant growth derived from epithelia and glandular tissues. The tumour has no capsule and spreads mainly by the lymphatics. The most usual sites are the skin, breast, alimentary tract, pancreas, and uterus. There are several different forms.

Carcinomatosis (kăr-sin-ō-ma-tō'sis). Generalized involvement by carcinoma.

Carcinosis (kăr-sin-ō'-sis). The production and development of carcinoma.

Cardamom (kăr'-da-mom). A drug derived from the dried ripe seeds of *Elettaria cardamomum*; carminative. Dose, tincture, 30-60 minims.

Cardiac (kăr'-di-ak). Pertaining to the heart.

Cardialgia (kăr-di-al'-ji-á). Gastric disturbance, sometimes associated with pain and heart-burn, in which there is a rush of acid watery fluid into the mouth; indigestion. Also, pain in the heart.

Cardiasthenia (kăr-di-as-thē'-ni-á). A neurasthenic cardiac weakness.

Cardinal (kăr'-din-al). Of the greatest consequence; very important.

Cardio (kăr'-di-ō). A prefix denoting relationship to the heart.

Cardiodynia (kăr-di-ō-din'-i-á). Pain in the heart.

Cardiogenic (kăr-di-ō-jen'-ik). Commencing within the heart itself.

Cardiogram (kăr'-di-ō-gram). A graphic tracing of the action of the heart.

Cardiograph (kăr'-di-ō-graf). An instrument for recording the force and form of heart-beat.

Cardiology (kăr-di-ol'-o-ji). The science dealing with the heart and its functions.

Cardio-omento-pexy (kăr'-di-ō-ŏ-men-tō-peks'-i). Operation for producing adhesions between the surface of the heart and the omentum brought up through the diaphragm; intended to provide a fresh vascular supply to the heart in cases of coronary artery disease.

Cardiopathy (kăr-di-op'-ath-i). Heart disease.

Cardiospasm (kăr'-di-ō-spazm). A spasmodic contraction of the cardiac end of the stomach.

Carditis (kăr-dī'-tis). Inflammation of the cardiac muscle.

Caries (kĕr'-i-ēz). Inflammatory decay of bone usually associated with pus formation. Dental C., decay of the teeth. Spinal C., Pott's disease; tuberculous disease of the vertebræ.

Carminative (kăr'-min-a-tiv). A substance which relieves flatulence and pain, *e.g.*, cinnamon, cloves, ginger, limewater, nutmeg, peppermint, etc.

Carmine (kăr'-mīn). A colouring matter derived from cochineal.

Carneous (kár'-ni-us). Fleshy.

Carotene (kar'-ō-tēn). Vegetable substances coloured yellow are thought to contain a yellow pigment known as *carotene*. These, when eaten, produce the effects of vitamin A, whereas colourless vegetables do not. Recent investigations have shown, however, that there is no carotene in animal fats rich in vitamin A. It is suggested that carotene is converted into vitamin somewhere within the body, and experiments strongly suggest that it is the precursor of vitamin A.

Carpal (kár'-pl). Pertaining to the carpus or wrist.

Carphology (kár-fol'-o-ji). A picking of the bedclothes. A very grave symptom found in persons who are acutely ill; is a sign of exhaustion.

Carpus (kár'-pus). The wrist, which is formed of eight small bones : (1) Scaphoid ; (2) semilunar ; (3) cuneiform ; (4) pisiform ; (5) trapezium ; (6) trapezoid ; (7) os magnum ; (8) unciform.

Carrel-Dakin Treatment. A method of wound irrigation first utilized by *Dr Alexis Carrel* and *Dr Henry Dakin* in 1915. The treatment is most suitable for deep septic wounds, and was therefore

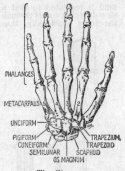

PHALANGES

METACARPALS 5 4 3 2

UNCIFORM

PISIFORM   TRAPEZIUM
CUNEIFORM   TRAPEZOID
SEMILUNAR   SCAPHOID
OS MAGNUM

The Carpus.

widely employed during the 1914-18 war. A special apparatus is necessary. This consists of a glass receptacle for the solution constructed on the principle of a thermos flask for maintaining a constant temperature. From this leads a rubber tube, which is attached to a glass connection piece, from which again are suspended several perforated fine gauge rubber tubes. Each is closed at the lower end, and is perforated for about half its length. Any number of tubes can be used, depending on the size of the wound. The flow of fluid is regulated so that a slow dropping occurs through the tubes continually, thus

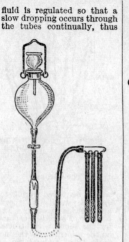

Carrel-Dakin Irrigation Apparatus.

keeping the wound constantly bathed. A Dakin's special solution is used.

Carrier (kar'-i-er). A person who harbours within his body a specific micro-organism, and while not manifesting any symptoms himself, can spread the in-

fection to other people. Some diseases which are conveyed by carriers are *typhoid fever, diphtheria, scarlet fever, cerebrospinal meningitis*, etc. The organism is commonly carried in the nose, throat, fæces, or urine.

Cartilage (kår'-til-åj). Gristle. There are three main varieties: (1) **Hyaline C.**, a semi-transparent substance with a granular matrix and elastic fibres; is a true cartilage. (2) **Yellow Elastic C.**; as the name implies, this is yellow in colour, elastic, and is a true cartilage. (3) **White Fibro C.**, a mixture of cartilage and fibrous tissue; is inelastic and not a true cartilage. **Articular C.**, that which covers the articulating surfaces of bone. **Temporary C.**, cartilage which later ossifies into bone. **Permanent C.**, the variety which normally is not subject to ossification.

Cartilaginous (kår-til-aj'-in-us). Consisting of or relating to cartilage.

Caruncle (ka'-rung-kl). A small bright red growth at the entrance to the urethra. Is very painful, and bleeds readily on being touched. **C. Myrtiformis**, the tag-like ends left after rupture of the hymen during coitus.

Cascara (kas-kår'-á). The

Spanish for bark. **C. Amarga,** Honduras bark; a drug obtained from the bark of *Picramnia antidesma*; used as an alternative and tonic. **C. Sagrada,** the Spanish sacred bark; derived from the bark of *Rhamnus purshiana*; is prepared as an *extract* and *fluid extract*; is a valuable laxative. Dose of liq. extract, 30-60 minims.

Cascarin (kas'-kár-in). A purgative preparation obtained from *cascara sagrada*.

Case. (1) A special instance of disease, *e.g.*, a case of mumps. (2) A person suffering from some special disease. **C. Book,** a book into which is entered particulars of cases; especially used by midwives.

Caseation (kā'-zi-ā'-shun). The formation of a soft, cheese-like mass.

Casein (kā'-zē-in). The main protein of clotted milk and cheese.

Caseinogen (kā-zē-in'-ō-jen). A protein of milk which is converted into casein by the addition of *rennin*. *See* Rennet.

Caseous (kā'-zi-us). Resembling cheese.

Cassava (kas-á'-và). A plant, the roots of which yield a starchy substance which, after passing through a purifying process, is known as *tapioca*.

Cast. A shape; a mould of a hollow cavity or tube. **Decidual C.,** the moulded mass of false decidua expelled from the uterus in a case of ruptured tubal pregnancy. **Blood C.,** a cast formed of coagulated albumin enclosing a number of blood-corpuscles; found in the urine. **Renal C.,** an albuminous cast of one of the uriniferous tubules of the kidney.

Castor Oil. *See* Oleum.

Castration (kas-trā'-shun). The removal of the testicles in the male, or of the ovaries in the female.

Casual (kas'-ū-al). Relating to accidents or accidental injuries. A person who occupies a bed in the casual ward.

Casualty (kas'-ū-al-tē). Accidental injury; one who has suffered such injury. **C. Department,** a department provided specially for the reception and treatment of accident cases.

Catalepsy (kat-à-lep'-si). An abnormal state in which the body remains insensible, the pulse and respirations become exceedingly slow and feeble, there is marked muscular rigidity, and the bodily functions are suspended. The condition may last from a few minutes to days, or even months.

Cataleptic (kat-á-lep'-tik). Pertaining to *catalepsy.*

Catalysis (kat-al'-i-sis). The process by which the velocity of a chemical action is increased through the medium of a catalyzer or catalyst.

Catalyzer (kat'-ah-li-zer). An agent which will hasten a chemical or physical reaction between two other substances without itself becoming altered or changed in the process, *e.g.*, the enzymes of the digestive tract, such as *ptyalin*, *pepsin*, etc., act in this way.

Catamenia (kat-á-mēn'-i-á). The monthly discharge of blood from the uterus ; menstruation ; the menses.

Cataplasm (kat'-á-plazm). A poultice.

Cataplexis (kat-á-pleks'-is). A condition of muscular rigidity induced by severe mental shock or fear.

Cataract (kat'-á-rakt). An opacity of the crystalline lens of the eye or of its capsule. There are many different varieties, which can be mainly divided into *hard* and *soft*. Hard C., one containing a hard nucleus, tends to be dark in colour, and occurs in persons who have reached or passed middle age. Soft C., one without a hard nucleus, met with at any age, but particularly in the young.

Cataract usually develops slowly, and when it becomes mature is known as a Ripe C. These cases are treated surgically, and require very careful post-operative nursing.

Catarrh (kat-ár'). Inflammation of a mucous membrane associated with an excess secretion of mucus.

Catarrhal (kat-ar'-al). Relating to catarrh.

Catechu (kat'-e-kū or kat'-e-choo). An extract from the leaves and young shoots of *unearia gambier* ; is used as an astringent in diarrhœa and dysentery.

Catgut (kat'-gut). A form of ligature prepared from sheep's intestines rendered aseptic. **Chromicized C.** is prepared by immersion in a solution of chromic acid for 24 hours, after being boiled for 20 minutes in a sat. sol. of am. sulph. **Formalin C.** is prepared by boiling in a solution of alcohol and formalin. **Iodine C.**, prepared by soaking in a solution of iodine and iodide of potassium.

Catharsis (kath-ár'-sis). (1) Purgation. (2) Freud's method of treating a psychoneurosis. *See* **Abreaction.**

Cathartic (kath-ár'-tik). A purgative drug.

Catheter (kath'-e-ter). A tubular apparatus used for the discharge of fluids from a body cavity, usually the

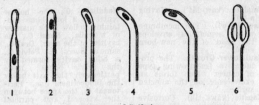

Types of Catheters.

1, Bulbous.   4, Coudé.
2, Ordinary.   5, Bi-Coudé.
3, Semi-Coudé.   6, Self-retaining.

bladder. **Bozeman's C.,** a two-way uterine catheter. **Eustachian C.,** used for passing into the Eustachian tube. **Coudé C.,** a gum-elastic urinary catheter with the tip bent at 45°; used for males. **Bi-Coudé C.,** a similar catheter, but with the tip bent twice. **Female C.,** one used for the female urethra. **C. Fever,** pyrexia caused by the improper use of a urinary catheter. **Self-retaining C.,** a rubber catheter with a soft enlargement at the end, which keeps it *in situ*, but allows drainage from the bladder. **Two-way** or **Double C.,** one which allows fluid passed into a cavity to run out again freely. **Urinary C.,** used for the urinary bladder; made of rubber,

glass, and silver for a female, and rubber, gum-elastic, and silver for males.

Catheterization (kath-e-te-rī′-zā′-shun). The act of passing a catheter.

Cathodal (kath-ō′-dal). Pertaining to a cathode.

Cathode (kath′-ōd). The negative pole of an electric circuit.

Cation (kāt′-I-on). The ion or element which passes to the negative electrode in an electrolyte.

Cauda Equina (kaw′-dă ĕ-kwī′-nă). The aggregation of lumbar and sacral nerves at the lower termination of the spinal column. (Latin for horse's tail.)

Caudal (kaw′-dal). Pertaining to the cauda or tail.

c*

73

Caudate (kaw-dāt'). Having a tail.

Caul (kawl). The membrane which sometimes envelops the head of the new-born child.

Cauliflower Growth. The proliferative free-growing type of cancer which forms an excrescence on the affected surface.

Caustic (kaws'-tĭk). Corrosive or destructive; the agent which produces such results.

Cauterization (kaw-ter-rī-zā'-shun). The destruction of living tissue by means of heat or caustics.

Cautery (kaw'-ter-rī). Any cauterizing agent. **Actual C.,** a heated iron for applying direct heat. **Paquelin's C.,** a form of actual cautery in which the hollow platinum point is kept at the required heat by a current of benzene vapour which is constantly pumped into it. **Galvanic C.,** a platinum wire cautery maintained at red heat by an electric current.

Cavernous Respiration. *See* **Respiration.**

Cavity. A hollow space; an enclosed area. **Abdominal C.,** the cavity below the diaphragm; the abdomen. **Buccal C.,** the mouth. **Cerebral C.,** the ventricles of the brain. **Cranial C.,** the brain box formed by the bones of the cranium.

Medullary C., the hollow centre of a long bone containing yellow bone marrow or medulla. **Nasal C.,** the cavities of the nose. **Oral C.,** same as *Buccal C.* **Pelvic C.,** a bony cavity formed by the pelvic bones; more particularly the part below the iliopectineal line. **Peritoneal C.,** the space between the visceral and parietal layers of the peritoneum. **Pleural C.,** the space between the visceral and parietal layers of the pleura. **Synovial C.,** the interior of a joint which is lined with synovial membrane. **Uterine C.,** the cavity within the body of the uterus.

Cedar Wood Oil. A volatile oil obtained from the cedar tree; much used in microscopy.

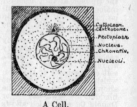

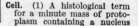

A Cell.

Cell. (1) A histological term for a minute mass of protoplasm containing a nucleus and other definite structures : the smallest particle of living matter known to the anatomist. (2) A jar or collection of jars containing chemicals, into which are placed two dissimilar metal plates which are connected by copper wire for the generation of electricity. **Voltaic C.** consists of a plate of copper and one of zinc in a bath of sulphuric acid (H_2SO_4). When Zn is placed in H_2SO_4, it forms zinc sulphate ($ZnSO_4 + H_2$). When Zn and copper are united by copper wire, an electric current flows from the copper to the zinc. The copper becomes the positive pole, and the zinc the negative. This is the simplest form of cell. **Daniell C.** consists of two parts : (1) An outer copper vessel which forms the positive pole ; (2) an inner porous vessel filled with H_2SO_4, and into which is fixed a zinc plate, forming the negative pole. The outer copper vessel contains copper sulphate ($CuSO_4$).

Cellular (sel'-ū-lar). Relating to or composed of cells.

Cellulitis (sel-ū-lī'-tis). Inflammation of cellular or connective tissue.

Cellulose (sel-ū-lōz). A carbohydrate forming the outer walls of plant and vegetable cells.

Celsius Thermometer (sel'-si-us). Same as *Centigrade*.

Centigrade Thermometer. A thermometer in which the freezing-point of water is fixed at 0° and boiling-point of water at 100°.

Centigram (sen'-ti-gram). The hundredth part of a gram.

Centilitre (sen'-ti-lē-ter). The hundredth part of a litre.

Centimetre (sen'-ti-mē-ter). The hundredth part of a metre.

Centrifugal (sen-trif'-ū-gal). Having a tendency to move outwards away from the centre.

Centrifuge (sen'-tri-fūj). A machine for separating solid and fluid constituents of a fluid by the centrifugal force of rotation.

Centripetal (sen-trip'-et-al). Having a tendency to move towards the centre.

Centrosome (sen'-trō-sōm). A minute spot in the cytoplasm of a cell supposed to be concerned with the division of the cell. *See* Mitosis.

Cephalhæmatoma (kef-al-hēm-a-tō'-mä). A collection of blood and clot which forms in the subcutaneous tissues of the scalp due to the rupture of small blood-vessels, caused by pressure of the head on its passage through the pelvis during delivery.

Cephalic (kef-al'-ik). Relating to the head. **C. Cry.** The

75

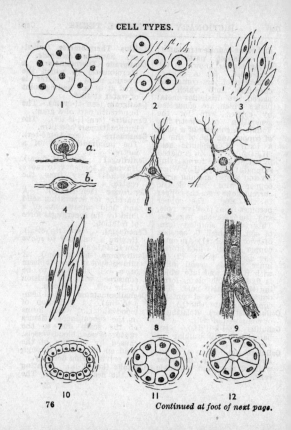

Continued at foot of next page.

typical loud cry heard in sufferers from tuberculous meningitis

Cephalotribe (kef'-al-ō-trīb). A heavy, two-bladed instrument working with a screw, which is used for crushing the fœtal head during obstructed labour.

Cera (sē'-rá). Wax or bees-wax.

Cerebellum (se-re-bel'-um). That part of the brain which lies behind and below the *cerebrum.* Its chief functions are the co-ordination of muscular movement and the control of bodily equilibrium.

Cerebrospinal (se-re-brō-spī'-nal). Pertaining to the brain and spinal cord. C. **Fluid,** the clear fluid filling the ventricles of the brain and neural canal, and also found beneath the cranial and spinal meninges in the pia-arachnoid space. C. **Fever,** an epidemic form of meningitis due to infection with the meningococcus ; is

sometimes accompanied by a purpuric rash, hence the name of *spotted fever.*

Cerebrum (se'-re-brum). The largest and uppermost part of the brain ; is divided into two hemispheres, by the longitudinal fissure, each containing a lateral ventricle. The internal substance is white, while the outer convoluted cortex is grey.

Cerium (sē'-ri-um). A metallic element.

Cerumen (se'-roo-men). A wax-like brownish substance secreted by the ceruminous glands of the ear ; ear-wax.

Cervical (ser-vī'-kal). Pertaining to the neck.

Cervicitis (ser-vis-ī'-tis). Inflammation of the cervix uteri.

Cervix (ser'-viks). A neck. C. **Uteri,** the neck of the uterus.

Chalazion (kal-ā'-zi-on). A small cyst on the edge of the eyelid which is the result

---

Cell Types.

1, Pavement epithelial cells.
2, Round or spheroidal cells.
3, Spindle cells.

Nerve Cells—
4, (*a*) Unipolar ; (*b*) Bipolar.
5, Pyramidal.
6, Ganglionic.

Muscle—
7, Involuntary or unstriped.
8, Voluntary or striped.
9, Cardiac.

10, 11, 12, Gland acini in various states of activity.

of blockage of the duct of a meibomian gland.

Chalicosis (chal- or kal-i-kō'sis). *See* Silicosis.

Chalybeate (kal-ē'-bi-āt). Containing steel or iron, or some preparation of iron.

Chamber (chăm'-ber). An enclosed space. **Anterior C. of the Eye,** the part between the iris behind and the cornea in front. **Posterior C.,** the part which lies behind the iris.

Chamomile (kam'-ō-mīl). An antispasmodic and carminative drug.

Champagne (sham-pān'). An effervescent, sparkling French wine, originally made in the district of Champagne, France, from which it derived its name.

Chancre (shang'-ker). The primary syphilitic lesion caused by the *Spirochæta pallidum.* Two main varieties of the sore are recognized. **Hard C.** is the primary sore of true syphilis. **Soft C.,** a non-syphilitic venereal sore caused by Ducrey's bacillus ; a chancroid.

Chancroid (shang'-kroid). Resembling a chancre ; the soft venereal sore.

Change of Life. The climacteric or menopause (*q.v.*).

Charbon (shàr'-bong.) A malignant pustule or anthrax boil.

Charcoal (chàr'-kōl). The residue left after burning organic substances, such as wood, at a very high temperature in an enclosed vessel. There are many varieties of charcoal ; it consists mainly of carbon. **C. Biscuits,** used in gastric disorders. **C. Poultice,** *see* Poultice.

Charcot's Disease (shàr'-kō). A wasting of the ends of the long bones, with erosion of the articular cartilage. There may be effusion into the joint. The disease occurs in tabes dorsalis.

Charpie (shar'-pē). Teazed out lint or linen threads used for dressing wounds. Obsolete.

Chaulmoogra Oil (shawl-moo'-grà). The oil expressed from the seeds of the chaulmoogra tree (*Taraktogenos kurzii*) which grows in the East. The oil is used in skin diseases and particularly in the treatment of leprosy. (*See also* Hydnocarpus Oil.)

Cheilitis (kī-lī'-tis). Inflammation of the lip.

Cheiloplasty (kī-lō-plas'-ti). Plastic operations on the lips.

Cheiloschisis (kī-lō-ski'-sis). Hare-lip.

Cheirospasm (kī'-rō-spazm). Writer's cramp.

Cheiropompholyx (kī-rō-pom'-fo-liks). A vesicular skin disease occurring on the hands.

Chemotaxis (kĕm-ō-taks'-is). The repulsion or attraction shown towards living cells by certain chemical substances.

Chemotherapy (kēm-ō-ther'-ap-i). The use of chemical compounds in treatment.

Chemotropism (kēm-ō-trō'-pizm). Tropistic action between chemicals and plants. Same as *Chemotaxis*.

Cherry-stalk Tea. A tea made from dried cherry stalks. The choke - cherry of North America has astringent properties. The wild cherry, *Prunus serolina*, is used as a sedative.

Cheyne-Stokes Respiration. An abnormal type of breathing in which the respirations are at first extremely quiet and shallow, but gradually increase in depth, loudness, and rapidity until a maximum is reached, gradually decreasing again until a minimum is reached, when the breathing becomes almost imperceptible. This is the *apnœic stage*. The symptom is a very grave one; most commonly met with in cases of head injuries and diseases, poisoning, acute nephritis, and uræmia.

Chiasm (kī'-azm). X-shaped crossing or decussation.

Chiasma Opticum. The meeting of the optic nerves; the optic commissure.

Chicken-pox. *See* Varicella.

Chilblain (chil'-blān). Localized inflammation of the superficial tissues due to imperfect circulation caused by cold or deficiency. Same as *Pernio*.

Childhood. The period between infancy and puberty, *i.e.*, from 2 to about 14 years.

Chill. A shivering attack associated with pallor and sensation of coldness.

Chimney-sweep's Cancer. Scrotal epithelioma.

Chiropodist (kī-rop'-o-dist). One skilled in the treatment of corns, bunions, and deformities of the hands and feet.

Chiropody (kī-rop'-o-di). The business of a chiropodist.

Chiropractic (kī-rō-prak-tik). The restoration of health by manipulative treatment of the spinal column.

Chirurgical (kī-rur'-jik-al). Relating to surgery.

Chitin (kī'-tin). The hard, horny outer covering which protects the bodies of some of the lower creatures, such as *lobsters, cray-fish, beetles*, etc.

Chloasma (klō-az'-mā). A term denoting various discolorations or pigmentation of the skin, such as may occur on the abdomen and face of a pregnant woman.

Chloral Hydrate (klor'-al hī'-drāt). A hypnotic antispasmodic drug; is also a heart depressant. Dose, 5-20 gr.

Chloralamide (klor-al'-am-Id). A hypnotic drug.

Chloramine-T (klor'-am-ēn-tē). A very efficient antiseptic and germicide much used for irrigating purposes and as a mouthwash. It is a white crystalline powder used in a 4% solution.

Chlorate (klor'-āt). A salt of chloric acid.

Chloretone (klor'-e-tōn). A hypnotic drug much used as a preventive of sea-sickness; also prescribed in cases of tetanus; is slightly soluble in water, but very much so in ether and alcohol. Dose, 5-20 gr.

Chlorine (klōr'-ēn or klawr'-ēn). Symbol, Cl. A greenish-yellow gaseous element; extremely irritating to the respiratory tract.

Chloroform ($CHCl_3$) (klor'-ō-fawm). A colourless, volatile liquid with a sweet, pungent odour; is used as an anæsthetic and administered by inhalation. Internally it is anodyne and carminative. Excreted mainly by the kidneys and lungs. Overdose produces excessive post-operative vomiting and pallor, and sometimes even causes death through heart-failure. Treatment consists in fresh air, artificial respiration, and stimulants.

Chloroma (klawr-ō'-má). Greenish-coloured tumour usually found under the periosteum of the bones of the face and skull. A form of sarcoma.

Chlorophyll (klor'-o-fIl). The green colouring matter contained in the cells of a plant.

Chloroplast (klor'-ō-plast). The special cells of a plant which contain the chlorophyll.

Chlorosis (klawr-ō'-sis). A variety of anæmia attacking adolescent girls. The skin assumes a greenish pallor, hence the name *green sickness*. The disease readily responds to fresh air, fruit, and vegetables. Sanitary surroundings, rest, and iron tonics form an important part of the treatment.

Choked Disc. Optic neuritis; papillitis.

Choking (chōk'-ing). Inability to breathe due to obstruction in the larynx, trachea, or bronchi.

Cholæmia (kōl-ēm'-i-á). The presence of bile in the blood.

Cholagogue (kōl'-a-gŏg). A drug which causes an increased flow of bile into the intestine, *e.g.*, podophyllum, aloes, and calomel.

Cholangitis (kōl-an-jī'-tis). Inflammation of the bile ducts.

Cholecystectomy (kōl-ē-sis-tek'-to-mi). Surgical removal of the gall-bladder.

Cholecystenterostomy (kōl-ē-sist-en-te-ros'-to-mi). The making of an artificial opening between the gall-bladder and small intestine.

Cholecystography (kŏl-ē-sis-tog'-ra-fi). Examination of the gall-bladder by means of the X-rays.

Cholecystostomy (kŏl-ē-sis-tos'-to-mi). An artificial permanent opening into the gall-bladder through the abdominal wall.

Choledochotomy (kŏl-ē-dō-kot'-o-mi). Incision into the bile duct in order to remove a stone.

Cholelithiasis (kŏl-ē-lith-ī'-a-sis). The formation of biliary concretions in the gall-bladder or its ducts.

Cholemesis (kŏl-ē-mē'-sis) The vomiting of bile.

Cholera (kol'-e-rà). An acute epidemic disease occurring in the East. The main symptoms are the evacuation of copious "rice-water" stools accompanied by agonizing cramp and severe collapse. The disease is spread mainly through contamination of the drinking-water and by overcrowding and insanitary conditions. The mortality is very high. **C. Infantum**, acute diarrhœa, occurring during the hot summer months in infants. Also known as *Summer Diarrhœa, Acute Enteritis*, etc.

Cholesteatoma (kŏl-es-tē-a-tō'-mà). A benign encysted tumour containing choles-terin crystals. Often occurs in the middle ear.

Cholesterin (kŏl-es'-te-rin). A crystalline substance of a fatty nature found in the brain, nerves, blood, and liver. It is excreted in the bile, and forms a large proportion of gall-stones.

Cholesterol (kŏl-es'-te-rol). Same as *Cholesterin*.

Cholesterosis (kŏl-es-te-rō'-sis). A chronic inflammation of the gall-bladder in which small collections of cholesterol form as yellow granules on the mucosal surface ; also known as strawberry gall-bladder.

Choletelin (kŏl-ĕt'-el-in). The end product formed during the oxidation of bilirubin.

Choluria (kŏl-ūr'-ĭ-à). The presence of bile in the urine.

Chondral (kon'-dral). Cartilaginous.

Chondrin (kon'-drin). A gelatinous protein obtained from cartilage.

Chondritis (kon-drī'-tis). Inflammation of cartilage.

Chondro- (kon'-drō). Relating to cartilage.

Chondroblast (kon'-drō-blàst) The embryonic cell which produces cartilage.

Chondrocostal (kon'-drō-kos'-tal). Pertaining to the costal cartilages and ribs.

Chondrocyte (kon'-drō-sīt). A cartilage cell.

Chondrodynia (kon-drō-din'-i-à). Pain in a cartilage.

Chondroma (kon-drō'-mà). A benign tumour composed of cartilage.

Chorda (kaw(r)'-dà). A collection of fibres forming a cord; also a tendon. **C. Achillis**, *see* **Tendo Achillis. C. Spermatica**, the spermatic cord. **Chordæ Tendinæ**, fine white glistening cords stretching between the valves and the ventricular walls of the heart. When stretched taut they enable the valves to close tightly, but prevent them from being pushed through into the auricles when the ventricle is filled with blood. **C. Tympani**, a branch of the facial nerve.

Chordee (kaw(r)-dē'). Painful erection of the penis due to urethritis; often caused by gonorrhœa.

Chorditis (kaw(r)-dī'-tis). Inflammation of the spermatic or vocal cords.

Chordoma (kaw(r)-dō'-mà). A tumour formed of the persistent remains of the notochord (*q.v.*), and usually found in the sacral region or on the surface of the basisphenoid.

C h o r e a (kawr-ē'-à). Involuntary muscular twitchings and contractions causing jerky, inco-ordinate movements. Most commonly seen in children, and is ascribed to rheumatism. Synonym, *St Vitus' Dance.*

Chorion (kawr'-i-on). The outer membrane forming the embryonic sac.

Chorionepithelioma (kawr'-i-on-ep-i-thē-li-ō'-mà). A malignant growth arising from the villi of the chorion. The tumour tends to grow through the wall of the uterus either during or after pregnancy; is extremely fatal. Treatment consists in immediate hysterectomy.

Chorionic (kawr-i-on'-ik). Pertaining to the chorion.

Choroid (kawr'-oid). The middle coat of the eye; so-called because of its resemblance to the vascularity of the chorion. It is highly pigmented, and forms the " dark " coat of the eye, the pigment preventing the passage of the light rays. It lies between the *sclera* and *retina.*

Choroiditis (kawr-oid-ī'-tis). Inflammation of the choroid.

Chromaffin(e) (krōm-af'-in). Pertaining to cells which stain yellow with chromic acid, *e.g.*, the cells of the adrenal which produce adrenalin.

Chromate (krōm'-āt). A salt of chromic acid.

Chromatic (krōm-at'-ik). Pertaining to chromatin; relating to or possessing colour.

Chromatin (krōm'-at-in). The network structure of the nucleus of a cell, so-called because it is the part of the cell which will receive a stain the most readily. *See* Chromosomes.

Chromatolysis (krōm-a-tol′-is-is or krōm-at-ō-lī′-sis). The fragmentation and disappearance of the Nissl granules in nerve cells.

Chromatophil(e) (krōm′-at-ō-fīl). Having an affinity for stains.

Chromic Acid. *See* Acid.

Chromidrosis (krōm-ī-drō′-sis). Coloured perspiration.

Chromogen (krōm-ō-jen). Producing a colouring matter.

Chromosomes (krōm-ō-sōms). The V-shaped thread-like bodies formed by the breaking up of the chromatin network in the nucleus of a cell during mitotic division. The number of chromosomes is constant for each species of animal. In man they number forty-eight. Their function is said to be concerned with the transmission of hereditary traits from the parents to their offspring.

Chronic (kron′-ik). A long-drawn-out morbid condition ; not acute.

Chrysarobin (kris-ar′-ō-bin). A powder obtained from a substance found in the trunk of *Andira Araroba* ; is much used in the form of an ointment in certain skin diseases, such as psoriasis and eczema.

Chvostek's Sign (shvos′-tek). Excessive twitching of the face when the facial nerve is mechanically irritated, *e.g.*, by tapping ; a sign of tetany.

Chyle (kīl). The fluid found in the mesenteric lymphatic vessels and formed chiefly of the emulsified fats which are absorbed from the intestines through the lacteals. After passing through the lymphatic glands, where it is filtered, it finally reaches the thoracic duct, and from thence enters the venous blood at the junction of the subclavian and internal jugular veins. Chyle owes its milky-white colour to its high percentage of fat. It has an alkaline reaction.

Chyluria (kīl-ūr′-i-á). The presence of chyle in the urine.

Chyme (kīm). A thick, creamy-yellow fluid resulting from the digestion of food in the stomach. It is acid in re-action. Chyme is gradually passed through the pyloric orifice of the stomach into the small intestine, where its digestion is completed.

Chymification (kīm-i-fi-kā′-shun). The transformation of food into chyme.

Cicatricial (sik′-a-trish-al). Pertaining to a cicatrix.

Cicatrix (sik-ā′-triks). A scar ; the healing of injured tissues.

Cilia (sil′-i-á). (1) The eye-lashes. (2) Microscopic vibratile hairs which project from certain epithelial cells. Membranes containing these cells are known as *ciliated membranes*. Examples are the lining of the trachea and Fallopian tubes.

Ciliary (sil'-i-a-ri). Pertaining to *cilia*; hair-like. **C. Body**, a specialized structure of the eye, consisting of the ciliary muscles and processes. **C. Muscles**, fine hair-like muscle fibres arranged in a circular manner between the edge of the *iris* and the *choroid* coat of the eye. **C. Processes**, a number of projections on the under surface of the choroid which are attached in a circular manner to the ciliary muscles.

Cinchona (sin-kō'-nä). A drug derived from the bark of a genus of rubiaceous trees growing in South America. Its action is tonic, antiperiodic, and antipyretic. The chief alkaloids are quinine, quinidin, and cinchonin.

Cinnamon (sin'-a-mon). An aromatic substance obtained from the cinnamon tree; is carminative and astringent, and much used in the early stages of a common cold. Dose: tincture, 30-60 minims; oil, 1-3 minims.

Circle of Willis. An anastomosis of arteries at the base of the brain formed by the union of the branches

of the internal carotids with the branches of the basilar artery.

Circulation (ser-kŭ-lā'-shun). As applied to the body fluids, the course and movement followed by them. There are four main parts of the blood circulation: (1) The Systemic C., the main flow to the whole body via the aorta and returning via the venæ cavæ; (2) Pulmonary C., that to the lungs for oxygenation, via the p. artery and returning by the p. veins; (3) Portal C., that from the gastrointestinal tract and spleen to the liver via the portal vein and then by the hepatic vein; (4) Coronary C., that to the heart itself via the coronary vessels. Collateral C., the continuation of the circulation through the smaller branches of a blood-vessel when the main branch is obstructed. **C. of Cerebrospinal Fluid**. The flow of C.S.F. from the ventricles of the brain, in which it is produced by the choroid plexuses, through the foramina of Magendie and Luschka to the cisterna magna of the subarachnoid space. From here it passes over the whole of the surfaces of the brain and cord. It also fills the central canal of the cord. It is absorbed back into the blood from the subarachnoid space through the arachnoid villi which project through the walls of the cerebral venous sinuses.

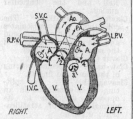

RIGHT.   LEFT.

Diagrammatic Section of the Heart showing Circulation. Arrows indicate direction of blood-stream.

1, Tricuspid valve.
2, Pulmonary valve.
3, Aortic valve.
4, Mitral valve.
A., A., Auricles.
V., V., Ventricles.
R.P.V., Right pulmonary veins.
L.P.V., Left pulmonary veins.
S.V.C., Superior vena cava.
I.V.C., Inferior vena cava.
Ao., Aorta.
P.A., Pulmonary artery.

C. of Bile. The passage of bile from the liver cells, where it is formed, via the gall-bladder and bile ducts to the duodenum and intestines in which its constituents are partly reabsorbed into the blood-stream and thus return in due course to the liver. Placental C., or Fœtal C., the circulation in the fœtus, umbilical cord, and placenta.

Circumcision (ser-kum-sizh-un). Removal of the prepuce by a circular incision.

Circumduction (ser-kum-duk'-shun). The action of swinging a limb, such as the arm, in such a manner that it describes a cone-shaped figure, the apex of the cone being formed by the joint at the proximal end, while the complete circle is formed by the free distal end of the limb.

Circumflex (ser'-kum-fleks). Winding around. C. Nerve, the nerve supplying the deltoid muscle.

Circumoral (ser-kum-awr'-al). Surrounding the mouth. C. Pallor, a pale appearance of the skin around the mouth ; symptomatic of scarlet fever.

Cirrhosis (sir-ō'-sis). A pathological change occurring in the tissues of certain organs, especially the lung and liver. The organ becomes contracted, granular, and hard. A liver showing this appearance is often known as *hobnail liver*, because of its knobbed surface.

Cirsoid (sir'-soid). Resembling

a varix. **C. Aneurysm**, a tangled mass of large pulsating blood-vessels, usually on the scalp.

Cisternal Puncture (sis-tern'-al). The withdrawal of cerebrospinal fluid from the cisterna magna, a subarachnoid space at the base of the brain. A hollow needle is introduced at the nape of the neck. The method is sometimes used when cerebrospinal fluid cannot be withdrawn through a lumbar puncture.

Citrate (sit'-rāt). A salt of citric acid.

Citric Acid. *See* **Acid.**

Cl. Symbol for chlorine.

Clamp. An apparatus used for holding a part as in a vice, or for compressing parts, such as an artery, hæmorrhoids, or the pedicle of an ovarian tumour.

Clap. The popular name for gonorrhœa.

Clarke's Column. A special column of nerve cells situated at the base of the posterior horn of grey matter in the spinal cord.

Claudication (klaw-di-kā'-shun). Lameness. **Intermittent C.**, spasm of the arteries, resulting in pain and cramp, and causing lameness; also known as "limping" disease.

Claustrophobia (klaws-trō-fō'-bi-à). A form of mental disturbance in which there is a morbid fear of enclosed spaces.

Claustrum (klows'-trum). The layer of grey matter in the brain between the Island of Reil and the lenticular nucleus.

Clavicle (klav'-ikl). The collar-bone. It articulates with the sternum at one end and the acromion process of the scapula at the other.

Clavus (klā'-vus). A corn.

Claw-hand. Muscular wasting of the hand and fingers.

Cleavage (klē'-vij). The splitting of a substance in an opposite direction to its normal plane of stratification; division.

Cleft Palate. A congenital defect of the hard palate or soft palate, in which the right and left halves remain separated instead of uniting in the median line during the normal process of development.

Cleidotomy (klī-dot'-o-mi). Division of the clavicle. Sometimes performed to facilitate delivery of the fœtus in a case of contracted pelvis.

Climacteric (klī-mak'-te-rik or klī-mak-te'-rik). The so-called *change of life*, *i.e.*, the period at about forty-five to fifty years when a woman ceases to menstruate. Other less marked changes, both physical and psychical, are also observed at this time. It is therefore a critical stage needing care and understanding; the menopause.

Climax (klī'-maks). The highest point; the moment of greatest intensity.

Clinic (klin'-ik). (1) The teaching of medical subjects at the bedside. (2) A place where patients attend for treatment and which is also a teaching centre.

Clinical (klin'-ik-al). Pertaining to a clinic. Practical observation and treatment of sick persons as opposed to theoretical study.

Clitoridectomy (klit-or-i-dek'-to-mi). Surgical removal of the clitoris.

Clitoris (klit'-or-is). A small erectile organ situated just below the mons veneris at the anterior junction of the labia majora; is the seat of sexual excitement in the female.

Cloaca (klō-ā'-kä). The common opening of the intestinal and urogenital tract in fishes and birds and reptiles; also found in some of the lower animals.

Cloacal (klō-ā'-kal). Pertaining to the cloaca.

Clonic (klon'-ik). Characterized by intermittent muscular contractions as opposed to tonic or continuous contractions.

Clonus (klō'-nus). Sudden jerky muscular contractions. **Ankle C.**, a state in which there are violent muscular contractions of the calf muscle when the foot is sharply flexed by pressure on the sole when the leg is extended. The condition is well marked in certain diseases of the brain and cord, particularly in disseminated sclerosis.

Clot. A coagulated mass of blood.

Clove Hitch. A species of knot; quickly made and useful as a first-aid sling; can be made of rope, thick string, or a strip of any material, such as a bandage.

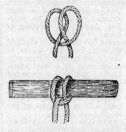

Clove Hitch.

Clovers' Crutch. An apparatus consisting of a long webbing shoulder-strap and two straps for controlling the legs; is used to keep the patient in the lithotomy position.

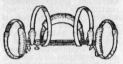

Clover's Crutch.

Club-foot. A congenital deformity of the foot. *See* Talipes.

Clyster (klis´-ter). An enema.

Coagulability (kō-ag-ūl-a-bil´-i-ti). Capable of being coagulated.

Coagulation (kō-ag-ū-lā´-shun). The conversion of a fluid substance into a firm jelly-like mass; the clotting of blood.

Cocaine (kō-kān´). An alkaloid derived from the leaves of the *Coca* plant. Formerly much used as a local anæsthetic, but now superseded by safer preparations. Overdose results in vomiting, delirium, asphyxia. Death results from paralysis of the respiratory centres.

Cocainism (kō-kān´-izm). Mental and physical degeneracy caused by a morbid craving for and excessive use of cocaine.

Coccus (kok´-us). A spheroidal shaped bacterium; a *micro-*

coccus. If occurring in pairs, is called a *diplococcus*; when in chain formation, a *strepto-coccus*; grouped together like a bunch of grapes, it is known as a *staphylococcus*.

Coccygeal (kok-si-jē´-al). Pertaining to the coccyx.

Coccyx (kok´-siks). The last bone of the vertebral column. It is triangular in shape and curved slightly forward. It is made up of four small bones which are separate in children but become fused together in the adult.

Cochlea (kok´-li-ă). The third section of the internal ear. It is a tube-like structure tapering towards the end, and having 2¼ spiral turns. It is named from its resemblance to the shell of a common garden snail.

Cochleare (kok-li-ā´-ri). A spoon. C. Magnum, a large spoon; a tablespoon. C. Medius, a dessertspoon. C. Minimus, a teaspoon.

Cocoa (kō´-kō). The seeds of *Theobroma cacao*. The powder is made into a nourishing, pleasant beverage. Contains theobromin and caffeine.

Cod-liver Oil. An oil obtained from the liver of cod-fish. Its beneficial action probably depends upon its rich content of vitamins A and D. It is therefore particularly good for children during the growing stage, as it helps to prevent rickets and promotes growth; is also given to consumptive patients. Should be given after meals. Dose, 30-120 minims.

Codeine (kō'-dē-ĭn). An alkaloid of opium; is a mild hypnotic, its action being much weaker than that of morphine; is given in diabetes, to allay cough, and for insomnia, etc. Dose, ½-1 gr.

Codex (kō-deks). The French pharmacopœia.

Cœliac (sē'-lĭ-ak). Relating to the abdominal cavity. C. Disease, an abnormal condition commencing in childhood and due to a defect in fat absorption from the intestines. It is characterized by the passage of large, pale, fœtid stools. The abdomen is enlarged, but the general nutrition and development are poor.

Cognition (kog-nish'-un). That part of a mental process which enables a person to recognize and become aware of certain objects; the perceptive mental processes.

Cohabitation (kō-hab-ĭt-ā-shun). The sexual relationship existing between a man and a woman; coition.

Cohesion (kō-hē'-zhun). The physical force which unites the particles of a body together.

Coitus (kō-ō'-tus or koi'-ĭ-tus). The act of sexual intercourse; copulation.

Colchicum (kol'-chi-kum). A drug obtained from certain plants of the Lillaceæ order. It is a gastric stimulant, lessens the blood-pressure, and is much used in gout and muscular rheumatism. Dosage: tincture, 5-15 minims.

Colectomy (kō-lek'-to-mi). Excision of part or the whole of the colon.

Coley's Fluid. A special fluid containing the toxins of *Streptococcus erysipelatis* and the *B. prodigiosus* is used in the treatment of certain forms of cancer, particularly sarcoma.

Colic (kol'-ik). Severe paroxysmal pain in the abdomen. Biliary C., acute pain caused by the passage of a gall-stone in the bile ducts. Cystic C., pain in the urinary bladder. Lead C., neuralgic pain in the intestines due to lead-poisoning. Painter's C., same as *Lead Colic*. Renal C., the severe pain caused by the passage of a calculus down the ureter.

Colicystitis (kō-lē-sis-tī'-tis). Inflammation of the urinary bladder due to infection with the *B. coli communis*.

Colitis (kō-lī'-tis). Inflammation of the colon.

Collagen (kol'-a-jen). The substance of which the white fibrous elements of connective tissue is composed; it yields gelatin when boiled.

Collapse (kol-aps'). (1) Approximation of parts that are normally separated, such as the walls of a hollow tube or cavity, *e.g.*, the walls of a vein collapse when cut across. (2) Sudden prostration and loss of vital activity due to severe injury, disease, or fright. Closely associated with shock (*q.v.*). *See also* **Atelectasis.**

Collar-bone. The clavicle.

Collargol (kol-ár'-gol). A soluble organic silver compound; is a germicide and antiseptic, and is used in the treatment of gonorrhœa.

Colles' Fracture (kol'-ēs). Fracture of the lower end of the radius. **C. Law**; a mother may breast-feed a syphilitic baby without herself becoming infected; the explanation being that she is already infected, but the symptoms are not manifested until much later in life.

Collodion (ko-lō'-di-on). A substance prepared by dissolving gun-cotton in alcohol and ether. When painted over skin abrasions it dries and forms a seal or air-tight skin over the wound. It is very inflammable, and since it readily dries in the air, must not be left uncorked.

Colloid (kol'-oid). A glue-like non-crystalline substance; matter in which the particles are larger than a molecule and are suspended in another substance. Colloids are diffusible but not soluble in water, and are unable to pass through animal membranes. Metals and other substances are now prepared in colloidal form for medical purposes, *e.g.*, gold, silver, lead, and iodine.

Collosol (kol-ō'-sol). A trade name for various colloidal preparations, *e.g.*, **C. Iodine** and **C. Argentum.**

Collutorium (kol-ū-tawr'-i-um). A mouth-wash; a gargle.

Collyrium (kol-lir'-i-um). A liquid used for bathing the eyes.

Coloboma (kol-ō-bō'-má). A congenital fissure or gap in the eyeball or one of its parts.

Colocynth (kol'-ō-sinth). A powerful, drastic purgative.

Colon (kō'-lon). The large intestine. That part of the bowel which extends from the *cæcum* to the *rectum*.

Colonic (kō-lon'-ik). Pertaining to the colon.

Colopexy (kōl-ō-peks'-i). The operation of stitching the colon to keep it in position.

Colorimeter (kul-or-im'-et-er). An instrument for measuring the colour value of a fluid against that of a standard solution in carrying out delicate biochemical analyses.

EYEPIECE

STANDARD SOLUTION

SOLUTION BEING TESTED

LIGHT
AS REFLECTED BY MIRROR

Colorimeter : General Principle.

Colostomy (kŏ-los'-tō-mi). The operation of making a permanent opening into the colon through the abdominal wall ; this acts as an artificial anus in cases of fistula, obstruction, and cancer.

Colostrum (kŏ-los'-trum). The milky-white fluid secreted in the breasts during the first three days after parturition, and before the true milk is established.

Colotomy (kŏ-lot'-o-mi). An operation for making a temporary opening in the colon.

Colour Index. The ratio of the hæmoglobin percentage to the number of red blood cells per c.mm. expressed as a percentage of the normal. In health the C.I. is 0·9 to 1·0 ; in pernicious anæmia it is above 1·0, and in the iron-deficiency anæmias it is less than normal.

Colpitis (kol-pi'-tis). Inflammation of the vagina.

Colpocleisis (kol-pō-klī'-sis). Occlusion of the vagina. Surgical closure of the vagina by stitching.

Colpoptosis (kol-pop-tō'-sis). Prolapse of the vaginal walls.

Colporrhaphy (kol-por'-a-fi). Surgical repair of a lacerated or prolapsed vagina. **Anterior C.**, the repair of a cystocele. **Posterior C.**, repairing of a rectocele.

Colpotomy (kol-pot'-ō-mi). Incision of the vagina.

Coma (kō'-mà). A state of deep insensibility from which the patient cannot be roused. Commonly seen in *alcoholism*, *apoplexy*, *diabetes*, and *uræmia.* **Vigil C.,** a form of coma in which the eyes are wide open instead of being closed.

Comatose (kōm'-a-tōz). In a state of coma.

Combustion (kom-bust'-yun). Burning; a chemical change in which heat is produced through oxidation of a substance, the end products being carbon dioxide and water.

Comedo (kom-ē'-dō). A plug of dried sebaceous matter filling the follicle of a sebaceous duct; a blackhead. Commonly seen on the face.

Comes (ko'-mēz). Pl. *comites.* A companion. In anatomy two or more veins which accompany an artery.

Comma Bacillus. The bacillus producing Asiatic cholera. *See* Spirillum.

Comminuted (kom'-in-ū-ted). Broken into many pieces. **C. Fracture,** a bone which is broken into several pieces; often caused by a crush, such as being run over.

Commissure (kom'-is-sūr). A connecting part. Used mainly of the brain and spinal cord, *e.g.,* the **Anterior C.,** the connecting strand of white matter in front of the central canal. **Posterior Grey C.,** that portion of the grey commissure of the spinal cord

behind the central canal. **Great C.,** *see* Corpus Callosum.

Compatible (kom-pat'-ib-il). Agreeable; not counteractive; the ability of one drug to mix with another without altering or lessening its efficacy.

Compensation (kom-pen-sā'-shun). The state of making up for a defect. **Cardiac C.,** hypertrophy and dilatation of the ventricular walls of the heart to overcome the defects of valvular incompetency.

Complement (kom'-pli-ment). A ferment-like substance existing in sera and cell-protoplasm which is capable of linking to a cell by means of an amboceptor, and is the active principle in producing *lysis. See* Ehrlich's Theory.

Complemental (kom-pli-men'-tal). Additional; making up a deficiency. **C. Air,** the extra air drawn into the lungs during an excessively deep inspiration.

Complex. In Freudian psychology a grouping of ideas with an emotional background. These may be harmless, and the individual fully aware of them, *e.g.,* an artist sees every object with a view to a possible picture, and is said to have established a complex for art. Often, however, the complex is aroused by some painful emotional reaction, such as fright or excessive grief, which, instead of being allowed a natural outlet, becomes unconsciously repressed, and later manifests itself in some abnormality of mind or behaviour. According to Freud, the best method of determining the complex is through the medium of psycho-analysis. *Jung* and *Rivers*, however, suggest finding out the complex by a series of time-and-reaction tests. *See* Psychoanalysis, Abreaction, and Test.

Complication. An added difficulty; a complex state. A disease or accident superimposed upon another without being specially related, yet affecting or modifying the prognosis of the original disease, *e.g.*, pneumonia is a complication of measles, and is the cause of many deaths from that disease.

Complicated Fracture. *See* Fracture.

Compos mentis (Latin). Of sound mind.

Compress (kom'-pres). (1) A fold of lint or gauze arranged in such a manner as to induce pressure. (2) A wet application, *e.g.*, Carbolic C., a piece of lint wrung out in carbolic lotion, 1-40, and applied to the head for 12 hours. It is covered with a jaconet cap to keep it moist, and is kept in position with a bandage. Its object is to destroy *Pediculi capitis* or head lice. Lead and Opium C., lint lightly wrung out in a solution of lead and opium (*lotio plumbi*), and allowed to evaporate; is a cooling lotion for strains, sprains, etc.; should be renewed frequently.

Compression (kom-presh'-un). A state of being compressed. Pressure on the brain caused by a depressed fracture, tumour, blood, or pus.

Compromise (kom'-pro-mīz). Incomplete adjustment of a mental conflict.

Conation (kō-nā'-shun). In psychology the third part of an instinct. That part of an instinct which impels to action or doing. *See also* Cognition and Affect.

Conception (kon-sep'-shun). The impregnation of the ovum by the spermatozoon.

Concha Auris (kong'-kä aw'-ris). The deepest hollow of the pinna of the external ear.

Concoction (kon-kok'-shun). The boiling of two or more substances together.

Concretion (kon-krē'-shun). A deposit of calcific or other hard material; a calculus.

Concubitus (kon-kū'-bit-us). Lying together; copulation.

Concussion (kon-kush'-un). A violent disturbance of the brain matter by which it ceases to function, and unconsciousness supervenes ; is caused through injury, such as a blow or fall.

Condenser (kon-den'-ser). An apparatus effecting condensation of light, etc. **Abbe's C.,** a specially constructed apparatus placed beneath the stage of a microscope which concentrates the lightrays reflected from the mirror.

Condome (kon-dōm). A thin sheath, usually of rubber, for the penis during copulation for the purpose of contraception.

Conduction (kon-duk'-shun). The transmission of heat, light, and sound ; also the passage of electrical currents and of nerve impulses. **Heat C.,** the transmission of heat by particles which are in contact with each other. Metals such as gold, silver, and copper are good conductors of heat ; liquids, except mercury, less good, while air and gases are distinctly poor ; also materials such as wood, porcelain, rubber, wool, silk, and sealing-wax are not good conductors.

Condyle (kon'-dĪl). A rounded protuberance at the articular end of a bone.

Condyloid (kon'-di-loid). Resembling a condyle in shape.

C o n d y l o m a (kon-dil-ō-má). Wart-like growths of the skin, especially the type round the anus and vulva, and usually due to venereal infection.

Condy's Fluid (kon'-dēz). A proprietary preparation consisting of a solution of sodium permanganate — *potassium permanganate* is commonly substituted for it ; is antiseptic, disinfectant, and deodorant.

Confection (kon-fek'-shun). Soft pasty preparations in which drugs are mixed with sugar, syrup, or honey.

Configuration (kon-fig-ū-rā'-shun). The general shape or outline of a body.

Confinement. *See* **Birth.**

Conflict. A psychological term denoting a state of mental disturbance in which the subconscious mind is in opposition to the ideals of the conscious mind.

Confluent (kon'-floo-ent). Running together. **C. Smallpox,** a severe type of smallpox in which the vesicles tend to coalesce, leaving no clear skin between.

Congenital (kon - jen' - it - al). Existing at the time of birth. **C. Heart Disease,** developmental abnormalities in the anatomy of the heart resulting in disturbance of the post-natal circulation. The blood is only imperfectly oxygenated, and therefore the skin of the individual is cyanosed. Breathlessness and clubbing of the fingers are also characteristic symptoms. A child with this disease usually dies before

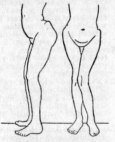

Bilateral Congenital Hip Disease.

puberty, although a few cases reach adolescence. Also known as *Blue Disease, Blue Baby*, etc. **C. Hip Disease**, dislocation of the hip joint occurring in childhood and due to faulty formation of the acetabulum.

Congestion (kon-jest'-shun). A condition characterized by the accumulation of blood in certain tissues of the body; hyperæmia. **Active C.**, that due to increased arterial flow to the part. **Passive C.**, congestion due to obstructed venous circulation.

Congress (kong'-gres). Assembling or gathering together. **Sexual C.**, coition.

Conium (kŏn'-i-um). Hemlock; a poisonous drug which acts as a depressant on the muscular and central nervous systems. The poison by which *Socrates* met his death.

Conjugate (kon'-joo-gāt). The most important pelvic measurement taken from the back of the symphysis pubis to the promontory of the sacrum. This is the **True C.** and measures not less than 4¼ in.; this measurement can only be taken under an anæsthetic. The **External C.** is taken from below the symphysis pubis to the spine of the last lumbar vertebra; this measures 8 in., but needs a pair of calipers for exactness. The **Diagonal C.** is taken from the inner side of the symphysis pubis to the sacro-iliac joints, and measures 5 in. **C. Deviation**, the turning of both eyes, as though coupled, from the normal line of vision.

Conjunctiva (kon-jungk-tī'-vă). The delicate transparent membrane which lines the inner surface of the eyelids, and reflects over the front of the eyeball.

Conjunctivitis (kon-jungk-tī-vī'-

tis). Inflammation of the conjunctiva.

Connective Tissue. The binding tissues of the body consisting of : (1) areolar tissue ; (2) adipose tissue ; (3) bone and dentine ; (4) lymphoid tissue ; (5) cartilage tissue. These tissues are mainly concerned in supporting and connecting other bodily structures.

Consanguinity (kon-sang-gwin'-i-ti). Blood relationship.

Consciousness. Awareness of oneself and surroundings.

Consolidation (kon-sol-i-dā'-shun). The act of becoming solid. Especially used in connection with the solidification of the lungs due to the cellular exudate into the alveoli which occurs in acute pneumonia.

Constipation (kons-ti-pā'-shun). Imperfect evacuation of fæcal matter. Sluggish action of the bowels.

Constitution. (1) In chemistry the structure of a substance with regard to the arrangements of its molecules. (2) The natural qualities or predisposition of a body.

Constricted (kon-strik'-ted). Tightened or contracted in the centre.

Consumption (kon-sump'-shun). (1) The act of consuming. (2) A common name for *pulmonary tuberculosis.* Galloping C., an acute form in which the patient loses weight and strength rapidly ; extremely fatal. *See* Tuberculosis, *also* Phthisis.

Contact (kon'-takt). (1) The point at which two or more bodies touch each other. (2) A means of spreading disease between persons in close association. Direct C., without the intervention of a third person or substance. Immediate C., *see* Direct C.

Contagion (kon-tāj'-'n). Infection conveyed from one person to another through direct contact.

Continued (kon-tin'-yūd). Without intermissions ; constant. C. Fever, a febrile attack in which the temperature does not reach the normal.

Contraceptive (kon-trā-sep'-tiv). Anything used to prevent conception.

Contra-indication. A sign suggesting that a certain line of treatment for a special disease should be discontinued or avoided.

Contraction (kon-trak'-shun). Shortening ; decrease in size.

Contre-coup (kong'-tre-koo). Injury or damage at a point opposite the impact resulting from transmitted force.

Contusion (kon-tū'-zhun). Injury of the subcutaneous tissues accompanied by slight hæmorrhage ; a bruise.

Convallaria. Lily of the valley. The drug obtained

is purgative, diuretic, and a cardiac stimulant.

Convergence (kon-ver'-jens). A turning towards each other, *e.g.*, of the eyes ; a coming together.

Convolutions (kon-vŏ-loo'-shunz). The folds and twists on the surface of the brain and intestines.

Convulsions (kon-vul'-shunz). A series of violent involuntary muscular contractions. **Clonic C.,** in which there is complete relaxation of the muscles between the spasms. **Tonic C.,** in which there is no intervening muscular relaxation ; a continuous contraction, as in tetanus.

Co-ordination (kŏ-awr-din-ā'-shun). Moving in harmony. **Muscular C.,** the harmonious action of muscles, permitting free, smooth movements under perfect control of the will.

Copaiba (ko-pī'-bä). An oleoresin obtained from the trunks of various species of *Copaifera.* Its action is chiefly diuretic, laxative, and stimulant ; is also used in the treatment of gonorrhœa. Dose : Copaiba balsam, 10–30 minims.

Coprolalia (kop-rŏ-lä'-li-ä). The insane repetition of obscene words in the course of ordinary conversation.

Copulation (kop-ū-lä'-shun). Sexual intercourse.

Copperas (kop'-er-as). Iron sulphate ; green vitriol.

Coracoid (kor'-a-koid). Shaped like the beak of a crow. The name given to a process having this shape on the *scapula.* It lies in front and below the acromion process.

Cord. A thread-like structure. The **Vocal C.,** the membranous bands in the larynx, vibrations of which are responsible for the voice. The **Spinal C,** a cord-like structure consisting of nervous tissue which lies in the spinal column, reaching from the *foramen magnum* to the first and second lumbar vertebræ ; it is a direct continuation from the *medulla oblongata.* **Spermatic C.,** the cord which suspends the testicles. **Umbilical C.,** the navel-string attaching the fœtus to the placenta.

Cordate (kaw(r)'-dät). Heart-shaped.

Core (kawr). The central part of anything.

Corium (kaw'-ri-um). The internal layer of the skin, lying immediately beneath the epidermis. The dermis or true skin.

Corn. A horny overgrowth of the epidermis with a hard core ; produced by friction or pressure. **Soft C.,** one developing between the toes, and softened by moisture ; to prevent their occurrence,

D

the area between the toes must be thoroughly dried, and powdered after washing.

Cornea (kaw(r)'-ni-á). The outwardly convex transparent membrane forming part of the outer coat of the eye. It is situated in front of the iris and pupil, and merges backwards into the *sclera*.

Corneal (kaw(r)'-ni-al). Pertaining to the cornea.

Cornu (kaw(r)'-noo). Any horn-shaped process or structure.

Corona (kor-ō'-ná). A crown; any structure resembling a crown.

Coronal (ko-rō'-nal). Pertaining to a corona. **C. Suture**, a suture joint of the skull formed by the articulation of the *parietal* and *frontal* bones.

Coronary (kor'-on-a-ri). Encircling, as of a vessel or nerve. **C. Arteries**, the arteries supplying the heart muscle. **C. Thrombosis**, infarction of the myocardium.

Coroner (kor'-o-ner). An officer who holds inquests on those dead from violence.

Coronoid (kor'-on-oid). Crown-like.

Corpora (kawr'-po-rá). Pl. of Latin *corpus*, a body. **C. Arantii**, minute bodies on the free margins of the semilunar valves of the heart. **C. Amylacea**, microscopical, hard, rounded bodies found in certain glandular structures and tumours, *e.g.*, prostate, pituitary, brain tumours.

Corpus (kawr'-pus). A body. **C. Arantii**, *see* **Corpora A**. **C. Callosum**, a band of white substance composed of nerve fibres which connects the two hemispheres of the cerebrum. **C. Luteum**, the yellow bodies formed in the ovary after the rupture of a Graafian follicle with expulsion of the ovum. The *false C. luteum* is formed in the non-pregnant state, and persists roughly for one month, at the end of which time it is reabsorbed by phagocytic action. The *true C. luteum* occurs in pregnancy, and persists for six months and has almost disappeared by the end of the ninth month.

Corpuscle (kawr-pus'-l). A microscopic mass of protoplasm. There are many varieties, but the term generally refers to the red and white blood cells. *See* **Erythrocytes** and **Leucocytes**.

Corpuscular (kawr-pus'-kū-lár), relating to the corpuscles.

Corrigan's Disease. An abnormal condition caused by aortic regurgitation, and recognized by visible pulsation in the main arteries. **C. Pulse**, a full bounding pulse, which appears to completely empty between the beats ; is associated with aortic insufficiency. Synonym, *Water-hammer Pulse.*

Corrosion (kor-rō'-zhun). Destruction through the action of chemicals ; eating away.

Corrosive (kor-rō'-ziv). Possessing the property of causing corrosion ; destructive in action. **C. Sublimate,** perchloride of mercury used in a strength of 1-1,000 to 1-4,000; is a powerful antiseptic; poisonous ; solutions are coloured blue as a distinctive mark.

Cortex (kawr'-teks). The outer bark or covering structures. **C. of the Brain,** the outer grey matter of the brain. **Renal C.,** the hard, firm outer layer of the kidney substance immediately under the capsule. **Suprarenal C.,** the outer capsule surrounding the medulla.

Cortical (kawr'-tik-al). Pertaining to the cortex.

Cortin (kawr'-tin). The extract of the suprarenal cortex.

Corynebacterium Diphtheriæ (kor-ī-nē . . .). The organism causing diphtheria. Also known as *Klebs - Loeffler bacillus.*

Coryza (kor-ī'-zà). The symptoms of a common cold ; nasal catarrh; also seen in syphilitic infants, the condition being known as *snuffles.*

Cosmetic (koz-met'-ik). (1) Making beautiful. (2) A remedy for beautifying the skin. **C. Operation,** an operation for lessening unsightliness.

Costal (kos'-tal). Relating to the ribs.

Costive (kos'-tiv). Constipated.

Cotyledon (kot-il-ē'-don). One of the raised subdivisions of the uterine surface of the placenta.

Cough. A sudden forced noisy expulsion of air from the lungs through the partially closed vocal cords ; *tussis.*

Coulomb (koo'-lom). The unit of electrical quantity. The quantity of electricity developed by a current of 1 ampere in 1 second.

Counteraction (kown-ter-ak'-shun). The action of one substance opposing the action of another.

Counter-extension. Extension applied both at the proximal and at the distal end of a limb simultaneously.

Counter-irritant (kown-ter-ir'-it-ant). An agent producing counter-irritation.

Counter-irritation (kown-ter-ir-it-ā'-shun). The application which, by inducing a superficial inflammation, relieves a more deep-seated inflammation.

Counter-opening (kown-ter-ō'-pen-ing). An opening made at a distance from the original incision, with a view to facilitating the drainage of pus or other secretion. Tubes inserted into such an opening are known as *counter-drainage tubes.*

Counter-stain (kown-ter-stăn). A stain applied to a microscope slide already stained, the second stain enhancing the clearness and colour of the first.

Counter-suggestion. A method of suggestion which produces action in an opposite direction. Same as *Contrasuggestion.*

Court-plaster. A form of sticking-plaster with a silk backing. Formerly used by Court ladies for patches worn on the face.

Courvoisier's Law (koor-voz'-i-erʒ). An enlarged and palpable gall-bladder in the presence of jaundice is not due to gall-stones. The "law" is often expressed in other forms all of which aim at indicating that obstructive jaundice is only associated with enlargement of the gall-bladder when this sac is not prevented from expanding by previous inflammatory thickening of its walls.

Cover-slip (kuv'-er-slip). A very thin square or circle of glass used for covering a prepared specimen on a microscope slide.

Cowpox. A specific infectious disease attacking milch cows. The lesions closely resemble those of smallpox, and occur chiefly on the udder. Vaccinia.

Coxa (koks'-à). The hip-joint.

Coxa Valga. A deformity of the neck of the femur in which the angle formed between the neck and the shaft is more than 130°, and resulting in decreased adduction of the limb.

Coxa Vara. A deformity of the neck of the femur in which the angle between the neck and the shaft is less than 130°, thus increasing adduction of the limb.

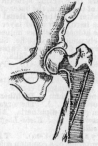

Coxa Vara.
(Shaded lines show normal.)

Coxalgia (koks-al'-ji-à). Pain in the hip.

Coxitis (koks-I'-tis). Inflammation of the hip joint.

Crab-louse (krab'-lows). The *pediculus pubis.*

Cracked Nipples. Fissures and cracks forming on the nipples of a nursing mother, generally caused by lack of care and cleanliness, or by too vigorous sucking of a strong infant. Since they are apt to cause breast abscesses, they must be healed with an application of tinct. benzoin compound, or by applying hot fomentations. A nipple shield should be used for feeding until the cracks have healed.

Cradle. A frame to prevent contact of some part of the patient with the bed-clothing.

Cramp (kramp). Painful spasmodic muscular contractions. **Occupational C.** may be caused by excessive use of certain groups of muscles, but more often is of psychic origin, and in addition to complete rest, needs psychotherapeutic treatment. Writers' C., Seamstresses' C., and Violinists' C. are common examples of this condition. Possibly the state is due to an unconscious defence mechanism.

Craniectomy (krān-i-ek'-to-mi). The operation of removing part of the cranium.

Cranioclast (krān'-i-ō-klåst). An instrument for crushing the fœtal head in difficult labour. *See* **Craniotomy**.

Craniometry (krān-i-om'-et-ri). The science which deals with the measurement of skulls.

Craniotome (krān'-i-ō-tōm). An instrument used for craniotomy.

Craniotomy (krān-i-ot'-o-mi). The operation of opening the fœtal skull to facilitate delivery. Never performed when any other method can be used, except in the case of a dead fœtus.

Cranium (krān'-i-um). The skull. Composed of eight bones, forming the cranial cavity for containing the brain and its meninges.

Creatin (krē'-a-tēn). A crystallizable nitrogenous substance found in muscular tissue.

Creatinin (kre - at' - in - ēn). Formed from creatin, and excreted in the urine.

Crèche (krāsh). A day nursery where the infants of working-class people may be cared for.

Credé's Method (krē'-dē). A method of delivering the placenta by gently rubbing the fundus uteri until it contracts, and then, by squeezing the fundus, expressing the placenta into the vagina from whence it is expelled. Also known as the *Dublin Method*.

Cremation (krē-mā'-shun). The method of reducing a dead body to ashes by burning.

Creolin (krē'-ō-lin). One of

101

the coal-tar products; is a good disinfectant and germicide. The solution is used from ½-2%.

Creosol (krē'-ō-sol). An antiseptic phenol derived from coal tar or wood tar.

Creosote (krē-ō-sōt). An oily transparent liquid obtained by the distillation of wood-tar. It turns from a yellowish to a brown or red colour on exposure to the air. It has a burning taste and a pungent odour; is said to be excellent for pulmonary diseases, especially *phthisis*, and for this purpose may be taken orally, or inhaled by adding 3l to boiling water 0l, and breathing in the vapour. Creosote is also a styptic, antispasmodic, and intestinal antiseptic.

Crepitation (krep-i-tā'-shun). The peculiar grating sound heard when the two ends of a broken bone are rubbed together. Also a similar sound heard on auscultation in a case of pneumonia, pleurisy, etc.

Crepitus (krep'-it-us). *See* **Crepitation.**

Crescentic (kres-sen'-tik). Shaped like a crescent or new moon. **C. Hymen,** one with an opening shaped like a crescent.

Creta (krē-tà). Chalk.

Cretinism (kret'-in-izm). A condition brought about by a deficiency in the secretion of the *thyroid gland*. The individual remains dwarfed in stature, feels the cold intensely, and has abnormal deposits of fat in the body. The hair is coarse and falls out readily. The mental faculties are undeveloped, so that the individual is practically an idiot. The condition is seen in young children. If puberty is reached, the normal sex functions do not appear. Fortunately, early treatment with *thyroid extract*, given orally, yields good results. A similar condition called *myxœdema* may occur in the adult, and is again due to thyroid insufficiency. **Sporadic C.,** occurring in a child born of normal parents, and living in a locality where goitre is not endemic.

Cricoid Cartilage (krī'-koid). The ring-shaped cartilage below the thyroid cartilage in front of the larynx.

Criminal Malpractice. The unlawful production of abortion.

Crisis (krī'-sis). (1) The turning-point of a disease; a very critical period. (2) The term used for the sudden descent of a high temperature to normal or below; generally occurs within 24 hours. A **True C.,** one accompanied by a fall in the pulse-rate. **False C.,** when the temperature falls and the pulse-rate remains high, suggesting that later on the temperature may rise again. (3) Sharp paroxysms of pain occurring over the course of a few days in certain diseases, *e.g.*, **Gastric C.**, **Vesical C.**, **Dietl's C.**, and **Laryngeal C.**, etc. (4) **Blood C.**, the appearance in the blood of large numbers of nucleated erythrocytes over the course of a few days.

Critical (krit'-ik-al). In a dangerous state.

Crohn's Disease. *See* **Regional Ileitis.**

Cross-birth. A transverse presentation.

Croton Oil (krō'-ton). A powerful purgative and poison; useful for unconscious patients. One minim is inserted in the centre of a small piece of butter and placed on the back of the tongue, where it melts and is automatically swallowed. Dose, ½-1 minim.

Croup (kroop). Acute laryngeal inflammation accompanied by spasm and dyspnœa. Synonym, *Spasmodic laryngitis.*

Crural (kroo'-ral). Pertaining to the thigh.

Cry. (1) Weeping. (2) A shriek. **Epileptic C.**, the peculiar shout uttered at the commencement of an epileptic fit. **Meningeal C.**, the dismal cry heard in children suffering from meningitis

Cryptomenorrhœa (krip'-tŏ-men-o-rē-ȧ). Retention of the menses due to a congenital obstruction, such as an imperforate hymen or atresia of the vagina.

Cryptorchid (kript'-awr-kid). A male whose testicles have not descended into the scrotum, *i.e.*, they are retained within the abdomen or inguinal canals.

Crystalline Lens. A biconvex body, oval in shape, which is suspended just behind the *iris* of the eye, and separates the aqueous humour from the vitreous humour. It is slightly less convex on its anterior surface than on the posterior. Its function is to refract the light-rays so that they focus directly on to the *retina.*

Crystalloids (kris'-tal-oidz). Substances of a crystalline nature which diffuse readily through a membrane and form true solutions in water.

Cuboid (kū'-boid). Shaped like a cube.

Culex (kū'-leks). A genus of two-winged insects, including mosquitoes and gnats.

Culture (kul'-tūr or kult'-cher). The growth and development of micro-organisms in artificial media. **C. Media,** various substances which are suitable for the artificial growth of bacteria, etc.; can be prepared from broth, beef extract, bouillon, peptone, agar-agar, milk, potato, etc. **Hanging Drop C.,** the organism is suspended in a hanging drop on a glass microscope slide and then inverted over the concave surface of another slide. It can then be examined under a microscope. **Negative C.,** when, after cultivation, suspected matter fails to show the presence of bacteria. **Positive C.,** one which reveals the presence of a suspected organism. **Pure C.,** a culture containing only one type of organism, uncontaminated by others. **Stab C.,** the introduction into solid media of bacteria by stabbing the media with the infected point of a platinum wire.

Cumulate (kŭ'-mū-lāt). To heap up; gather together.

Cumulative (kŭ'-mū-la-tiv). Increasing; gathering strength. Certain drugs which after being received into the body in small doses, often repeated, are not immediately eliminated, but tend to accumulate in the system and suddenly produce symptoms of poisoning. *Carbolic acid* and mercurial preparations are examples of drugs which act in this way.

Cuneiform (kŭ'-nē-i-form). Wedge-shaped; the name of the *third carpal bone* and *three of the tarsal bones,*

all of these being wedge-shaped.

Cupping (kup'-ping). A method of inducing hyperæmia by the use of bell-shaped glasses from which the air is exhausted. **Dry C.,** cupping over an unbroken skin. **Wet C.,** the skin is first scarified with a scalpel or scarifier, in which case blood exudes into the glass.

Cuprum (kŭp'-rum). Copper; symbol, Cu; atomic weight, 63·6. A red metallic element. **C. Acetate,** a green copper salt used as an astringent. **C. Sulphate,** a crystalline salt used as caustic and astringent. Synonyms, *Blue Stone* and *Blue Vitriol.*

Curare (kŭ-rá'-ri). A poisonous drug obtained from a South American plant. There are several varieties. Used by the natives for arrow poison. It paralyses the motor nerves and also the respiratory centre, thereby causing death; is sometimes used to control the convulsions of *tetanus,* but otherwise is of very little therapeutic value.

Curative (kūr'-a-tiv). Making well; restorative, not palliative.

Curettage (kŭ-ret'-āj). The surgical operation of scraping out the interior of a cavity with a curette, most commonly the uterine cavity.

Current. A flowing, as of liquid,

gas, electricity, or nerve impulse. **Alternating C.,** one in which the direction is periodically reversed. **Constant C.,** a current which is produced without interruption. **Direct C.,** one continually passing in the same direction. **Faradic C.,** an alternating current of induced electricity. **Galvanic C.,** a direct current produced from a battery.

Curvature (kurv'-a-tūr). A bend. **Greater C.** of the stomach ; the lower convex border of the stomach. **Lesser C.** of the stomach ; the smaller upper concave border of the stomach. **Spinal C.,** an exaggeration of the normal curves of the spinal column. Lateral or towards one side, is known as *scoliosis.* An exaggerated dorsal curve is called *kyphosis,* or hump-back. An exaggerated lumbar curve is known as *lordosis.*

Cusp (kusp). A projecting point, such as the edge of a tooth or the segment of a heart-valve. The *tricuspid* valve has three cusps ; the *mitral* valve only two.

Cutaneous (kū-tān'-i-us). Relating to the skin.

Cuticle (kū'-tik-l). The epidermis or outer skin layer. *See* Epidermis.

Cutis (kū'-tis). The skin. **C. Vera,** the true skin which lies beneath the epidermis. **C. Anserina,** "goose - skin" formed by the contraction of the minute capillary muscles of the skin, due to cold, fright, etc.

Cyanic (sī-an'-ik). (1) Blue. (2) Pertaining to cyanogen.

Cyanide Gauze (sī'-an-id). A disinfectant gauze impregnated with a mercuric cyanide, and coloured mauve to distinguish it. Wool can also be treated in this way.

Cyanogen (sī-an'-ō-jen). ON. An extremely poisonous gas if inhaled ; has a bluish colour.

Cyanosis (sī-an-ō'-sis). Blueness of the skin due to venous engorgement ; is caused by insufficient oxygenation, such as might result from (1) *blue disease, strangulation, hanging,* or *acute dyspnœa* ; (2) anything interfering with the circulation of the blood, respiration or exchange of gases in the lungs.

Cycle (sī'-kl). A series of movements or events ; a sequence. **Cardiac C.,** the series of movements through which the heart passes in performing one heart-beat ; it includes contraction or *systole,* relaxation or *diastole,* and a short rest pause, the *diastase* ; a complete cycle corresponds to one pulse-beat, and takes 0·8 of a second.

Cyclical Vomiting (sī'-kli-kl).

D *

Periodical and recurring attacks of vomiting met with in children of a nervous temperament. The condition is usually associated with acidosis.

Cyclitis (sī-klī′-tis). Inflammation of the ciliary body.

Cycloplegia (sī-klō-plē′-ji-ȧ). Paralysis of the ciliary muscles.

Cyesis (sī-ē′-sis). Pregnancy. **Pseudo-C.**, an imaginary pregnancy, caused by an overwhelming desire for children in a childless person.

Cylinder (sil′-in-der). An elongated body of an equal diameter in the whole of its length in transverse section.

Cylindrical. Pertaining to a cylinder. *See also* Axon.

Cyst (sist). A hollow sac or mass containing fluid or semi-solid matter.

Cyst-adenoma (sist-ad-e-nō′-mȧ). A glandular tumour also containing cysts.

Cystic (sis′-tik). Resembling or consisting of cysts.

Cysticercus (sis-ti-ser′-kus). The larval stage in the development of a tape-worm.

Cystin (sis′-tēn). A sulphur containing amino-acid, produced by the breaking down of proteins during the digestive process.

Cystitis (sis-tī′-tis). Inflammation of the urinary bladder ; may be acute or chronic.

Cystocele (sis′-tō-sēl). Hernia

or prolapse of the posterior wall of the urinary bladder into the vagina.

Cystolithiasis (sis-tō-lith-I′-a-sis). The presence or formation of calculi in the bladder.

Cystoscope (sis′-tō-skōp). A special instrument for viewing the interior of the bladder. It also enables fine gum-elastic catheters to be passed into the ureters. The appar-

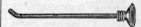

Cystoscope.

atus may be connected to an electric battery which lights a small bulb at the end of the instrument, thus illuminating the bladder.

Cystoscopy (sis-tos′-ko-pi). Examination of the bladder by means of a cystoscope.

Cystotomy (sis-tot′-o-mi). Surgical opening of the bladder. **Suprapubic C.**, incision into the bladder just above the symphysis pubis. **Perineal C.**, an opening into the bladder through the perineum.

Cytology (sī-tol′-o-ji). The science which deals with the structure of cells.

Cytolysis (sī-tol′-i-sis). The destruction of cells.

Cytoplasm (sī′-tō-plazm). The protoplasmic structure of a cell in which the nucleus is supported.

Cyton (sī'-ton). A nerve cell; may be bipolar, multipolar, or unipolar.

D.

Dacryadenalgia (dak-ri-ad-en-al'-ji-à). Pain of the lachrymal gland.

Dacryadenitis (dak-ri-ad-en-ī'-tis). Inflammation of the lachrymal gland.

Dacryocyst (dak'-ri-ō-sist). The tear-sac.

Dacryocystitis (dak-ri-ō-sis-tī'-tis). Inflammation of the tear-sac.

Dacryolith (dak'-ri-ō-lith). The presence of a calculus in the lachrymal duct.

Dacryoma (dak-ri-ō'-má). Blockage or obstruction of a tear-duct, causing the tears to overflow down the cheek.

Dactyl (dak'-til). A finger or toe; one of the digits.

Dactylion (dak-til'-i-on). The growth of a skin between the fingers or toes; may be congenital or the result of burns, etc.; webbing.

Dactylitis (dak-til-ī'-tis). Inflammation of the digits; generally observed in syphilitics, tuberculous subjects, or in poorly nourished persons.

Dactylology (dak-til-ol'-ō-ji). A means of communication between deaf and dumb persons, the words being represented by signs made with the fingers; the deaf and dumb language.

Dakin (dā'-kin). See Carrel-Dakin Treatment.

Daltonism (dawl'-ton-izm). A congenital inability to distinguish colours or the shades of a particular colour. Named after John Dalton, English chemist and physicist, who suffered from this disability.

Dandruff (dand'-ruff). A disease affecting the hair and skin of the scalp. The epidermis is shed in fine powdery scales. The exact cause is uncertain. If neglected, may lead to baldness and various skin complaints.

Dandy Fever (dan'-di). See Dengue.

Darwin, Charles. English naturalist and scientist, born in Shrewsbury on 12th February 1809; is famous for his work on the subject of evolution. His writings include "The Origin of Species," "The Descent of Man," "The Voyage of the Beagle," etc.

Darwin's Tubercle. A small prominence on the helix of the ear. According to *Darwin*, the vestigial remains of the pointed ear of a simian ancestor; usually more marked in males than in females.

Darwinism (dár'-win-izm). The

theory of human evolution as taught by Darwin. The evolution of mankind from the lower to the higher animals through a process of variation and *natural selection*. He suggests also that man and monkeys descend from a common ancestor.

Daturine (da´-tū-rin). An alkaloid of the common thorn-apple or *D. stramonium*; has a similar action to atropine.

Deaf-mute. A person who is both deaf and dumb.

Deaf-mutism. The state of dumbness resulting from congenital or acquired deafness.

Deafness. Loss of ability to hear. May occur from several causes, such as (1) injury or disease of that part of the cortex controlling the centre for hearing; (2) hysteria, without any abnormality of the ear or brain; (3) injury to the ear itself, *e.g.*, from loud noises, such as the firing of a gun at close range; (4) disease of the labyrinth of the internal ear; (5) an abnormal mental state which may produce auditory aphasia, a condition in which, although sounds are understood, they cannot be construed into their meaning. This state is called *Mind* or *Psychic D.*

Dealcoholisation (dē-al-kŏ-hol-i-zā´-shun). The removal

of alcohol from a substance; generally used in connection with the preparation of microscope slides.

Deaminated (dĕ-am´-in-ā-ted). The splitting off of ammonia from an amino-acid.

Debility (de-bil´-it-ī). Weakness or loss of tonicity in the functions of the body; a lowering of vitality.

Decalcification (dē-kal-si-fi-kā´-shun). The removal of lime salts from a bone.

Decalitre (dek-ă-lē-ter). Ten litres.

Decapitation (dē-kap-i-tā´-shun). The removal of the head from the body.

Decay (de-kā). Gradual decomposition and disintegration of matter; deterioration; also a gradual decline in health and vigour, as commonly accompanies old age; senility.

Decerebrated (dē-se´-ri-brā-ted). Deprived of the cerebrum.

Decidua (de-sid-ū-ă). The membranous structure which develops in the gravid uterus, so-called because after parturition it is expelled from the uterus. The D. Vera is that part which remains adherent to the wall of the uterine cavity. The basal part, which also is firmly attached and which later forms the placenta, is known as the D. Basalis, while that part which reflects over the embryo, forming a complete membranous sac, is the D. **Capsularis** or **D. Reflexa**.

Deciduoma Malignum (de-sid-ū-ō-má mal-ig-num). *See* **Chorion-epithelioma**.

Deciduous (de-sid'-ū-us). A term denoting structures which are shed or given off from the body during life. **D. Teeth**, the *milk teeth* or *temporary teeth*, which are shed about the age of seven years.

Decigram (des'-i-gram). One-tenth of a gram.

Decilitre (des'-i-lē-ter). One-tenth of a litre.

Decimetre (des'-i-mē-ter). One-tenth of a metre.

Decline (de-klīn'). (1) The descent of a high temperature to the normal line. *See* **Crisis** and **Lysis**. (2) Diminution in power and activity; said of a disease when the acute stage is over. (3) A popular term for *phthisis* or any disease marked by emaciation and weakness.

Decoction (dē-kok'-shun). The preparation of a drug by boiling the substance in water.

Decoloration (dē-cul-er'-rā'-shun). The removal of colour by chemical agents or by bleaching.

Decomposition (dē-kom-pō-zish'-un). (1) The occurrence of putrefactive changes in a substance. (2) The reduction of a complex substance into its constituent parts, *e.g.*, the splitting of a compound into its chemical elements.

Decompression (dē-kom-presh'-un). An operation performed for removing pressure on the brain by trephining the skull.

Decrement (dek'-re-ment). The defervescent period of a disease.

Decubitus (de-kū'-bit-us). (1) The posture assumed in lying. (2) A bed-sore.

Decussation (dē-kus-ā'-shun). The crossing of certain structures, *e.g.*, the D. of the Pyramids, the crossing of the bundles of motor nerve fibres as they pass through the medulla oblongata.

Defæcation (dē-fē-kā'-shun). The act of expelling fæces from the bowel.

Defective (de-fek'-tiv). Imperfect. **Mental D.**, one who is lacking in mental ability; an idiot.

Defervescence (dē-fer-ves'-ens). (1) The decline of a disease. (2) The period during which a temperature is falling to normal.

Defibrinated (dē-fī'-brin-ā-ted or dē-fib'-rin-ā-ted). Deprived or rendered free of fibrin, *s.g.*, **serum** is defibrinated *plasma*.

Degeneracy (dē-jen'-e-ra-si).

109

Inability to maintain a certain standard; the act of becoming poorer in type; a loss of those qualities which have been built up and developed by one's ancestors; a reversion to a primitive form.

Degeneration (dē-jen-e-rā´-shun). A loss of quality; retrogression. **Amyloid D.**, the deterioration of tissue with a deposit of waxy substance. *See* **Lardaceous Disease. Calcareous D.**, degeneration associated with the deposition of lime salts in the tissues. **Caseous D.**, an alteration in the tissues into cheesy material; commonly seen in tuberculous inflammation. **Colloid D.**, the appearance of colloid material in tumours and growths. *See* **Colloid. Fatty D.**, condition in which the normal tissues become infiltrated with fat, often observed in the heart and the liver. **Fibroid D.**, the formation of fibrous material in muscular tissue. **Hyaline D.**, the deposit of hyaline matter which gives the tissue a transparent, smooth, shining appearance. **Senile D.**, the bodily and mental changes which occur in old age. **Waxy D.**, *see* **Amyloid D.**

Deglutition (dē-gloo-tish´-un). The act of swallowing; is partly voluntary and partly involuntary.

Dehiscence (dē-his´-enz). The rupture of a follicle. The term is particularly applied to the rupture of a *Graafian follicle*.

Dehydration (dē-hī-drā´-shun). The removal or withdrawal of water from a compound substance, organ, or body.

Dejecta (dē-jek´-tá). Fæces.

Dejection (dē-jek´-shun). A state of being cast down. **Mental D.**, a feeling of sadness or of inferiority.

Deleterious (del-e-tē´-ri-us). Harmful; liable or tending to cause deterioration.

Deliquescence (del-i-kwes´-ens). The liquefaction of a substance by its ability to absorb water from the atmosphere.

Delirious (de-lir´-i-us). In a state of delirium.

Delirium (de-lir´-i-um). A state of mental confusion and excitement. The mind wanders, speech is incoherent, and the patient is in a state of continual, aimless physical activity. There are many forms of delirium, depending mainly upon the cause, but two main types are generally recognized: (1) The **Wild Maniacal D.**, often associated with high temperature and acute illness; (2) the low, muttering type accompanied by great physical exhaustion, as seen in cases of typhoid fever. The main causes of delirium are: acute alcoholism, resulting in the condition known as **D. Tremens**; acute insanity, hysteria, long continued exhausting illnesses, nervous shock and toxæmia. The patient should never be left alone for an instant, since attempts at suicide are frequent in such cases. The nursing of delirium calls for the highest attributes of a good nurse, and needs endless patience, tact, and understanding.

Deliver (de-liv´-er). To yield up or set free.

Delivery. Expulsion of the child from the uterus of a pregnant woman. *See* **Parturition**.

Deltoid (del´-toid). Resembling the shape of the Greek letter Δ (delta). Triangular shaped. **D. Muscle**, the large muscle covering the prominence of the shoulder.

Delusion (de-loo´-zhun). A false belief which is impervious to the most complete demonstration of its impossibility, and unshaken by the presence of incompatible and obviously contradictory facts. There are three main types of delusion: (1) **Grandiose D.**, in which the individual is firmly convinced he is an important personage, such as the King of England, even though he may be actually living in very poor circum-

stances. (2) **D. of Persecution**, a morbid state in which the patient imagines he is being subjected to persecution. (3) **D. of Reference**, in which ordinary actions and conversations are misconstrued as referring to the individual without any foundation in fact; a morbid state in which a man imagines other persons are talking about him; the delusion becomes fixed, and the patient will not listen to reason; the condition sometimes affects conduct.

Demagnetize (dē-mag´-net-Iz). To remove the magnetic properties of a substance.

Demarcation (dē-mår-kā´-shun). The sharply defined line between diseased and healthy tissue; used most commonly in connection with the division between gangrenous and normal tissue, and also with reference to the raised inflamed edge of erysipelas.

Demented (de-men´-ted). Afflicted with dementia.

Dementia (de-men´-shi-å). A form of insanity; mental deterioration and loss of intellectual power.

Demulcent (de-mul´-sent). A soft, soothing substance, useful for alleviating an inflamed membranous surface. Examples are: white of egg, milk, barley water.

111

Denature (dē-nā'-tūr). To deprive a substance of its nature. In connection with alcohol, to render it unfit to drink.

Dendrite (den'-drīt). One of the branched filaments which are given off from the body of a nerve cell.

Dengue (deng'-gū). A tropical infectious disease transmitted by the mosquito *Stegomyia fasciata*, and occurring in epidemic form. It is associated with severe myalgia and pain in the joints and limbs, and the appearance of a rash somewhat resembling measles. Synonyms, *Dandy Fever*, *Break-bone Fever*.

Dens (dens). A tooth.

Density (den'-sit-i). The mass per unit volume.

Dental (den'-tal). Pertaining to the teeth.

Dentaphone (den'-ta-fōn). An apparatus for the use of deaf persons. When placed between the teeth, the sounds are transmitted through them to the bones of the head, and so to the labyrinth.

Dentiform (den'-ti-fawm). Tooth-like.

Dentifrice (den'-ti-fris). A substance in the form of a powder, paste, or solution used for cleansing the teeth.

Dentine (den'-tēn). The hard outer substance of a tooth ; that part forming the crown of the tooth is covered by enamel. Dentine is one of the hardest substances in the body.

Denture (den'-tūr). A set of teeth, whether natural or artificial.

Deodorant (dē-ōd'-or-ant). An agent which destroys or neutralizes foul odours. Those in common use are : chloride of lime, creolin, izal, iodoform, permanganate of potash, and sanitas.

Deoxidation (dē-oks-i-dā'-shun). The removal of oxygen from a substance.

Depilation (dē-pil-ā'-shun). The procedure of removing hair by plucking it out.

Depilatory (dē-pil'-a-tor-i). Any substance which will remove hair.

Deplete (de-plēt'). To empty, as by bleeding the body, or by purgation ; to lessen the fluid contents of a cavity or structure.

Deposit (de-poz'-it). The falling or settlement of a substance to the bottom of a fluid ; a sediment or precipitate.

Depressant (de-pres'-ant). A drug which acts by lessening the force and activity of an organ or system.

Depression (de-presh'-un). (1) A hollow place or indention. (2) Diminution of power. (3) A low condition, either mental or physical.

Derangement (de-rānj'-ment).

A state of disorder. **Mental D.**, unbalanced state ; insanity.

Dermatitis (der-ma-tī'-tis). Inflammation of the skin.

Dermatoid (der'-mat-oid). Resembling the skin.

Dermatology (der-mat-ol'-o-ji). The science which deals with the structure, functions, and diseases of the skin.

Dermis (der'-mis). The true skin ; the *Cutis vera*.

Dermographia (der-mō-grăf'-i-ă). Literally, writing on the skin. A condition in which when the nail is drawn lightly over the skin it leaves a raised red line, which later becomes white, and lasts for some minutes.

Dermoid (der'-moid). Pertaining to or like skin. **D. Cyst**, a sac-like structure filled with a semi-fluid or thickish sebaceous matter. It occurs chiefly in the skin of the head, face, and back. The **D. Cyst of the Ovary** is a cystic teratoma and often contains hair, bone, teeth, etc., in addition to sebaceous matter.

Descemet's Membrane (des'-e-mă or des'-e-met). The membrane lining the posterior surface of the cornea.

Desiccation (des-ik-ā'-shun). The process of drying a substance, especially used in connection with the drying of certain drugs.

Desquamation (des-kwa-mă'-shun). The shedding or falling off of the epidermis as fine particles or flakes.

Detergent (de-ter'-jent). Cleansing by rubbing or wiping.

Determinism (de-ter'-min-izm). A psycho-analytical term, indicating that all mental activity is controlled by the unconscious as well as by the conscious mind.

Detritus (det'-ri-tus). The powdery accumulation resulting from the rubbing down of a solid substance; waste matter.

Dettol. A saponaceous, non-poisonous germicide, containing a halogenated xylenol. Three times as strong as carbolic acid but non-irritant on normal skins. Employed full strength in thin films in emergencies, 30% in water (sparingly) for midwifery, and 2-10% for treating septic wounds. The clear fluid forms emulsions with water.

Deviation (dē-vi-ā'-shun). Turning away from the normal course ; lack of alignment ; divergence.

Devitalization (dē-vīt-al-i-zā'-shun). The act of removing life ; the destruction of vitality in a part.

Dexter (deks'-ter). Right ; pertaining to the right-hand side.

Dextrin (deks'-trin). The name given to one of the polysaccharide group of carbohydrate substances, formed by the hydrolysis of starch and also by the action of certain ferments. The enzyme of saliva converts starch into dextrins known as *erythro-dextrin* and *achroo-dextrin*, and if the action is further continued, into a form of sugar called *maltose.*

Dextrose (deks'-trōz) ($C_6H_{12}O_6$). A carbohydrate substance belonging to the monosaccharide group, is white and crystalline, and is soluble in water. Its presence in urine is detected by the Fehling's or Benedict's test; also known as Glucose and Grape-sugar.

Dextrous (deks'-trus). Skilful in manipulation or expert in movement; not clumsy.

Dhobie Itch (dō'-bē). An irritating infection of the skin of the groins, etc., due to growth of an epidermophyton fungus.

Diabetes (dī-a-bē'-tēz). A disease characterized by the voidance of an excessive amount of urine. There are several varieties of diabetes. **D. Insipidus,** often associated with pituitary disease; large quantities of pale-coloured urine with a low specific gravity are passed; there is no glycosuria; thirst is extreme on account of the great amount of body fluid which is lost; emaciation and asthenia are marked. **D. Innocens,** the sudden appearance of glycosuria, which

clears up in a short time, is not due to disease but to the intake of too much carbohydrate, which is eliminated in the urine. **Lipogenic D.,** a form of diabetes associated with excessive fatness. **D. Mellitus,** this is the most usual form of diabetes; the symptoms include polyuria, persistent glycosuria, hyperglycæmia, excessive hunger and thirst, emaciation and weakness; various complications may arise, each producing its own particular symptoms; this type of diabetes is essentially a disease due to faulty metabolism, and results in the insufficient utilization and oxidation of carbohydrate substances in the body; the essential cause is the defective production of insulin by the Islands of Langerhans in the pancreas. **Renal D.,** a form of diabetes associated with marked glycosuria, but with no other abnormal symptoms; is possibly due to a low renal threshold for sugar. **True D.,** *see* **D. Mellitus.**

Diabetic (dī-a-bet'-ik). Relating to, or pertaining to diabetes. **D. Puncture,** an experimental puncture of the floor of the fourth ventricle in animals; it results in glycosuria.

Diacetic Acid (dī-a-sē'-tik). A

precursor of acetone in diabetic urine.

Diachylon Plaster (dī-ak'-il-on). Lead plaster ; an adhesive plaster containing lead oxide : 1 part of oxide is boiled in 2 of olive oil and 1 of water.

Diagnose (dī'-ag-nōz). To make a diagnosis.

Diagnosis (dī-ag-nō'-sis). The art of recognizing a disease from a study of the signs and symptoms it presents. Careful observation and minute attention to detail is necessary for an accurate diagnosis. **Differential D.**, arriving at a correct decision between diseases presenting similar symptoms.

Diagnostician (dī-ag-nos-tish'-i-an). One who is skilful in diagnosis.

Dialysed (dī'-al-īzd). Separation by dialysis.

Dialysis (dī-al'-i-sis). The separation of colloid from crystalline substances in solution by the passage of the latter through a porous membrane.

Dialyzer (dī'-al-ī-zer). The apparatus used in the process of dialysis.

Diameter (dī-am'-et-er). The distance traversed by a straight line from one side of a rounded object to the other and passing through the centre.

Diapedesis (dī-ap-e-dē'-sis). The passage of red corpuscles and white cells through the intact walls of a blood-vessel.

Diaphoresis (dī-af-or-ē'-sis). Perspiration.

Diaphoretic (dī-af-or-et'-ik). An agent which produces diaphoresis.

Diaphragm (dī'-a-fram). The dome-shaped muscular partition between the thorax above and the abdomen below.

Diaphragmatocele (dī-a-frag-mat-ō-sēl). Protrusion of a viscus through the diaphragm. Diaphragmatic hernia.

Diaphysis (dī-af'-i-sis). The shaft of a long bone.

Diaphysectomy (dī-af-i-sek'-to-mi). Excision of the shaft of a long bone.

Diarrhœa (dī-a-rē'-à). Loose and frequent evacuation of the bowels. **Summer D.**, an acute form which affects infants during hot weather ; is very fatal.

Diarthrosis (dī-ár-thrō'-sis). A freely movable articulating surface, e.g., the ball and socket joints of the body.

Diastase (dī'-as-tās). (1) An enzyme present in malt, which, during the process of brewing, liquefies the grain, converting the starch into soluble compounds, namely, sugar, dextrins, and maltose. A similar starch-splitting ferment produced by the pancreas and present in the urine. (2) A term sometimes used for the cardiac rest-pause.

Diastasis (dĭ-as′-ta-sĭs). Forcible separation of bones without fracture ; dislocation.

Diastole (dĭ-as′-to-lĭ). The relaxation period of the cardiac cycle, as opposed to *systole*.

Diastolic (dĭ-as-tol′-ĭk). Relating to the diastole. D. Murmur, a murmur produced during the diastole, heard during auscultation.

Diathermy (dĭ-a-ther′-mĭ). A form of electrical treatment in which high frequency currents are passed through an electrode in contact with the tissues, whereby the temperature of the latter is considerably raised ; is used in many conditions, but chiefly in inflammation or its results. Surgical D., electrical treatment in which the temperature is increased sufficiently high to cause destruction of the tissues, as in the removal of a neoplasm.

Diathesis (dĭ-ath′-e-sĭs). A constitutional predisposition to certain diseases.

Dichotomy (dĭ-kot′-o-mĭ). Dividing into two parts, such as the halving of professional fees ; a form of bribery.

Dick Test. A skin test for scarlet fever performed in a similar manner to the Schick Test (*q.v.*). The *positive* reaction appears in 6 to 12 hours reaching its maximum

in 24 hours, as a reddened area, ¼ in. or more in diameter. It fades rapidly and is only very rarely followed by pigmentation or desquamation.

Dicrotic (dĭ-krot′-ĭk). Usually referred to a pulse which has a double beat.

Didactyl (dĭ-dak′-til). The possession of only two fingers or toes.

Didymitis (did-i-mī′-tis). Inflammation of the testicle ; orchitis.

Didymodynia (did-i-mō-din′-ĭ-ă). Pain in the testicle.

Dietetics (dĭ-e-tet′-ĭks). The science concerned with the study of foodstuffs and their nutritional values, and preparations of special diets and their effect in disease.

Dietitian (dĭ-e-tish′-un). One who is especially concerned with the study of diets ; a food expert.

Dietl's Crises (dēt′-l). Paroxysmal attacks of pain in the abdomen due to the presence of ureteral calculus or to nephroptosis ; severe gastric pain associated with vomiting may also occur.

Diffusion (dif-fū′-zhun). (1) The process by which gases and liquids intermingle when brought into contact with each other. (2) The process which occurs when the molecules of crystalloids in solution penetrate a permeable membrane, so that the solution on each side of the membrane becomes equal.

Digestion (di-jest'-chun). The changing of food into such a form that it can readily be absorbed into the blood-stream and utilized by the tissue cells.

Digit (dij'-it). A finger or a toe.

Digital (dij'-it-al). Pertaining to a digit.

Digitalis (dij-it-à'-lis). A drug obtained from the foxglove; cardiac stimulant and diuretic; poison. Overdose must be watched for. The symptoms include slow intermittent pulse, diminution of urine excretion, headache, dizziness, and nausea. Dose: digitalis recens, repeat dose, 90-300 minims; single dose, 1-4 fl. oz.; tincture, 5-15 minims, repeat dose.

Digitus (dij'-it-us). A finger or toe.

Dilatation (di-la-tā'-shun). Stretching or enlargement of an organ or cavity.

Dilator (di-lā'-tor). An instrument used for performing dilatation of a cavity.

Diluent (dil'-ū-ent). An agent added to another substance to make it weaker or less potent.

Dilution (dil-oo'-shun). Weakening a substance with an inert or less potent substance.

Dioxide (di-oks-īd). A compound containing two atoms of oxygen and a base.

Diphtheria (dif-thēr'-i-à). A disease caused by the *Corynebacterium diphtheriœ*. It commonly attacks the nose, throat, and fauces, and is recognized by the formation of a greyish-white membranous patch which may produce suffocation by blocking the air-passage. The mortality, which was formerly very high, has been greatly reduced by the introduction of an antidiphtheritic serum. The disease more rarely develops on the cornea, mucous wall of the vagina, and in open wounds.

Diphtheroid (dif'-the-roid). Resembling diphtheria; applied particularly to relatively harmless bacteria which resemble the diphtheria bacilli.

Diplegia (di-plē'-ji-à). Paralysis occurring on both sides symmetrically.

Diplococcus (dip-lō-kok'-us). Micrococci whose bodies are joined in pairs.

Diploë (dip-lō'-ē). The bony cancellous tissue situated between the inner and outer table of the cranial bones.

Diplopia dip-lō'-pi-à). Double vision.

Dipsomaniac (dip-sō-mān'-i-ak). One who suffers from an overwhelming desire for alcohol.

Director (di-rek'-tor). A grooved instrument for directing a surgical knife.

Disarticulation (dis-art-ik-ū-lā'-

shun). Disconnecting two articulating surfaces; amputation through a joint.

Discission (dis-si'-shun). The operation used for rupturing the capsule of the lens in cases of cataract ; needling.

Discrete (dis-krēt'). Apart ; separate. Opposite of confluent.

Disinfectant (dis-in-fek'-tant). An agent which destroys bacteria.

Disintegration (dis-in-te-grā'-shun). A destructive process ; breaking up of a substance into its constituent parts, as, for example, the disintegration of erythrocytes, thereby setting free hæmoglobin, iron, etc.

Dislocation (dis-lō-kā'-shun). The displacement or putting out of position, as the displacement of the head of one bone out of the socket of another ; such a dislocation may be partial or complete.

Dispensing (dis-pens'-ing). The art of preparing drugs and medical preparations.

Dissection (dis-sek'-shun). Separation of tissues by cutting for detailed study. *See* **Anatomy**.

Disseminated (dis-sem'-in-ā-ted). Distributed or scattered. **D. Sclerosis**, a disease of the nervous system caused by scattered areas of destruction and scarring in the spinal cord.

Dissociation (dis-sō-si-ā'-shun). The separation of the parts of a compound. In psychological terms it signifies disunion of the mind, of which the person is unaware. Dual personalities, fugues, somnambulism, etc., come under this heading. Dissociation is probably an attempt on the part of the individual to find a solution for a repressed complex. *See* **Complex** and **Conflict**.

Dissolution (dis-sō-loo'-shun). Death.

Distal (dis'-tal). Farthest from the head or centre ; towards the periphery.

Distillation (dis-til-ā'-shun). The conversion of liquids into

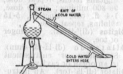

Distillation (Liebig's Condenser).

vapour, with subsequent condensation back into fluid. **Destructive D.**, a process of destruction of a substance in a closed vessel, whereby new products are evolved. **Dry D.**, the distillation of solid substances, *e.g.*, of coal which leaves coke, produces gas and various coal-tar distillates.

Diuresis (dī-ū-rē'-sis). Excessive urinary secretion.

Diuretic (dī-ū-ret'-ĭk). A drug or other agent which excites an excessive flow of urine. Examples of drugs acting in this way are: digitalis, strophanthus, juniper, copaiba, etc.

Diver's Paralysis. Same as *Caisson Disease.*

Divergence (dī-ver'-jens). Deviation from a common centre; the act of branching off in opposite directions.

Divergent (dī-ver'-jent). Pertaining to divergence.

Diverticulitis (dī-ver-tik-ū-lī'-tis). Inflammation of a diverticulum.

Diverticulum (dī-ver-tik'-ū-lum). A blind end or pouch-like projection; a cul-de-sac.

Dolichocephalic (dol-i-kŏ-kef'-al'-ĭk). Having a long or tall head.

Dolor (dŏ'-law(r)). Pain.

Domette (dŏ-met'). A loosely woven woollen material used for bandages.

Dorsum (daw(r)'-sum). The back.

Dosage (dŏ'-sāj). The regulation of the doses of drugs.

Dose (dōs). The quantity of a drug which will combine efficiency with safety; the amount given at one time. **Fractional D.**, a dose which is divided into small portions

to be taken at stated intervals. **Lethal D.**, a dose sufficiently strong to cause death. **Maximum D.**, the greatest dose which may be administered with safety. **Minumum D.**, the smallest dose which will produce any effect.

Double. Two-fold; a pair. **D. Consciousness**, dual personality. **D. Uterus**, *see* **Bicornuate Uterus**. **D. Vision**, same as *Diplopia.*

Douche (doosh). The introduction of a stream of fluid into a cavity. Douches are used for cleansing purposes, to relieve inflammation and

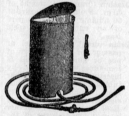

Douche Can.

congestion, for the arrest of hæmorrhage, and also as an astringent application (*q.v.*). **D. Can**, an irrigator or vessel used specially for douching. **D. Pan**, a large slipper-shaped bed-pan used for receiving the fluid after vaginal douching.

Douglas's Pouch. A cul-de-sac of the pelvic cavity in the female which lies between the posterior surface of the uterus and the anterior surface of the rectum. The cavity is lined with peritoneum which is much less absorptive than that of the abdominal peritoneum.

Dover's Powder. A powder which is diaphoretic and sedative in its action. Two of its main ingredients are opium and ipecacuanha. Dose, 5-10 gr.

Drachm (dram). A weight of 60 gr. Fluid D., a measure of 60 minims ; the eighth part of an ounce ; also spelt *dram*.

Drain (drān). A channel or passage for the discharge of pus or fluid, etc. This is sometimes accomplished by inserting a length of rubber tubing into a cavity or sinus. Glass drainage tubes are also used, such as those of *Paul* or *Keith*. The former is used for drainage of the intestines in acute obstruction, while the latter is for abdominal drainage. Cigarette D., a wick of gauze surrounded by rubber dam or oil-silk.

Drastic (dras'-tik) Severe ; very powerful.

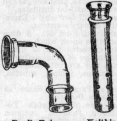

Paul's Tube.   Keith's Tube.

Glass Drainage Tubes.

Draught (drăft). A dose of medicine.

Draw-sheet. A sheet arranged across the bed and covering a mackintosh similarly placed. It should be *wide* enough to stretch from below the shoulder-blades to below the knees, and *long* enough to tuck well under the mattress on both sides. It should be drawn through at intervals so that the patient can lie on a cool, clean part ; hence its name.

Dressing. (1) The technique of renewing or applying a covering or appliance for an open wound. (2) Gauze, lint, or other substance used to cover a wound.

Drop. A spherical particle of

120

fluid; approximately equivalent to a minim. **Hanging D.,** *see* Culture. **D. Hand or Wrist,** a form of paralysis in which the hand hangs limp; caused by lead-poisoning, etc. **D. Lid,** ptosis of the eyelid.

Dropsical (drop'-sik-al). Pertaining to dropsy.

Dropsy (drop'-sǐ). Œdema; the collection of fluid in the cellular tissues and cavities of the body as the result of disease. *See* Œdema.

Drug. A substance used as a medicine.

Drum. The membrana tympani (*q.v.*).

Dublin Method. *See* Credé. Also known as the *Rotunda Method*.

Ducrey's Bacillus. A small oval bacillus, the causative agent of chancroid.

Duct (dukt). A canal or tube; alimentary canal.

Duodeno-cholecystostomy (dū-ŏ-dē-nŏ-kŏ-lē-sis-tos'-to-mi). The formation of a fistula between the duodenum and the gall-bladder.

Duodenojejunal (dū-ŏ-dē'-nŏ-je-joo'-nal). Relating to both duodenum and jejunum.

Duodenostomy (dū-ŏ-dē-nos'-to-mi). The making of an artificial opening into the duodenum.

Duodenum (dū-ŏ-dē'-num). The first part of the small intestine. It measures 10 in. or 12 finger-breadths in length.

Dupuytren's Contracture (dū'-pwi-trong). Flexion of the third and fourth digits towards the palm, due to contraction of the palmar ligaments and fascia.

Dura Mater. The outer membrane of the meninges which surround the brain and spinal cord.

Dwarf. A person of stunted growth.

Dynamic (dī-nam'-ik). Relating to force or power.

Dynamics. The science dealing with force and movement.

Dynamo (dī'-na-mō). A machine for generating electricity.

Dysæsthesia (dis-ăs-thēz'-i-à). Dullness of sensation.

Dyscrasia (dis-krā'-zi-à). An abnormal or diseased state.

Dysentery (dis'-en-ter-ĭ). Inflammation of the intestinal mucous membrane with bloody and mucoid evacuations, abdominal pain, and tenesmus. There are two kinds of dysentery. **Amœbic D.,** caused by the *Entamœba histolytica*, also known as *Amœbiasis*. **Bacillary D.,** caused by the *B. dysenteriæ*. There are several varieties of these, but those of *shiga* and *flexner* are the chief.

Dyskinesia (dis-kĭn-ēz'-i-à). Pain and discomfort on movement.

Dysmenorrhœa (dis-men-o'-rē'-à). Painful menstruation; three main varieties are recognized. **Congestive D.**, due to some congestion in the pelvis. **Membranous D.**, a painful form of dysmenorrhœa, in which shreds of membrane are cast in the menstrual fluid. **Spasmodic D.**, a type accompanied by severe colicky pain and vomiting, due to spasmodic uterine contraction.

Dysopia (dis-ō′-pi-à). Defective or painful vision.

Dysorexia (dis-o-reks′-i-à). A craving for unnatural or unsuitable food.

Dyspareunia (dis-pàr-ū′-ni-à). Painful coitus.

Dyspepsia (dis-pep′-si-à). Indigestion.

D y s p h a g i a (dis-fā′-ji-à). Difficulty in swallowing.

Dysphasia (dis-fā′-zi-à). Difficulty in speech.

Dyspnœa (disp-nē′-à). Difficulty in breathing.

Dystocia (dis-tōs′-i-à). Difficult parturition.

Dystrophia (dis-trō′-fi-à). Imperfect nutrition. *Also* **Distrophy.**

Dysuria (dis-ū′-ri-à). Difficult and painful micturition.

E.

Ear. The organ of hearing.

Easton's Syrup. A tonic containing iron, phosphates, quinine, and strychnine.

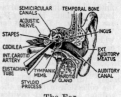

The Ear.

Eberth's Bacillus. The *B. typhosus.*

Ebullition (eb-ū-li′-shun). Boiling.

Eburnation (ē-bur-nā′-shun). Changes occurring in bone in which it becomes hardened and dense like ivory.

Ecbolic (ek-bol′-ik). A drug which tones up the uterine muscle, thus facilitating the expulsion of the fœtus.

Ecchondroma (ek-kon-drō′-mà). A cartilaginous tumour.

Ecchymosis (ek-i-mō′-sis). An extravasation of blood under the skin; a bruise.

Echinococcus (ē-kīn-ō-kok′-us). The hydatids or daughter cysts of the tapeworm, *Tœnia echinococcus.*

Echolalia (ek-ō-lāl′-i-à). The repetition of questions asked, repeating the words like an echo.

Echophony (ek-of′-o-ni). The echo of a vocal sound heard during auscultation of the chest.

Eclampsia (ĕ-klamp-si-ȧ). A severe convulsive seizure affecting pregnant women. May occur either before, during, or after labour. Fits occurring during the puerperium are generally considered to have the worst prognosis. The condition is usually associated with high blood-pressure and albuminuria.

Eclamptic (ĕ-klamp'-tik). Pertaining to eclampsia.

Eclectic (ek-lek'-tik). Selecting or choosing.

Ecmnesia (ek-nē'-zi-ȧ). A loss of memory for events covering a certain period, the memory being normal both before and after. A vacant space in the memory, during which time certain events are completely forgotten.

Ecraseur (ā'-krȧ-zūr). A surgical instrument consisting of a wire loop used for the amputation of small pedunculated tumours, by passing the loop over them and crushing the pedicle or stem.

Ecstasy (eks'-ta-si). A state of high mental exaltation; a sense of uplift and joyfulness.

Ecthyma (ek-thē'-mȧ). A non-contagious pustular skin disease.

Ectoblast (ek'-tō-blast). *See* **Ectoderm.**

Ectoderm (ek'-tō-derm). The external primitive germ layer of the embryo. From it are developed the skin structures, the nervous system, organs of special sense, pineal gland, and part of the pituitary and suprarenal glands.

Ectodermal (ek-tō-der'-mal). Relating to the ectoderm.

Ectopia (ek-tō'-pi-ȧ). A congenital malposition of an organ or structure. **E. Vesicæ,** an abnormally placed urinary bladder which protrudes through or opens on the abdominal wall.

Ectopic (ek-top'-ik). Relating to ectopia. **E. Gestation,** development of the fœtus outside the uterus; **extra-uterine.**

Ectosarc (ek'-tō-sȧrk). The outer transparent layer of a protozoa, *e.g.,* the outer delicate covering of the amœba.

Ectozoa (ek-tō-zo'-ȧ). External parasites.

Ectropic (ek-trop'-ik). Everted or turned out.

Ectropion (ek-trō'-pi-on). Eversion of the eyelid.

Eczema (ek'-ze-mȧ). An inflammatory cutaneous eruption often accompanied by an exudation of lymph.

Edible (ed'-ib-l). Suitable for food.

Effector (ef-fek'-tor). Productive of movement or effect.

Efferent (ef'-er-ent). Passing outwards from the centre;

opposite to afferent. **E. Nerves**, motor nerves, *i.e.*, nerves which convey impulses outward from the nerve centre to the periphery.

Effervescent (ef-fer-ves'-ent). Bubbling due to the presence of gas.

Effleurage (ef-flûr'-ǎzh). A movement in massage in which the stroke is made from the periphery towards the heart.

Effluvium (ef-floo'-vi-um). An odour or exhalation.

Effusion (ef-fū'-zhun). Extravasation of fluid into the body tissues or cavities.

Ehrlich's Theory of Immunity. A theory which attempts to explain the formation of antitoxin in the blood; is also known as *E. Side-chain Theory*, because the protoplasmic cell is said to possess certain receptors or "side-chains" which are capable of becoming fixed to certain protein groups with which they have a chemical affinity. This "fixation" is of value to the cell in that it enables it to attach the various food-substances which it needs for its nourishment. The molecules of a toxin also, according to this theory, contain two groups for attachment to the cell: (1) The *Haptophore group* which becomes fixed to a suitable cell receptor. When this happens, the receptor

detaches from the cell and floats in the blood-stream. The cell responds to this loss by producing more effectors, which are again liberated into the blood, where they combine with toxins and thereby render them inert, and so form free antitoxin. (2) A *Toxophore group*; toxicity results when this becomes attached to certain receptors of the cell called toxiphiles, and this union is prevented by rendering the haptophore group inert.

Ejaculation (ē-jak-ū-lā'-shun). A sudden emission of semen.

Ejecta (ē-jek'-tǎ). Bodily excretions; waste matter.

Elastic Bandage. A rubber bandage.

Elasticity (ē-las-tis'-i-ti). The property possessed by certain substances of returning to their original size or shape after the deforming force is removed.

Elastoplast (ē-las'-tō-plast). A resilient, adhesive dressing for surgical and orthopædic purposes. It consists of a medicated gauze and lint pad, containing bismuth subgallate, 5%, combined with an elastic and adhesive base. *E. Bandages*, these are 3 yds. long, but stretchable to 6 yds.: (*a*) one side is entirely covered with plaster, and when applied permits bathing without removal;

(*b*) covered on one side with adhesive in strips, allowing for ventilation. These bandages are applied in the treatment of varicose ulcer, and for the injection treatment of veins. The bandage is applied firmly, as compression reduces œdema and pain and promotes healing. It is renewed once a week, and when re-

moved must be unwound, but not cut.

Electric Rectoscope (rek′-tō-skōp). For illuminating the anal canal and rectum; used in the diagnosis and injection treatment of hæmorrhoids. The torch is detachable so that the instrument may be sterilized. When the *obturator* is withdrawn, the *protective cover* over the light

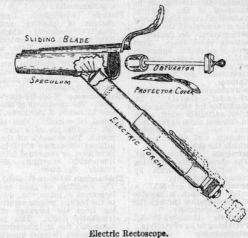

SLIDING BLADE

SPECULUM

OBTURATOR

PROTECTOR COVER

ELECTRIC TORCH

Electric Rectoscope.

prevents fluid fæces from soiling the lamp. The speculum can then be thoroughly cleaned, and the *protector cover* removed.

Electricity (ē-lek-tris′-it-i). A natural force which can be produced by chemical, mechanical, and magnetic means.

Electrocardiograph (ē-lek-trō-kâr′-di-ō-graf). An apparatus by means of which a photographic tracing can be obtained of the electrical variations taking place during the movements of the heart.

Electrocautery. *See* **Cautery.**

Electrode (ē-lek′-trōd). That part of an electric apparatus which is in actual contact with the skin during electrical treatment. *See* **Anode** and **Cathode.**

Electroencephalograph (ē-lek-trō-en-kef′-a-lō-graf). An apparatus for recording electrical variations which occur in different parts of the brain and used for localizing tumours and other lesions within the skull.

Electrolysis (ē-lek-trol′-is-is). The chemical decomposition of certain compounds by means of electricity.

Electrolyte (ē-lek′-trō-līt). A substance which is capable of disintegration through the action of electricity.

Electrolytic (ē-lek-trō-lit′-ik). Pertaining to an electrolyte.

Electromagnetic (ē-lek-trō-mag-net′-ik). Relating to electromagnetism.

Electromagnetism (ē-lek-trō-mag′-ne-tizm). The production of magnetic action by means of electricity.

Electromotive Force (abbreviation, E.M.F.). That which produces or tends to produce movement of electricity. The unit of E.M.F. is the volt, and this is measured by means of a galvanometer.

Electron (ē-lek′-tron). Unit charges of positive and negative electricity which form an atom. The central positive electrons form a nucleus or proton, while the negative electrons are grouped about it in sufficient numbers to render the atom neutral or stable.

Electrotherapy (ē-lek-trō-ther′-a-pi). The treatment of disease by means of electricity.

Element (el′-e-ment). One of the constituents of a compound. The elements are the primary substances which in pure form or combined into compounds constitute all matter. *See* **Atom.**

Elephantiasis (el-ef-an-tī′-a-sis). The condition of gross enlargement of limbs, etc., due to the brawny œdema resulting from the blockage of lymphatic ducts. This is commonly due to infestation by parasites (worms) known as *Filaria*, but may be due to other causes.

Elevation (el-e-vā′-shun). The act of being raised or exalted.

Elevator (el′-e-vā-tor). That which raises, *e.g.*, a muscle which raises a limb. **Periosteal E.**, a surgical instrument used for raising the periosteum of bone.

Elimination (ē-lim-in-ā′-shun)· The giving off of waste matter from the body.

Emasculation (ē-mas-kū-lā′-shun). The production of impotence by removal of the testicles.

Embed (em-bed′). To fix in firmly ; to insert in a solid substance.

Embolism (em′-bo-lizm). The presence in the blood-stream of a detached part of a thrombus or other foreign body which travels with the stream until it reaches a vessel too small to allow it to pass, with the result that the circulation becomes obstructed.

Embolus (em′-bo-lus). A clot or other foreign body which travels in the blood-stream.

Embryo (em′-bri-ō). The term applied to the developing ovum during the first three months of gestation.

Embryology (em-bri-ol′o-ji). The science which deals with the growth and development of the embryo.

Embryonic (em-bri-on′-ik). Pertaining to the embryo.

Emesis (em-ē′-sis). The act of vomiting.

Emetic (ē-met′-ik). An agent which causes vomiting. They are of two kinds. **Direct E.**, those acting directly on the gastric nerves, *e.g.*, mustard, sodium chloride, copper sulphate, etc. **Indirect E.**, those which act on the vomiting centre in the brain ; examples are apomorphine, antimony, and ipecacuanha.

Emetine (em′-e-tēn). An alkaloid of ipecacuanha ; it is both expectorant and emetic ; specific for amœbic dysentery. Emetin hydrochlor. Emetic dose, $\frac{1}{2}$-1 gr. by injection.

Emigration (em-i-grā′-shun). The passage of a leucocyte through the wall of a blood-vessel into a surrounding tissue.

Eminence (em′-in-ens). A projection or tuberosity.

Emission (ē-mish′-un). An ejaculation or sending forth. An involuntary ejaculation of semen.

Emmenagogue (em-men′-a-gōg). A drug which stimulates the menstrual flow.

Emmet's Operation (em′-et). A method of repairing a lacerated uterine cervix.

Emollient (ē-mol′-i-ent). A softening and soothing agent.

Emotional (ē-mō′-shun-al). Pertaining to mental agitation ; a state of being easily upset ; excitable.

Emphysema (em-fĭ-sē'-mȧ). The presence of air in the cellular tissues. **Cutaneous E.**, the presence of air in the subcutaneous tissues, with consequent distension. **Gangrenous E.**, malignant œdema. **Pulmonary E.**, excessive distension of the alveoli of the lung with air, caused by strain during blowing a musical instrument, or in coughing, and in persons suffering from asthma. In severe cases the thin partitions between the air-sacs break down, with loss of elasticity in the lung tissue, with the result that the blood becomes insufficiently aerated ; the condition is often associated with a chronic bronchitis. **Surgical E.**, the presence of air in the subcutaneous tissues, the result of an injury, or occasionally due to a surgical operation. It occurs especially after wounds to the respiratory organs.

Empiric, Empirical (em-pĭr'-ĭk). (1) A quack doctor. (2) Treatment based on the results of experience rather than on scientific knowledge.

Emplastrum (em-plas'-trum). A plaster.

Emprosthotonos (em-pros-thot'-o-nos). Muscular contractions of a violent nature which bend the trunk of the body

forwards, seen in strychnine poisoning and tetanus.

Empyema (em-pī-ē'-mȧ). A collection of pus, especially in the pleural cavity, but may also occur in other closed body cavities, *e.g.*, the antrum of Highmore, gall-bladder, etc.

Emulsification (e-mul-si-fĭ-kā'-shun). The process of making an emulsion.

Emulsion (e-mul'-shun). A fluid containing fat or oil particles in a state of fine subdivision and suspension, so that a smooth milky white fluid results.

Enamel (ē-nam'-el). The hard external covering of a tooth.

Enarthrosis (en-ȧr-thrō'-sis). A ball and socket joint.

Encanthis (en-kan'-this). A growth in the inner canthus of the eye.

Encapsulation (en-kap-sū-lā'-shun). Enclosure within a capsule.

Encephalitis (en-kef-a-lī'-tis). Inflammation of the brain.

Encephalitis Lethargica (en-kef-a-lī'-tis leth-ȧr'-jĭ-kȧ). An infective disease which first appeared in England in 1918. Generally occurs in sporadic form. It is characterized by stupor, ocular paralysis, tremor, nocturnal wakefulness. The face becomes expressionless and grave. Moral changes may result. The symptoms vary in different individuals. The disease is notifiable. Synonym, *Sleepy Sickness.*

Encephalocele (en-kef'-al-ō-sēl). Hernia of the brain.

Encephaloid (en-kef'-a-loid). Resembling brain substance.

Encephalomyelitis (en-kef-al-ō-mī-e-lī'-tis). Inflammation of the brain and spinal cord.

Encephalon (en-kef'-a-lon). The brain.

Enchondroma (en-kon-drō'-mă). A cartilaginous tumour.

Enciente (ong'-sant). Pregnant.

Encysted (en-sis'-ted). Enclosed in a sac or cyst.

End. A termination. **E. Artery,** an artery which does not anastomose directly or indirectly with other arteries, *e.g.,* in kidney and spleen, etc. **E. Bud,** the terminal of a cutaneous nerve. **E. Plate,** the distal end of a motor nerve. **E. Result,** the ultimate or final result.

Endarteritis (end-árt-e-rī'-tis). Inflammation of the intima or lining coat of an artery.

Endemic (en-dem'-ik). Recurring frequently in the same locality. **E. Diseases,** infectious diseases constantly appearing in a particular area.

Endemiology (en-dēm-i-ol'-o-ji). The special study of endemic diseases.

Endo (en'-dō). A prefix indicating within.

Endocarditis (en-dō-kár-dī'-tis). Inflammation of the endo-

cardium and valves. The commonest causes are rheumatic fever and septicæmia.

Endocardium (en-dō-kár'-di-um). The lining membrane of the heart. It not only lines the cavities, but covers the valves and is also continuous with the intima or internal coat of the arteries and veins which open into or from the heart.

Endocervicitis (en-dō-ser-vi-sī'-tis). Inflammation of the mucous lining of the cervix uteri.

Endocrine Glands (en'-dō-krin or en'-dō-krīn). The ductless glands of the body, those which possess an internal secretion or hormone, *e.g.,* the pineal, pituitary, thyroid, parathyroids, thymus, suprarenals, ovaries, testes, and pancreas. The latter has both an internal and external secretion.

Endocrinology (en-dō-krin-ol'-o-ji). The science which deals with the study of the ductless glands and the function of their internal secretions.

Endogenous (en-doj'-en-us). Commencing or occurring within the body.

Endolymph (en'-dō-limf). The fluid contained in the membranous labyrinth of the internal ear.

Endometritis (en-dō-me-trī'-tis). Inflammation of the endometrium.

Endometrium (en-dŏ-mē'-tri-um). The lining mucosa of the uterus.

Endoneurium (en-dō-nū'-ri-um). The delicate connective tissue surrounding the nerve fibres.

Endosarc (en'-dō-sàrk). The inner dense mass of protoplasm forming the body of the protozoa.

Endosteum (end-os'-ti-um). The thin lining of the medullary cavity of bone.

Endothelial (en-dō-thē'-li-al). Pertaining to the endothelium.

Endothelioma (en-dō-thē-li-ō'-mà). A growth of the endothelium, generally of a malignant nature.

Endothelium (en-dō-thē'-li-um). The lining membrane of serous cavities, blood-vessels, and lymph vessels.

Endotoxin (en-dō-toks'-in). The toxin which is contained within the body of a bacterium. When the latter disintegrates the toxin is set free in the tissues or blood-stream, thereby causing the specific symptoms manifested by the particular infection.

Enema (en'-e-mà). The fluid or mixture introduced into the intestine through the rectum; there are several varieties. **Anthelmintic E.,** one given especially to destroy and expel worms, *e.g.*, an enema made from an infusion of *quassia chips*; 1 oz. of the infusion is added to 1 pint of water; aloes and hypertonic saline solution are also used; anthelmintic drugs are sometimes ordered per mouth, such as *santonin* and *filix mas*. **Nutrient E.,** one given for nourishing purposes when food cannot be taken by the mouth; milk, beef tea, egg and milk, chicken broth, etc., can be used; but this method of feeding has become obsolete, since it is realized that the colon, while absorbing large quantities of water and a little sugar and salt, does not absorb the heavier foodstuffs. **Purgative E.,** one given in order to procure an evacuation of the bowel, *e.g.*, (a) E. Saponis, 1 oz. of ordinary yellow soap or soft soap is added to 1 pint of warm water (temp. 103° F.); 2 pints of solution are given with a tube and funnel or Higginson syringe. (b) *Castor Oil E.,* 1 oz. each of castor oil and yellow soap, mix well in a mortar; add 1 pint of warm water and administer with a tube and funnel. (c) *Glycerine E.,* 1 oz. of glycerine is warmed by adding an equal quantity of warm water; it is injected per rectum with a glycerine syringe. (d) E. Magnesii

Sulphatis, 1-2 oz. of sulphate of magnesia is added to mucilage of starch or warm water, and 6 oz. given with a tube and funnel. (*e*) *Olive Oil E.*, warm 7 oz. of olive oil and inject slowly; is given for constipation; the oil lubricates the hard fæcal masses, which in half an hour's time are evacuated by giving a simple enema (the oil must not be more than 100° F., and must be tested with a thermometer, as oil absorbs heat rapidly). **Simple E.**, *see* E. Saponis. **Turpentine E.**, take ʒi of turpentine, add ʒi of olive oil or the white of an egg; beat these well together to form an emulsion, then add 1 pint of warm enema saponis; or the turpentine can be added

Glycerine Syringe.

to starch mucilage, 10 oz.; the turpentine stimulates peristaltic action and expels flatus; since turpentine is liable to burn the intestinal mucosa, oil is added as an emollient. **Sedative E.**, prepare 2-4 oz. of thin mucilage of starch, and add the prescribed amount of opium (usually not more than ℳxxx). (*N.B.*—The starch should be boiled in order to burst the starch granules.) The enema is given tepid with a catheter and funnel and retained. **Stimulative E.**, ordered for patients suffering from shock or collapse, may consist of normal saline solution, glucose and saline (*see* Saline), strong black coffee, ℥v, strained, and to which may be added brandy, ℥ss, if ordered by the physician. A **High E.**, is *one in which the rubber tube* is introduced past the sigmoid flexure, so that fluid reaches the higher parts of the colon; the tube must be carefully inserted in order to prevent "kinking." A **Low E.** is the more usual method, in which the tube merely enters the rectum. A high enema is only administered on the special orders of the physician. A **Gravity E.** is one in which the fluid is introduced by means of a long rectal tube

131

and a glass funnel (*see Diagram*). The force and flow of the fluid can be regulated by raising or lowering the funnel. **E. Syringe,** an apparatus used for giving enemata; the most usual

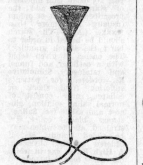

Rectal Tube and Funnel.

one is that known as *Higginson's syringe*, consisting of a rubber tube with a bulb in the centre; at one end of the tube is an ivory nozzle for inserting into the rectum, and at the other end is a suction apparatus which is kept immersed in the fluid to be injected; this syringe is being largely superseded

by the use of the tube and funnel, *i.e.*, the *gravity* method. The *glycerine syringe* is small, capable of holding 2 oz., and having a nozzle and fittings of vulcanite, with a glass barrel and piston of glass. *Ball syringe*, a thick rubber ball with an ivory nozzle about 2½ in. long, and used for giving nutrient enemata; the syringe is now obsolete, being replaced by a small funnel and catheter.

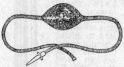

Higginson Enema Syringe.

Energen (en'-er-jen). The principle of starch reduction with increase of protein embodied in the standardized dietary foods marketed under this registered trade name; used in the diet for diabetes, obesity, high blood-pressure, r h e u m a t i s m, indigestion, constipation, underweight, catarrh, gastritis, nephritis, skin disorders, etc. Every package bears a guaranteed statement as to contents in

132

grams of protein and carbohydrate and calorie value.

Energy (en'-er-ji). Activity; the power of doing work. **Kinetic E.**, the energy produced during movement or work. **Potential E.**, the energy contained within a body by virtue of its position; the energy which a resting body is capable of producing. Synonym, *Latent E.*, *Static E.*

Enervating (en'-er-vā-ting). Weakening.

Engorgement (en-gawrj'-ment). (1) Filled to repletion. (2) Congested and distended with blood, as in *venous* congestion.

Ensiform Process (en'-si-fawm). The sword-shaped tip of the sternum. The small process below the gladiolus of the sternum. Also known as the *Xiphoid Process*.

Entamœba Coli (en-ta-mē'-bà kō-li). A more or less harmless parasitic form of amœba found in the large intestine. **E. Histolytica**, the pathogenic form of amœba which causes amœbic dysentery.

Enteralgia (en-te-ral'-ji-à). Intestinal pain.

Enterectomy (en-te-rek'-to-mi). Excision of a part of intestine.

Enteric Fever (en-te'-rik). An acute infectious disease affecting the small intestine, particularly the Peyer's patches, which become inflamed and ulcerated. The term is synonymous with *typhoid fever*, but is also used to cover the *paratyphoid fevers A* and *B*.

Enteritis (en-te-rī'-tis). Inflammation of the intestines.

Enterocele (en'-te-rō-sēl). The protrusion of a portion of intestine into a hernial sac.

Enteroclysis (en-te-ro-klī'-sis). The administration of an intestinal enema.

Enterokinase (en-te-rō-kī'-nāz). One of the enzymes of the succus entericus, which has the power of activating trypsinogen by converting it into trypsin.

Enterolith (en'-te-rō-lith). A fæcal stone or intestinal concretion.

Enterolithiasis (en-te-rō-lith-ī'-a-sis). The formation of intestinal calculi or concretions.

Enteropexy (en-te-rō-peks'-i). Suturing of the intestine to the abdominal wall.

Enteroptosis (en-te-rop-tō'-sis). Prolapse of the intestines.

Enterorrhaphy (en-te-ror'-ra-fi). Stitching of the intestines.

Enterostomy (en-te-ros'-to-mi). The formation of an opening into the intestine by surgical means.

Enterotomy (en-te-rot'-o-mi). A temporary incision or opening into the intestines.

Enterozoa (en-te-rō-zō'-à). Protozoic parasites of the intestines.

133

Entrails (en'-trālz). The intestines.

Entropion (en-trō'-pi-on). Turning inwards of the margins of the eyelids.

Enucleation (ē-nū-klē-ā'-shun). The operation of removing a tumour or other mass by shelling it out of the surrounding tissues, as of a fibroid from the uterine muscle, or of the eye from its socket.

Enuresis (en-ū-rē'-sis). Incontinence of urine, especially bed-wetting.

Enzyme (en'-zīm). A ferment; an organic catalyst, destroyed by heating; the active principle of the digestive juices; a chemical capable of hastening changes in other substances without itself becoming altered.

Eosin (ē'-ō-sin). A red staining agent used in histology.

Eosinophile (ē-ō-sin'-ō-fīl). A term used for certain cells which readily take an eosin stain, *e.g.*, a variety of leucocyte possessing this property.

Ependyma (e-pen'-di-mà or ep-en-dī'-mà). The membrane lining the ventricles of the brain, and also the central canal of the spinal cord.

Ephedrine (ef'-ed-rin). An alkaloid obtained from *Ma huang*, a species of *Ephedra*, first isolated by Nagai in 1887. *Ma huang* had a reputation in ancient Chinese medicine as a diaphoretic and antipyretic. It was not until recent times, however, that its action was studied and its valuable therapeutic properties made known. The action of ephedrine is similar to that of adrenalin. Its effects, although less powerful, are more prolonged, and it exerts an action when given orally, whereas adrenalin is effective only by injection. Ephedrine orally (or by injection) dilates the bronchial muscles, contracts the nasal mucosa, and raises the blood-pressure. It is chiefly used for its broncho-dilator effect in asthma, and for its constricting effects on the nasal mucosa in hay fever. Dose, $\frac{1}{4}$-$1\frac{1}{2}$ gr. It is found that some patients need carefully regulated doses. The least dose which will give the specific desired effect is desirable. Two strengths of " Tabloid " Brand Ephedrine Hydrochloride products are issued, $\frac{1}{4}$ and $1\frac{1}{2}$ gr.

Ephidrosis ((ef-id-rō'-sis). A pathological increase of sweat secretion.

Epicanthus (ep-i-kan'-thus). A fold of skin passing from the side of the nose to the inner border of the eyebrow, hiding the canthus; a congenital defect.

Epicardium (ep-i-kár'-di-um).

The visceral layer of the pericardium.

Epicondyle (ep-i-kon'-dīl). The bony projection above a condyle.

Epicranium (ep-i-krăn'-i-um). The soft structures covering the cranium.

Epicritic (ep-i-krit'-ik). The term applied to the finer sensations of heat, touch, etc.

Epidemic (ep-i-dem'-ik). The appearance of infectious disease attacking a large number of persons within a certain period and in the same area. Such epidemics are mostly caused by infected water, milk, and food supplies, dust, flies, and carriers, and by droplet infection.

Epidemiology (ep-i-dem-i-ol'-o-ji). The science which deals with the causes, symptoms, and treatment of epidemic diseases, and of their seasonal rise and fall.

Epidermis (ep-i-der'-mis). The external layer of the skin ; the cuticle ; also known as the *Scarf-skin*.

Epidermophyton (ep-i-der-mō-fī-ton). A fungus which affects the skin, producing such common conditions as athletes' foot, Dhobie itch, etc.

Epidiascope (ep-i-dī'-as-kōp). An optical lantern which will project opaque objects as well as prepared slides on to an illuminated screen. The pictures are shown in their natural colours.

Epididymis (ep-i-did'-i-mis). A small oblong body attached to the posterior surface of the testes. It consists of the tubules which convey the spermatozoa from the testes to the vas deferens.

Epididymitis (ep-i-did-i-mī'-tis). Inflammation of the epididymis.

Epidural (ep-i-dūr'-al). Upon or external to the dura.

Epigastric (ep-i-gas'-trik). Pertaining to the epigastrium.

Epigastrium (ep-i-gas'-tri-um). The abdominal region lying directly over the stomach.

Epiglottis (ep-i-glot'-is). The thin leaf-shaped flap of cartilage which closes the opening leading into the larynx during the act of swallowing.

Epiglottitis (ep-i-glot-ī'-tis). Inflammation of the epiglottis.

Epilation (ē-pīl-ā'-shun). Ridding the skin of superfluous hair.

Epilatory (ē-pīl'-a-tor-i). An agent for procuring epilation.

Epilepsy (ep-i-lep'-si). A nervous disease characterized by attacks of unconsciousness, and often convulsions of both tonic and clonic type. *Petit mal* is a slight attack which only lasts a moment or two and is not accompanied by convulsions.

Grand mal is a severe form of the disease. *Status epilepticus*, a grave form of epilepsy in which the fits follow each other in rapid succession; generally fatal. **Idiopathic E.**, the usual type of epilepsy of unknown origin. **Jacksonian E.**, fits caused by a local lesion of the brain, *e.g.*, a depressed fracture of the skull.

Epileptic (ep-i-lep'-tĭk). Pertaining to epilepsy. **E. Aura**, premonitory symptoms experienced by an epileptic prior to the attack. **E. Cry**, the peculiar shout which characterizes the onset of an epileptic convulsive attack. **E. Mania**, insanity resulting from an epileptic seizure.

Epileptiform (ep-i-lep'-tĭ-fawm). Resembling epilepsy.

Epilose (ep'-i-lōz). Bald; hairless.

Epinephrine (ep-i-nef'-rēn). The hormone of the supra-renal glands; the same as adrenalin.

Epineurium (ep-i-nūr'-i-um). The sheath of a nerve.

Epiphora (ē-pif'-o-rà). Excessive lachrymation so that the tears run down the cheeks.

Epiphysis (ē-pif'-i-sis). The ends of a long bone which in children are separated from the shaft by cartilage which in time becomes completely ossified. **Separation of E.**, the separation or tearing

away of the epiphyseal cartilage from the bone.

Epiphysitis (e-pif-i-sī'-tis). Inflammation of the epiphysis.

Epiploic (ep-i-plō'-ik). Pertaining to the omentum.

Epiploon (ep-i-plō'-on). The omentum.

Epispadias (ep-i-spā'-di-as). A congenital opening of the urethra on the dorsum of the penis.

Epispastic (ep-i-spas'-tik). A blister.

Epistaxis (ep-i-staks'-is). Bleeding from the nose.

Epithelial (ep-i-thēl'-i-al). Relating to epithelium.

Epithelioma (ep-i-thēl-i-ō'-mà). A malignant growth arising in epithelial tissue, usually the skin; a squamous cell carcinoma.

Epithelium (ep-i-thēl'-i-um). The surface layer of cells covering cutaneous, mucous, and serous surfaces.

Epsom Salts. Magnesium sulphate; used for many purposes medicinally, but chiefly as a purgative. Dose, 30-240 grs.

Epulis (ep'-ū-lis). A tumour growing on or from the gums.

Equation (ē-kwā'-zhun). A collection of symbols which are so arranged as to represent the nature of a chemical reaction.

Equilibrium (ek-wi-lib'-ri-um). A state of balance.

Equivalent (e-kwiv'-a-lent).

1

2

3

4

5

Histological Cell Types of
Epithelium.

1, Squamous stratified.
2, Transitional stratified.
3, Columnar ciliated.
4, Cubical.
5, Flattened (pavement).

Of equal strength or value.
In chemistry: of equal
valency: then pronounced
(ē-kwi-vā'-lent).

Erasion (ē-rā'-zhun). An efface-
ment or rubbing out.

Erb's Paralysis. Paralysis of a
group of muscles of the
shoulder and upper arm in
which the cervical roots of the
fifth and sixth spinal nerves
are involved. Those muscles
affected are the *deltoid*,
biceps, *brachialis anticus*, and
supinator longus. The arm
hangs limp and the hand is
rotated inwards, while the
normal movements are lost.

Erectile (ē-rek'-tīl). Upright;
capable of being elevated.

Erepsin (ē-rep'-sin). One of the
enzymes of the succus
entericus. It has a slight
action in splitting peptone
into amino-acids during intestinal digestion.

Ergometrine (ur'-gō-met-rēn).
The principal alkaloid in
ergot; is obtainable as a
pure and standardized product. It exerts a rapid and
powerful effect (contractions)
on the parturient and post-
partum uterus, and is of use
particularly in post-partum
hæmorrhage.

Ergosterol (ur'-gō-ste-rol or
ur-gos'-te-rol). A sterol that
was first isolated from ergot
of rye. On irradiation it is
transformed into sterol called
"Calciferol," or D_2. This

E *   137

has antirachitic properties, like vitamin D_1 which is present in cod-liver oil, etc.

Ergot (ur'-got). A fungus which attacks rye and other cereals and from which a drug is obtained. It causes contraction of uterine muscle. Dose : Liq. extract of ergot, 10-20 minims.

Ergotin (ur'-got-in). Extract of ergot ; used hypodermically for the arrest of uterine hæmorrhage.

Ergotism (ur'-got-izm). Poisoning by ergot.

Erosion (ē-rō'-zhun). Ulcerative destruction of tissues ; corrosion.

Erratic (e-rat'-ik). Irregular or uncertain.

Eructation (e-ruk-tā'-shun). Noisy expulsion of gas from the stomach ; flatulence.

Eruption (e-rup'-shun). A breaking out, as of a skin rash, whether vesicular, papular, or pustular.

Erysipelas (e-ri-sip'-e-las). An acute inflammatory disease of the skin caused by the *Streptococcus erysipelatis*, a pyogenic organism. The affected skin is swollen, red, and shiny, with a definite raised edge where the healthy and diseased tissues are in contact. There is much constitutional disturbance and fever.

Erysipeloid. An infective dermatitis due to a streptothrix infection, resembling erysipelas but without its fever.

Erythema (e-ri-thē'-mà). A redness of the skin. **E. Infectiosum**, a mildly contagious disease of children associated with a rose-coloured maculo - papular rash. **E. Nodosum**, an acute inflammatory type characterized by raised red painful nodules occurring on the extensor surfaces of the lower limbs. There is marked local tenderness on pressure. The disease is said to be associated with rheumatism and, according to some authorities, with tuberculosis.

Erythematous ((e-ri-them'-at-us). Pertaining to erythema.

Erythroblast (e-rith'-rō-blast). A nucleated red blood cell found in the red bone marrow, and from which the erythrocytes are derived.

Erythrocytes (e-rith'-rō-sīts). The normal non-nucleated red cells of the circulating blood ; the red blood corpuscles.

Erythrodextrin (e-rith-rō-deks'-trin). A dextrin formed by the action of ptyalin on starch. It gives a red reaction with iodine, hence the prefix.

Erythropoiesis (e-rith'-rō-poi-ē-sis). The production of red blood cells.

Erythropsia (e-rith-rop'-si-à).

Abnormal vision in which everything appears to be red.

Erythropsin (e-rith-rop'-sin). *See* **Rhodopsin.**

Erythruria (e-rith-rū'-ri-à). Red urine.

Esbach's Method (es'-bak's). A method of estimating the quantity of albumin in urine. *See* p. 384.

Eschar (es'-kàr). A hard, dry slough or scab, such as forms on the summit of the *malignant pustule* of anthrax.

Escharotic (es-kàr-ot'-ik). A caustic or other agent which will produce an eschar.

Eserine (es'-e-rēn). A drug obtained from the Calabar bean. It causes contraction of the pupil. Synonym. *Physostigmine.* Eserine sulphate, 1/64-1/32 gr.

Es'march's Bandage. A rubber bandage used for controlling bleeding. Before the operation commences, the bandage is applied tightly to the limb, commencing at the distal end and reaching above the site of operation, where a rubber tourniquet is firmly applied. The bandage is then removed. This method renders the operative area absolutely bloodless.

Esoteric (es-ō-te'-rik). Arising from within.

Essence (es'-ens). A solution of a volatile oil in rectified spirit.

Essential (es-sen'-shal). (1) Pertaining to an essence. (2)

Necessary. (3) The important part or active principle of a substance. **E. hypertension.** Primary and persistent raised blood-pressure not due to recognizable causes.

Estlander's Operation (est'-lander's). Removal of portions of several ribs to allow of the collapse of part of the chest wall.

Ether, also **Æther** (ē'-ther). A volatile, inflammable liquid used as a general anæsthetic, and often administered by inhaling the ether sprinkled on a face-mask. This is known as the *open method.* In the *closed method* the patient breathes into a rubber bag, known as *Clover's inhaler,* into which ether is admitted. Ether is considered to be a much safer general anæsthetic than chloroform in the majority of cases. It is very highly inflammable, and is never used near a naked light. It is sometimes given hypodermically as a heart stimulant.

Ethmoid (eth'moid). A bone which enters into the formation of the nose. It resembles a sieve, and is also known as the cribriform bone.

Ethyl Chloride (eth'-il), C_2H_5Cl. An anæsthetic fluid which may be used for general or local anæsthesia. When used locally it is used to " freeze " the tissues by spraying.

139

Ethylene (eth'-il-ēn), C_2H_4. A poisonous inflammable gas; is anæsthetic and sedative.

Etiology (ē-ti-ol'-o-ji). The science treating of the causation of disease.

Eucain (ū-kān). A proprietary local anæsthetic.

Eucalyptus (ū-ka-lip'-tus). A colourless, aromatic, and antiseptic oily fluid distilled from the leaves of *E. globulus*, *E. amygdaline*, and other species of the gum-tree. It can be used in the form of an ointment, and is also inhaled for common colds, bronchitis and phthisis.

Eudrenin (ū-drē'-nin). A preparation of eucain to which adrenalin is added; used as a local anæsthetic.

Eugenics (ū-jen'-iks). The science which deals with the physical, moral, and intellectual improvement of the human race by careful and judicious mating. It is also concerned with (1) the sterilization of mental defectives; (2) intermarriages; (3) restriction of marriage between persons physically unfit; (4) birth control and allied problems.

Eunuch (ū'-nuk). A human male from whom the testes have been removed; a castrated male.

Eupad (ū'-pad). A powder consisting mainly of fine bleaching powder and boracic acid. The name means Edinburgh University Pathological Department, where the mixture was first produced.

Eupepsia (ū-pep'-si-à). Normal digestion.

Euphoria (ū-faw'-ri-à). The sense of well-being.

Eupnœa (ūp-nē'-à). Normal breathing.

Eusol (ū'-sol). An antiseptic solution containing hypochlorous acid. It is prepared from Eupad by adding 25 grm. of the powder to 1 litre of water, after which it is carefully filtered and left to stand. Since it is unstable it should be freshly prepared at frequent intervals.

Eustachian (ūs-tā'-shi-an). Named after B. Eustachius, an Italian anatomist of the sixteenth century. E. Catheter, an instrument used for dilating the Eustachian tube when it becomes blocked. E. Tube, a canal measuring about 4 inches, extending from the throat near the tonsils to the middle ear. It allows air to pass into the middle ear, so that the air-pressure is kept even on both sides of the ear-drum. E. Valve, the valve guarding the entrance of the inferior vena cava into the right auricle of the heart.

Euthanasia (ū-than-ā'-zi-à). An easy or painless death.

Eutocia (ū-tō'-si-à). A natural

and normal labour without any complications.

Evacuant (e-vak'-ū-ant). An agent which causes an evacuation.

Evacuation (e-vak-ū-ā-shun). The act of emptying a cavity ; generally referred to the discharge of fæcal matter from the rectum.

Evaporate (e-vap'-o-rāt). To convert from the liquid into the gaseous state by means of heat.

Evaporating Lotion (e-vap'-o-rāt-ing lō'-shun). A cooling lotion such as lead lotion. A piece of lint is dipped in the lotion and applied to the part ; as soon as it dries it must be renewed.

Eventration (ē-ven-trā'-shun). An abdominal hernia ; protrusion of the abdominal viscera.

Eversion (ō-ver'-shun). A turning outwards.

Evipan (ev'-i-pan). A general anæsthetic introduced by the intravenous method in amounts varying from 1 to 4 c.c.

Evisceration (ē-vis-e-rā'-shun). Removal of the viscera.

Evolution (e-vo-loo'-shun). A gradual change from the primitive and simple to a highly complex specialized form. **Spontaneous E.**, the sudden, unaided expulsion of a fœtus in the transverse presentation. The fœtus is small, premature, and usually dead.

Evulsion (e-vul'shun). Forcible tearing away of a structure.

Exacerbation (eks-as-er-bā'-shun). Increased severity, as of symptoms.

Exanthem, Exanthema (eks-an'-them (á)). A cutaneous eruption. Pl. *exanthem'ata.*

Excavation (eks-ka-vā'-shun). A hollowing out.

Excipient (eks-sip'-i-ent). A vehicle or medium for administering drugs.

Excision (ek-sizh-un). Removal, or the act of cutting away.

Excitability (eks-sīt-a-bil'-i-ti). Rapid response to stimuli ; a state of being easily irritated.

Exclusion (eks-kloo-zhun). Shutting out.

Excoriation (eks-kor-i-ā'-shun). An abrasion or rubbing off of the skin.

Excrement (eks'-kre-ment). Fæces (*q.v.*).

Excrementitious (eks-kre-men-tish'-us). Pertaining to, or resembling fæces.

Excrescence (eks-kres'-ens). An abnormal protuberance or growth of the tissues.

Excreta (eks-krē-tá). The waste matter which is normally discharged from the body, particularly urine and fæces.

Excretion (eks-krē'-shun). The act of eliminating waste material from the body, and also the matter so discharged.

Exenteration (eks-en-te-rā'-shun). Evisceration or disembowelment in embryotomy.

Exfoliation (eks-fō-li-ā-shun). The scaling off of dead tissues.

Exhalation (eks-hal-ā'-shun). The emission of body vapours.

Exhaustion (egz-awst'-yun). Fatigue ; loss of vitality ; the limit of endurance.

Exhumation (eks-hū-mā'-shun). Disinterment of the body.

Exophthalmia (eks-of-thal'-mi-à). Same as exophthalmos.

Exophthalmic (eks-of-thal'-mik). Relating to exophthalmos. **E. Goitre,** exophthalmos associated with enlargement of the thyroid gland and other symptoms of a nervous character. Synonym, *Graves' Disease.*

Exophthalmos (eks-of-thal'-mos). Protrusion of the eyeballs.

Exostosis (eks-os-tō'-sis). An overgrowth of bone tissue forming a tumour.

Expectant (eks-pek'-tant). Hopeful ; full of anticipation. **E. Treatment,** a method of treating disease by alleviating the main symptoms, and then waiting and watching the course of the disease before more drastic methods are adopted.

Expectorant (eks-pek'-to-rant). A drug which promotes or increases expectoration.

Expectoration (eks-pek-tor-ā'-shun). The act of clearing

secretion from the respiratory tract by coughing. *See* **Sputum.**

Expert (eks'-pert). A skilled person ; an authority in a special subject.

Expiration (eks-pi-rā'-shun). (1) The exhalation of air from the lungs. (2) Death. (3) The finish.

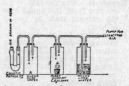

Apparatus to demonstrate that Plants yield CO_2 in expiration.

Exploration (eks-plaw-rā'-shun). The making of an examination as an aid to diagnosis.

Exploratory Laparotomy (eks-plor'-a-tor-i lap-a-rot'-o-mi). A median-line incision into the abdominal cavity to ascertain the cause of disease.

Expression (eks-presh'-un). Expulsion by force ; a pressing out, as of the placenta from the uterus. *See* **Dublin Method.**

Exsanguinate (eks-sang'-gwin-āt). To render bloodless.

Extension (eks-ten'-shun). (1) A method of treating fractures by applying a pulling force or weight to the distal part, so that the broken ends of the bone are brought into apposition. (2) The opposite to flexion, *i.e.*, straightening into alignment of two bones which hinge at a joint.

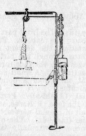

Extension Apparatus.

Extensor (eks-ten'-sawr). A muscle which causes extension of a part.

External (ex-ter'-nal). On the outside. **E. Os**, the external mouth of the canal of the cervix uteri which opens into the vagina.

Extirpate (ex'-ter-pāt). To remove completely.

Extra-articular (eks-trā-ăr-tik'-ū-lăr). Outside the joint.

Extracapsular (eks-trā-kap'-sū-lăr). Outside the capsule.

Extract (eks'-trakt). A prepa-ration obtained by evaporating a solution of a drug.

Extraction (eks-trak'-shun). The drawing out or removal, as of a tooth from its socket.

Extractive (eks-trak'-tiv). Relating to an extract; a substance which has been extracted from another.

Extradural (eks-trā-dūr'-al). External to the dura mater.

Extraneous (eks-trā'-ni-us). Foreign; superfluous or unnecessary to the matter in hand; not essential.

Extra-uterine. Gestation. Pregnancy occurring outside the uterus. *See* **Ectopic.**

Extravasation (eks-trav-a-sā'-shun). An escape of fluid from its normal enclosure into the surrounding tissues. Thus **E. of Blood**, effusion of blood into the tissues as the result of the rupture of a blood-vessel. **E. of Urine**, escape of urine into the tissues.

Extremity (eks-trem'-it-i). The limb. **Upper E.**, the arm. **Lower E.**, the leg.

Extrinsic (eks-trin'-sik). Developing or having its origin from without; not internal.

Exudate (eks'-ū-dāt). The product of exudation.

Exudation (eks-ū-dā'-shun). The oozing out of fluids, as of blood through the capillary walls, or of sweat through the pores of the skin.

Eye. The organ of vision.

143

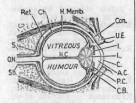

The Eye.

Ret., Retina.
Ch., Choroid.
H. Memb., Hyaloid membrane.
Con., Conjunctiva.
U.E., Upper eyelid.
I., Iris.
L., Lens.
C., Cornea.
A.C., Anterior chamber.
P.C., Posterior chamber.
C.B., Ciliary body.
S., Sclerotic.
O.N., Optic nerve.
Sh., O.N. sheath.
H.C., Hyaloid canal.

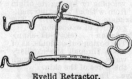

Eyelid Retractor.

144

Eyeball. The globe of the eye.
Eyelid. The covering of the eyeball.
Eye-teeth. The canine teeth in the superior maxillæ. *See* **Teeth.**

F.

F. Abbreviation for *Fahrenheit* and *fiat*.
Face (făs). The front part of the head ; the features. F. Presentation, the descent of the fœtus through the birth passages with the face foremost.
Facet (fas'-et). A small, smooth, flat surface of a bone or a calculus.
Facial (fā'-shi-al). Pertaining to the face. F. Nerve, seventh pair of cranial nerves.
Facies (fas'-i-ēz). The appearance ; particularly applied to the face as an indicator of disease or other abnormal state. Abdominal F., an anxious facial expression seen in patients suffering from acute abdominal symptoms ; the face may be flushed or pale, according to the state of the temperature ; the eyes are dull and heavy. F. Hippocratica, the drawn, pale, pinched appearance seen in patients who are likely to die ; the nose becomes thin, pointed, and pinched about the nostrils, while the ears, nose, and lips assume a cyanotic appearance, and the

face is very pale ; the condition is named after Hippocrates, who first described it.

Faculty (fak´-ul-ti). The innate ability to perform some special function ; mental power ; also the name given to a body of professors or teachers in a special university department, such as medicine, law, science, etc.

Fæcal (fē´-kal). Pertaining to or resembling fæces.

Fæces (fē´-sēz). The waste matter ejected from the bowel through the anus. It consists of 50% bacteria. The colouring matter is a pigment called *stercobilin*, derived from bilirubin. Other constituents include water, cholic acid, indol, skatol, and epithelial cells, fat, and roughage ; there may be also some undigested foodstuffs. In *shape* and *consistency* the fæces should be a soft cylindrical mass ; about 4½ oz. are evacuated daily.

Fahrenheit Thermometer (făr´-en-hīt). The thermometric scale used in England. The freezing-point of water is fixed at 32°, and its boiling-point at 212°. Named after the German physicist, *Gabriel Fahrenheit*, who invented it.

Faint (fānt). A swoon ; a state of temporary unconsciousness due to cerebral anæmia.

Falciform (fal´-si-fawm). Shaped like a sickle. The name given to certain ligaments.

Falling of the Womb. Uterine prolapse. **F. Sickness,** epilepsy. **F. Temperature,** one that is descending to normal.

Fallopian Tubes (fal-lō´-pi-an). Two tubes opening out of the upper part of the uterus. Each measures 4 in., and the distal end is fimbriated and lies near the ovary. Their function is to convey the ova into the uterus.

Familial (fam-il´-i-al). Relating to the family, as of a disease affecting several members of the same family.

Faraday (far´-a-dā). Michael Faraday, a famous English physicist.

Faradic (far-ad´-ik). Pertaining to the scientist Faraday. **F. Current,** an induced electrical current.

Farinaceous (far-in-ā´-shi-us). Pertaining to cereal substances, *i.e.*, made of flour or grain.

Fascia (fash´-i-ä). A connective tissue sheath consisting of fibrous tissue and fat which unites the skin to the underlying tissue. It also surrounds and separates many of the muscles, and, also, in some cases, holds them together.

Fasciculus (fas-sik´-ū-lus). A little bundle, as of muscle or nerve fibres.

Fast. (1) To abstain from food.

145

(2) Resistant, as certain forms of bacteria which are acid-fast after certain forms of staining.

Fastigium (fas-tij′-i-um). The highest point ; the greatest height of the temperature during a febrile disease.

Fat. An oil which may be either solid or liquid and of animal or of vegetable origin. A molecule of fat is constituted of one molecule of glycerine and three of a fatty acid, *e.g.*, oleic, stearic, or palmitic acids.

Fatal (fā′-tal). Causing death.

Fatigue (fa-tēg′). A sense of weariness due to the presence of poisons or toxins in the muscles caused by excessive mental or physical activity. These toxins are therefore known as fatigue poisons, as their accumulation in the body gives rise to the discomfort of excessive tiredness.

Fauces (faw′-sēz). The structures dividing the posterior part of the mouth from the pharynx. It comprises structures formed by the soft palate, including the uvula, and the anterior and posterior arches.

Faucial (faw′-si-al). Relating to the fauces.

Favus (fā′-vus). An infectious skin disease caused by a fungus, most commonly found on the scalp. The for-

mation of yellow cup-shaped scabs are characteristic.

Febrifuge (feb′-ri-fūj). An agent which reduces temperature.

Febrile (feb′-rīl). Feverish ; accompanied by fever.

Fecundation (fe-kun-dā′-shun). Impregnation.

Fecundity (fe-kun′-di-ti). The power of reproduction ; fertility.

Fehling's Solution (fā′-ling). An alkaline copper solution used for the detection and estimation of sugars (*see* Appendix—Urine Testing).

Fel. Bile. **F. Bovis,** ox-bile ; it causes an evacuation of the bowel by stimulating peristalsis.

Felix-Weil Reaction (fē-liks-vīl). A test for typhus fever in which the infected patient's serum agglutinates a suspension of "bacillus proteus ×19."

Felon (fel′-on). (1) Suppuration of the terminal joint of a finger ; a whitlow. (2) One guilty of a felony or grave crime.

Female (fē′-māl). A woman.

Femoral (fem′-or-al). Pertaining to the femur or thigh-bone. **F. Artery,** the artery commencing from the *external iliac artery* and terminating behind the knee as the *popliteal artery* ; it lies on the inner side of the femur. **F. Vein,** the continuation of the *popliteal vein* upwards towards the *external iliac vein*.

Femur (fē'-mur). The thigh-bone ; the longest and strongest bone in the body.

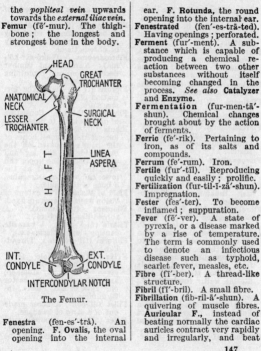

The Femur.

Fenestra (fen-es'-trá). An opening. F. Ovalis, the oval opening into the internal

ear. F. Rotunda, the round opening into the internal ear.

Fenestrated (fen'-es-trä-ted). Having openings ; perforated.

Ferment (fur'-ment). A substance which is capable of producing a chemical re-action between two other substances without itself becoming changed in the process. *See also* **Catalyzer** and **Enzyme**.

Fermentation (fur-men-tä'-shun). Chemical changes brought about by the action of ferments.

Ferric (fe'-rik). Pertaining to iron, as of its salts and compounds.

Ferrum (fe'-rum). Iron.

Fertile (fur'-tīl). Reproducing quickly and easily ; prolific.

Fertilization (fur-til-ī-zä'-shun). Impregnation.

Fester (fes'-ter). To become inflamed ; suppuration.

Fever (fē'-ver). A state of pyrexia, or a disease marked by a rise of temperature. The term is commonly used to denote an infectious disease such as typhoid, scarlet fever, measles, etc.

Fibre (fī'-ber). A thread-like structure.

Fibril (fī'-bril). A small fibre.

Fibrillation (fib-ril-ä'-shun). A quivering of muscle fibres. **Auricular F.,** instead of beating normally the cardiac auricles contract very rapidly and irregularly, and beat independently of the ventricles ; treatment consists mainly in rest and in the administration of digitalis.

Fibrin (fī'-brin or fib'-rin). A protein formed from the fibrinogen of blood plasma when blood clots.

Fibrinogen (fī-brin'-ō-jen). The precursor of fibrin.

Fibrinous (fī'-brin-us). Composed of, containing, or resembling fibrin.

Fibroadenoma (fī-brō-ad-e-nō'-mä). A benign tumour containing fibrous and glandular tissue.

Fibrocartilage (fī-brō-kár'-til-āj). Cartilage containing fibrous tissue.

Fibrochondritis (fī-brō-kon-drī'-tis). Inflammation of fibrocartilage.

Fibroid (fī-broid). The common name given to the fibromyoma of the uterus. F. Degeneration, the conversion of membraneous tissue into fibrous tissue. Uterine F., a fibromyoma developing from the unstriped muscle and fibrous tissue of the uterine wall. Interstitial F., a tumour in the muscular wall of the uterus ; this may grow inwards and form a Polypoid F., or grow outward and become a Subperitoneal F. or Subserous F.

Fibroma (fī-brō'-mä). A be-

nign tumour composed of fibrous tissue.

Fibromyoma (fī-brō-mī-ō'-mä). A benign tumour consisting partly of muscle and partly of fibrous tissue.

Fibrosarcoma (fī-brō-sár-kō'-mä). A malignant tumour derived from and containing fibrous tissue.

Fibrosis (fī-brō'-sis). The formation of fibrous tissue in a structure.

Fibrous (fī'-brus). Consisting of or pertaining to fibres.

Fibula (fib'-ū-lä). One of the longest and thinnest bones of the body ; situated on the outer side of the leg and articulating at the upper end with the tibia and at the lower end with the astragalus, a bone of the ankle.

Field of Vision. The extent of vision while the eyes are fixed.

Filament (fil'-a-ment). A thread-like structure.

Filaria (fil-ē-'-rī-ä). A parasite causing elephantiasis (*q.v.*).

Filiform (fil'-ī-form). Threadlike.

Filix Mas. Male fern ; destroys the tape-worm ; is given on an empty stomach, and followed later by castor oil. Dose of Ext. Filicis., 45-90 minims.

Fillet (fil'-et). A noose made out of a strip of bandage.

Filter (fil'-ter). A porous substance through which lightrays, air, or liquid may be passed in order to eliminate certain unwanted elements or particles.

Filtrate (fil'-trāt). That part of the substance which passes through the filter. The residue left behind is the precipitate.

Filtration (fil-trā'-shun). The act of passing fluid through a porous medium.

Fimbria (fim'-bri-à). A fringe or frond; resembling the fronds of a fern, as, for example, the fimbria of the Fallopian tubes.

Fimbriated (fim'-bri-ā-ted). Fringed; possessing fimbria.

Finger (fing'-ger). A digit. **F. Stall,** a tubular covering for the finger; sometimes cut from an old glove; may be made of rubber, stockinette, chamois leather, silk, etc.

Finsen Light Treatment. A method of treating skin diseases, particularly lupus, by means of violet and ultra-violet light-rays.

Fission (fish'-un). A splitting directly into two or more parts; a method of reproduction in the lower forms of life.

Fissure (fish'-ur). A split or cleft. **Anal F.,** a linear ulcer on the margin of the anus. **Longitudinal F.,** the deep cleft between the two hemispheres of the cerebrum. **Occipito-parietal F.,** the fissure between the occipital and parietal lobes of the brain. **Palpebral F.,** the opening between the eyelids. **Portal F.,** the opening into the liver on its under surface; continues into the liver as the portal canal. **Transverse F.,** the fissure between the cerebellum and cerebrum of the brain.

Fistula (fis'-tū-là). An unnatural communication between two different structures. **Anal F.,** a tubular passage extending from the skin surface just beyond the anus to the deeper structures; it may or may not communicate with the bowel. **Fæcal F.,** one in which there is a discharge of fæces through the opening. **Biliary F.,** one which discharges bile; occurs after operations on the gall-bladder or bile ducts. **Parotid F.,** an abnormal leakage of saliva on to the external surface of the cheek. **Vesico-vaginal F.,** one opening from the bladder into the vagina.

Fit. A sudden paroxysmal attack.

Fixation (fiks-ā'-shun). Causing to remain firm or to adhere.

Flaccid (flak'-sid). Soft, flabby; not firm.

Flagellum (fla-jel'-um). A fine hair-like appendage with a lashing movement; many of the bacteria are flagellated.

Flap-amputation. A method

of amputating so that the raw end surface is covered by a flap of skin.

Flash-point. The temperature at which an oil or other combustible fluid gives off vapour which will then fire if exposed to a naked light.

Flat Foot. An abnormality of the foot in which the muscles and ligaments become weakened, allowing the arches of the foot to become flattened.

Flat Pelvis. A common pelvic deformity in which the antero-posterior diameter is shortened.

Flatulence (flat'-ū-lens). Gastric and intestinal distension with gas.

Flatulent (flat'-ū-lent). Producing or evincing flatulence.

Flatus (flā'-tus). Air or gas in the stomach or intestines.

Flesh. The body tissues. Proud F., excessive overgrowth of granulation tissue.

Flex. To bend.

Flexion (flek'-shun). The act of bending.

Flexure (fleks'-ūr). A bend. **Hepatic F.**, the bend of the colon beneath the liver. **Splenic F.**, that part of the colon which bends near the spleen. **Sigmoid F.**, the S-shaped bend at the lower end of the descending colon : is situated in the *left iliac fossa.*

Floccillation, Floccitation (flok-

sil-ā'-shun, flok-sit-ā'-shun). Same as *Carphology.*

Floccule (flok-ūl). A flake.

Fluctuation (fluk-tū-ā'-shun). A rising and falling with a wave-like motion. Oscillation. Felt on digital examination of a tumour which contains fluid, *e.g.*, an abscess.

Fluid Ounce. A liquid measure of the value of 8 drachms ; or 480 minims ; or 30 c.c. approximately.

Fluorescence (floo-or-es'-ens). The property of certain fluids and solids of exhibiting a bluish or greenish sheen in addition to its ordinary colour.

Fluorescent (floo-or-es'-ent). Having the property of fluorescence. **F. Screen**, an opaque screen will fluoresce when exposed to X-rays.

Fluorescine (floo-or-es'-sēn). A coal-tar product used in ophthalmology ; it has no effect on a healthy cornea, but will stain an ulcer or other abrasion a bright green colour.

Flux (fluks). A flow of fluid. **Bloody F.**, dysentery.

Focal (fō'-kal). Pertaining to the focus of anything.

Focus (fō'-kus). The point which gives the maximum definition. When an object is *in focus*, a sharp, clear, bright image is seen. When it is *out of focus*, the image becomes blurred and is only seen indistinctly.

Fœtal (fē'-tal). Pertaining to the fœtus.

Fœtid (fet'-id). Pertaining to fœtor.

Fœtor (fē'-taw(r)). A bad smell as of decaying matter.

Fœtus (fē'-tus). The child after the first four months of intra-uterine life. **F. Papyraceous**, a dead fœtus, one of a twin, which has become flattened and mummified.

Fold. The doubling of one part over another ; a pleat. **Gluteal F.**, the crease in the skin where the buttock meets the thigh.

Follicle (fol'-ikl). A small secreting sac. **Graafian F.**, minute vesicles contained in the stroma of an ovary each containing a single ovum.

Follicular Tonsillitis. Inflammation of the follicles on the surface of the tonsil ; these become filled with pus, and the tonsil is therefore seen to be covered with yellow pustular spots ; the constitutional symptoms are usually severe.

Folliculin (fol-ik'-ū-lin). A hormone, produced by the ripening Graafian follicle, which controls the changes in the uterine endometrium in the post-menstrual phase ; also known as œstrin.

Fomentation (fō-men-tā'-shun).

A hot wet application for the relief of pain or inflammation. **Surgical F.**, one applied to an open wound. Cut a double thickness of surgeon's lint, slightly larger than the size of the wound ; be sure to see that the cotton side is external. Now place it in the centre of a linen wringer, place both in a sterilizer, and boil them for seven minutes. The fomentation is wrung out as tightly as possible by twisting the ends of the wringer in opposite directions. Having shaken the lint lightly to allow the steam to escape, it is placed over the wound, covered with a piece of jaconet, cut half an inch larger than the lint ; then an equal-sized piece of absorbent wool, and lastly a bandage to keep the whole in position. Some authorities prefer to do without the jaconet, in which case non-absorbent brown wool must be used. **Boracic F.**, this may be prepared with boracic lint, which is already impregnated with boracic, and is coloured pink as a distinguishing mark ; or boracic may be added to surgeon's lint, either in the form of powder or crystals, and then wrung out of boiling water as before. **Eusol F.**, lint is wrung out of equal parts of eusol solution and warm

151

water; applied to septic wounds. **Saline F.,** add sodium chloride to the lint and wring out of boiling water. **Medical F.,** instead of lint, two or three thicknesses of flannel are used, and the fomentation is applied to unbroken skin, otherwise the procedure is the same as for a surgical fomentation; it is unnecessary to boil it; flannel is used because it retains the heat better than lint. This fomentation is also called a *Stupe.* **Turpentine F.,** sprinkle ʒi of turpentine evenly over the dry flannel and then wring out of boiling water. **Opium F.,** for this wring out the fomentation first and then sprinkle tr. of opium ♏xxx over the flannel, and apply.

Fomites (fō-mīt'-ēz). Articles which are capable of carrying infection, such as clothing, books, toys, etc.

Fontanelle (fon-ta-nel'). Spaces in the skull, covered by membrane and formed by incomplete ossification of the junction of the cranial bones. There are two main fontanelles : the diamond-shaped Anterior F., or bregma, at the junction of the sagittal, frontal, and coronal sutures ; and the triangular Posterior F. formed by the junction of the sagittal and lambdoidal sutures.

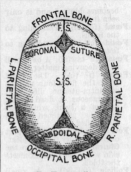

The Fontanelles.

A.F., Anterior fontanelle.
P.F., Posterior fontanelle.
F.S., Frontal suture.
S.S., Sagittal suture.

Foot. The extreme end of the lower limb. **F. Drop,** inability to *flex* the foot ; caused by damage to the nerves, the pressure of tightly tucked-in bed-clothes, or imperfect application of a splint, particularly when the heel does not fit properly into the angle of a back-splint. **F. Presentation,** the descent of the fœtus through the genital tract, with one or both feet appearing first. **F.-pound,** the amount of force required to raise one pound to the height of one foot.

Foot and Mouth Disease. A contagious disease occurring in epidemic form among cattle. It is characterized by the appearance of vesicles in the mouth and on the feet.

Foramen (for-ā'-men). A hole or opening. Generally used in connection with bones.

Forceps (faw(r)'-seps). A surgical instrument resembling a pair of tongs. *Artery F.,* forceps used for compressing a bleeding blood-vessel; there are several different patterns, but *Spencer-Wells'* and *Kocher's* are in common use. *Delivery F.,* forceps used for facilitating the delivery of the child during difficult child-birth. *Dental F.,* forceps used for the extraction of teeth. *Dissecting F.,* forceps shaped like sugar-tongs. They may be "plain" or "rat-toothed," the latter having two small-pointed prongs at the tip which prevent the forceps slipping when holding tissues. *Dressing F.,* this type is used for ordinary ward dressings. *Sinus F.,* used for enlarging a sinus in surgical dressings. *Tongue F.,* used for holding the tongue forward during states of unconsciousness. *Towel F.,* also known as *Towel Clips.* Used for keeping towels in position during operations or surgical dressings.

Forcipressure (fawr'-si-presh'-ur). Arrest of hæmorrhage by the application of artery forceps.

Foreign Body. Any substance which is not normally present.

Foreskin (faw(r)'-skin). The prepuce or skin covering the glans penis.

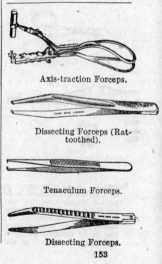

Axis-traction Forceps.

Dissecting Forceps (Rat-toothed).

Tenaculum Forceps.

Dissecting Forceps.

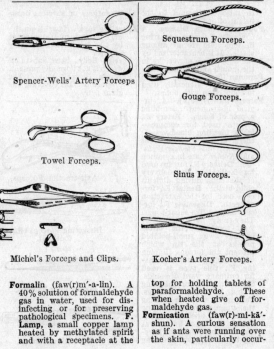

Spencer-Wells' Artery Forceps

Sequestrum Forceps.

Gouge Forceps.

Towel Forceps.

Sinus Forceps.

Michel's Forceps and Clips.

Kocher's Artery Forceps.

Formalin (faw(r)m´-a-lin). A 40% solution of formaldehyde gas in water, used for disinfecting or for preserving pathological specimens. **F. Lamp**, a small copper lamp heated by methylated spirit and with a receptacle at the top for holding tablets of paraformaldehyde. These when heated give off formaldehyde gas.

Formication (faw(r)-mi-kā´-shun). A curious sensation as if ants were running over the skin, particularly occur-

154

ring during nerve regeneration.

Formula (faw(r)m′-ū-là). A prescribed method for solving problems, or a series of symbols denoting the chemical composition of a substance.

Fornix (faw(r)′-niks). An arch; particularly referred to the vagina, *i.e.*, the space between the vaginal wall and the cervix of the uterus. Pl. *fornices*.

Fossa (fos′-sà). A depression or furrow.

Fourchette (foor′-shet). A membranous fold connecting the posterior ends of the labia minora.

Fourth Disease. The name given to a contagious exanthematous condition, having points of similarity with measles, scarlet fever and rubella. Also known as *Duke's Disease*.

Fovea (fō′-vi-à). A small fossa or depression.

Fowler's Position. The patient is propped up with pillows in the sitting position. The small of the back and nape of the neck must be well supported. An air-ring is placed beneath the buttocks, and the knees are flexed over a knee-pillow, the ends of which are tied to the head of the bed to prevent the patient from slipping. The position is adopted (1) for

drainage purposes ; (*a*) after child-birth, to allow for the free escape of lochia from the vagina ; (*b*) in cases of acute abdominal disease, so that fluid or pus may collect in the pelvis (pouch of Douglas), where the peritoneum is less absorptive than that in the abdomen. (2) To facilitate breathing in cases such as pneumonia, heart disease, or any other condition characterized by respiratory distress.

Fowler's Solution. Liquor arsenicalis. Dose, 2-8 minims.

Fractional Distillation. A method which affords the means of separating, more or less, the several constituents of mixed and instillable liquids, by collecting the portions or fractions which pass over at varying temperatures.

Fractional Test Meal. A method of examining the gastric contents by withdrawing samples at intervals after a standard meal and subsequently submitting them to chemical analysis. The data so gained are often of diagnostic importance.

Fracture (frakt′-ūr). A breach in the continuity of a bone ; a break. A fracture is named according to the direction of the break, thus : *transverse*, *oblique*, *spiral*, *stellate*, *T-shaped*. The symptoms of fracture are pain and swelling, unnatural mobility, loss of power, shortening, bruising, and crepitus. **Simple F.,** one in which the bone is broken, but there is no injury to the surrounding tissues or skin. **Compound F.,** the jagged ends of the bone protrude through the skin; this is a much more serious type, since sepsis of the wound may delay union of the bones. **Complicated F.,** the broken ends of bone have caused injury to adjacent organs or structures, e.g., the lung may be pierced by a broken rib. **Comminuted F.,** one in which the bone is broken into several pieces; often caused by a crush, such as being run over. **Depressed F.,** caused by direct violence on a part such as the skull, when a portion of the inner table of the cranium becomes depressed on to the surface of the brain. **Impacted F.,** when one end of a broken bone is driven into, and firmly wedged into, the opposite end, usually in a bad position. **Incomplete F.,** when the bone is only cracked or fissured. When it splits and bends like a green twig, it is known as a **Greenstick F.,** this only occurs in young bones containing a greater proportion of organic than of inorganic matter. **Intracapsular F.,** one in which the break occurs within the capsule of the joint. **Pathological F.,** one caused by local disease of the bone, particularly by presence of cancer secondary deposits. **Spontaneous F.,** one caused by the pull of the muscles on brittle or diseased bones; is not due to violence. *See* **Fragilitas Ossium.** *See also* **Colles' F.** and **Pott's F.**

Frænum (frē'-num). A fold of membrane which passes from the under-surface of the tongue to the floor of the mouth.

Fragilitas Ossium (fraj-il'-i-tas os'-i-um). Brittleness of the bones due to an abnormal deposit of mineral matter.

Framboesia (fram-bē'-zi-à). Yaws.

Fremitus (frem'-it-us). Thoracic vibrations observed on auscultation or palpation.

Frenum. *See* **Frænum.**

Freud, Sigmund (froid). A famous Austrian psychoanalyst whose teachings stress the theory: (1) of the existence of a subconscious mind; (2) that psychical processes are never accidental or due to chance, but are determined by laws, as are physical events; (3) that emotional processes have the attributes of quantity, and can be displaced from one idea to another; (4) that the sex instinct does not develop at puberty, but that the child experiences a rich sexual life, and from this is derived the later stages of *narcissism* or self-love, *homosexuality* or attraction to the same sex, *heterosexuality*, which is the normal attraction to the opposite sex) (*see* Œdipus and **Complex**); (5) that dreams are fulfilments of wishes which find no realization in waking hours ; theories are also formulated with regard to the importance of sex in dreams ; (6) that forgetting, misplacing articles, and slips of the tongue or pen are the outward manifestation of repression. *See also* **Psycho-analysis, Abreaction,** etc.

F r i a b l e (frī-ab'l). Easily crumbled ; readily pulverized.

Friars' Balsam. Compound tincture of benzoin.

Friedreich's Ataxia. A form of paralysis of hereditary origin, and commencing at about the same age in each generation.

Frigotherapy (frij-ō-the´-ra-pi). The treatment of disease by cold.

Frontal (frun´-tal). Pertaining to the front. **F. Bone,** the bone forming the forehead.

Frost-bite (frost´-bīt). Freezing of the skin and superficial tissues due to extreme cold.

In severe cases the parts become gangrenous.

Fructose (fruk´-tōz) ($C_6H_{12}O_6$). One of the hexoses belonging to the monosaccharide group. Synonyms, *Lævulose* and *Fruit Sugar.*

Fuchsine (fook´-sin). A red staining agent used in microscopy.

Fulgurant (ful´-gū-rant). Suddenly severe and agonizing ; a darting, momentary pain.

Fulminating (ful´-min-ā-ting). Developing quickly and with an equally rapid fatal termination.

Fumigation (fū-mi-gā´-shun). A method of disinfection for destroying bacteria by filling the room, etc., with gas, such as sulphur dioxide or formaldehyde.

Function (fungk´-shun). The special work performed by an organ or structure in its normal state.

Functional (fungk´-shun-al). Pertaining to function. Disorder of an organ which is not due to an organic disease.

Fundus (fun´-dus). The basal portion of a hollow structure ; the part which is distal to the opening.

Fungiform (fun´-ji-form). Resembling a fungus.

Fungus (fung´-gus). A low form of vegetable life, including mushrooms. Pl. *fungi* (fun´-ji) or *funguses* (fung-gus-ez).

Funic Souffle (fū'-nik soof'-l). A
sound heard on abdominal
auscultation in a pregnant
woman, believed to be due
to the flow of blood through
the umbilical cord.

Funiculus (fū-nik'-ū-lus). A
cord-like structure.

Fur. (1) Coating of the tongue
due to ill-health. (2) A
deposit formed on the walls
of kettles, boilers, etc., in
which hard water has been
boiled.

Furuncle (fū-rung'-kl). A localized abscess or boil.

Furunculosis (fū-rung-kū-lō'-
sis). A condition characterized by boil formation.

Fusiform (fū'-zi-form). Resembling a spindle.

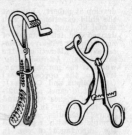

Ferguson's   Doyen's
   Gag.   Gag.

G.

Gadus Morrhua (gā'-dus mor-
rū'-á). The cod-fish. *See*
Oleum Morrhua.

Gaertner's Bacillus (gĕrt'-nerz).
An organism found in con-
taminated meat. A common
cause of food-poisoning.

Gag. An apparatus for keeping
the jaws open.

Gait (gāt). The individual
manner of walking or run-
ning. **Ataxic G.,** the jerky,
irregular walk of a person
suffering from *locomotor
ataxy*; the feet are lifted
high and jerked forward,
with the heel reaching the

ground first with a stamp.
Spastic G., movement with
the limbs held stiffly, with
the feet dragging.

Galactagogue (ga-lak'-ta-gog).
An agent for increasing the
flow of milk.

Galactocele (ga-lak'-tō-sēl). A
milk-containing cyst of the
female breast, formed as the
result of blockage of a milk
duct.

Galactorrhœa (gal-ak-tō-rē'-á).
Excessive milk secretion.

Gall. Bile secreted in the liver.
G.-bladder. A pear-shaped
organ about 4 in. in length
situated on the under-surface
of the liver. Its function is
to concentrate and store the
bile. **G.-duct,** the cystic
duct leading from the gall-
bladder. **G.-stones,** concre-

tions formed within the gall-bladder; they are often multiple and facetted.

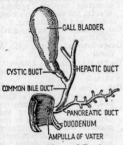

CALL BLADDER

CYSTIC DUCT — HEPATIC DUCT

COMMON BILE DUCT

PANCREATIC DUCT

DUODENUM

AMPULLA OF VATER

Gall-bladder and Ducts.

Gallic Acid (gal'-ik). Obtained from nutgall.

Gallon (gal'-on). A liquid measure equal in value to 8 pints, or 4 qts., or 32 gills, or 160 oz., or 1,280 drachms, or 76,800 minims. In the metric system it equals 4,000 c.c. (approx.).

Galvanism (gal'-van-izm). *See* Current.

Galvanometer (gal-van-om'-e-ter). An instrument for measuring an electrical current.

Galyl (gal'-il). A preparation of arsenic used for the treatment of syphilis. It is pre-

pared in three forms : **(1)** G. (simple), for intravenous injection in a concentrated form. Doses, 0·20, 0·25, 0·30, 0·35, 0·40 grm. (2) **G.** (with sodium carbonate), this is a soluble preparation like neo-salvarsan, and is administered intravenously in a diluted form dissolved in sterile water. Same dose, (3) **G.** (in oil emulsion), for intramuscular injection. Doses, 0·20, 0·30, 0·40 grm.

Gamgee (gam'-jē). A surgical dressing consisting of absorbent wool covered with a fine absorbent gauze mesh; used for many purposes in medicine and surgery, one of the best known and most useful of these being the pneumonia jacket. The tissue was first suggested and used by *Mr Joseph Sampson Gamgee* after whom it is named.

Ganglioma (gang-li-ō'-mä). A swelling consisting of lymphoid tissue.

Ganglion (gang'-li-on). (1) A mass of nerve tissue which receives and sends out nerve fibres ; *e.g.*, the ganglionic masses forming the sympathetic nervous system. (2) Cystic tumours developing on a tendon or aponeurosis ; sometimes occur on the back of the wrist due to strain such as excessive practice on the piano. (3) An enlarge-

159

ment on the course of a nerve such as is found on the receptor nerves before they enter the spinal cord. (4) An enlarged lymphatic gland.

Ganglionic (gang-li-on'-ik). Pertaining to a ganglion.

Gangrene (gang'-grēn). Death of a portion of the tissues of the body. Gangrene is the result of obstruction in the normal flow of blood to a part, thereby causing the death of the tissues. It may therefore be caused by (1) constriction and pressure, as by prolonged application of a tourniquet ; (2) embolism, infarcts, or diseases of the blood-vessels ; (3) the action of certain drugs such as ergot ; (4) extreme cold, affecting the fingers, toes, nose, and cheeks ; (5) very rarely the cause is unknown, and this is then known as *Idiopathic G.* ; (6) when gangrene is the result of extensive injuries it is called *Traumatic G.* Carbolic G., a form of gangrene resulting from indiscriminate use of a carbolic compress. Diabetic G., that which affects the fingers and toes as a complication of diabetes mellitus. Dry G., so-called when the tissues are depleted of blood, and in consequence become black, hard, and shrunken. Gas G., *see under* Gas. Hospital G., a type of gang-rene formerly rampant in overcrowded hospital wards due to inefficient antiseptic methods. Senile G., gangrene occurring in old persons. Wet G., the tissues are moist, rotten, and foul-smelling.

Gangrenous (gang'-gre-nus). Relating to gangrene.

Gargarisma (går-gå-ris'-må). A gargle.

Gargle (går'-gl). An antiseptic solution for washing the throat.

Gas. One of the three states of matter ; it retains neither volume nor shape when released. A number of the natural elements exist in the gaseous state at ordinary temperatures and pressures, but when the latter is increased the gas can be converted into liquid. G. Gangrene, a special form of gangrene caused by a bacillus producing gas bubbles in the tissues ; infection with the *Cl. welchii* group of anaerobic bacilli.

Gasserian Ganglion (gas-ēr'-i-an). The ganglion of the sensory root of the *trigeminal nerve* (fifth cranial).

Gastralgia (gas-tral'-ji-å). Pain in the stomach.

Gastrectomy (gas-trek-to-mi). Partial or complete removal of the stomach.

Gastric (gas'-trik). Relating to the stomach. **G. Juice**, the digestive juice secreted by the gastric glands.

Gastritis (gas-trī'-tis). Inflammation of the stomach.

Gastrocele (gas-trō-sēl). Hernia of the stomach.

Gastrocnemius (gas-trok-nē'-mi-us). The large two-headed muscle of the calf; it terminates in the *tendo Achilles*, which inserts in the os calcis of the heel; the muscle is innervated by the internal popliteal nerve; the function of the gastrocnemius is to raise the heel off the ground.

Gastroduodenostomy (gas-trō-dū-ō-den-os'-to-mi); the production of an artificial passage between the stomach and duodenum.

Gastro-enterostomy. Gastrojejunostomy (-en-te-ros'-to-mi. -je-joo-nos'-to-mi). An artificial communication between the stomach and jejunum of the small intestine.

Gastropexy (gas-trō-peks'-i). Surgical fixation of a displaced stomach by stitching.

Gastrophotography (gas-trō-fō-tog'-ra-fi). The technique of using the gastrophotor.

Gastrophotor (gas-trō-fō'-tor). An instrument designed to take photographs of the stomach wall in the living subject. It consists essentially of (1) two miniature steroscopic cameras attached to the distal end of a rubber

tube like a stomach-tube, and (2) a transformer. No lenses are used, but miniature pin-holes ensure that the cameras are properly focused under all conditions and that distortion is avoided. Each camera has four little films, each ¼ in. wide by ¾ in. long, placed behind four pairs of pinholes in such a way that with each exposure four pairs of stereoscopic photographs of the interior of the stomach are obtained. The insertion of the tube must be achieved without using any lubricant, such as glycerine, which might obscure the glass cylinder round the camera. The shutters of the camera are two sliding rings. Approximately 75% of the stomach wall can be photographed. The *light* consists of a special filament lamp, 5/16 in. in diameter, arranged between the cameras, and producing an instantaneous blue light of 12,000 candle-power in 1/120 second. The filament is burnt out at each exposure, but does not become hot.

Gastrophrenic (gas-trō-fren'-ik). Relating to the stomach and diaphragm.

Gastroplasty (gas-trō-plas'-ti). A plastic operation for the cure of hour-glass stomach (*q.v.*).

Gastroplication (gas-trō-plik-ā'-shun). An operation for the cure of dilated stomach by making a pleat in the wall by means of sutures.

Gastroptosis (gas-trop-tō'-sis). Falling of the stomach from its normal position.

Gastropylorectomy (gas-trō-pī-lor-ek'-to-mi). Excision of the pyloric end of the stomach.

Gastrorrhagia (gas-trō-rā'-ji-à). Bleeding from the stomach. *See* **Hæmatemesis.**

Gastrorrhaphy (gas-tror'-a-fi). Suturing the stomach.

Gastroscope (gas'-trō-skōp). An apparatus for examining the interior of the stomach.

Gastroscopy (gas-tros'-ko-pi). The procedure of using the gastroscope.

Gastrostaxis. *See* **Gastrorrhagia** and also **Hæmatemesis.**

Gastrostomy (gas-tros'-to-mi). An artificial opening into the stomach through the abdominal wall, used for introducing food into the stomach by means of a rubber tube in conditions of obstruction of the œsophagus commonly resulting from malignant growths, or from stricture due to the scar formation after burns and scalds, syphilitic lesions, swallowing of acids, etc.

Gastrotomy (gas-trot'-o-mi). A temporary opening into the stomach.

Gaucher's Splenomegaly (gow'-sher). A familial anæmia

characterized by histological changes in the reticulo-endothelial system. The enlarged spleen shows large cells distended with lipoid.

Gaultheria (gawl-thēr'-i-à). Oil of winter-green ; antipyretic and antirheumatic.

Gauze (gawz). A thin, loosely woven material used as a dressing for wounds. If used plain, it is sterilized by being subjected to great heat in an autoclave. Antiseptic gauze is impregnated with chemicals such as carbolic, iodoform (coloured yellow), double cyanide gauze (mauve), sal alembroth (sky-blue). Thin strips of gauze are also used for plugging cavities and for draining a wound.

Gavage (gav'-àzh). Forcible feeding with a stomach-tube.

Gelatine (jel'-a-tēn). A jelly-like substance obtained by boiling animal tissues such as cartilage, bone, etc. It is a protein substance, but since it does not contain certain essential amino-acids, notably tryptophane, it cannot serve as the sole source of protein ; but it is a wholesome food, especially valuable when it is desired to add variety to the diet as in soups or deserts.

Gelatinous (jel-at'-in-us). Resembling jelly.

Gelsemium (jel-sem'-i-um). A drug obtained from the root of the yellow jasmine ; is a powerful depressant of the motor parts of the spinal cord, and is therefore prescribed in tetanus, mania, and trigeminal neuralgia.

Gemmation (jem-ā'-shun). A method of reproduction by a process of budding.

General (jen'-er-ral). Not local ; diffused.

Generate (jen'-er-rāt). To give birth ; to reproduce.

Generation (jen-er-rā'-shun). (1) The act of giving life or reproducing. (2) An age or period.

Genetic (jen-et'-ik). (1) Relating to the origin or cause. (2) Congenital.

Genital (jen'-it-al). Pertaining to organs of generation.

Genitalia (jen-it-ā'-li-á). The organs of generation.

Genito-urinary (jen-it-ō-ū'-rin-a-ri). Pertaining to the reproductive and urinary organs.

Gentian (jen'-shi-an). The dried root of *Gentiana lutea*. The drug obtained is bitter, tonic, and stomachic. Dose : *Extract*, 2-8 gr. ; *infusion*, co. conc., 30-60 minims ; *tincture*, 30-60 minims.

Genu (jen-ū). The knee. **G.-pectoral Position**, a position sometimes adopted during labour, when the patient rests on her chest and knees. **G. Valgum**, knock-knee. **G. Varum**, bow leg.

Germ. A microscopic organism ; bacterium ; an ovum

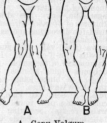

A, Genu-Valgum.
B, Genu-Varum.

or spore. **G. Cell**, the cells concerned with reproduction. **G. Plasm**, the protoplasm of the cell. **G. Theory**, the theory that all infectious diseases are caused by their particular germ.

Germicide (jer'-mi-sīd). An agent which will destroy germs.

Germination (jer-min-ā'-shun). The development of a seed of germ.

Gestation (jes-tā'-shun). Pregnancy. **G. Sac**, the contents of the pregnant uterus.

Gigantism (jī-gan'-tizm). An abnormal overgrowth due to disturbance of the pituitary gland. *See* **Acromegaly**.

Gill (jil). Quarter of a pint.

Gilliam's Operation. A method of correcting retroversion by shortening the round ligaments of the uterus.

Ginger (jin'-jer). The dried rhizome of *Zingiber officinale*; used for flavouring and as a carminative.

Gingiva (jin-jī-và). The gum.

Gingivitis (jin-jī-vī'-tis). Inflammation of the gums.

Ginglymus (ging'-gli-mus or jing-). A hinge joint, *e.g.*, the elbow and knee.

Girdle. A belt. **G. Pain,** a constricting pain round the waist region, occurring in tabetic persons. **Pelvic G.,** the bones of the pelvis. **Shoulder G.,** the girdle formed by the clavicles and scapulæ.

Glabrous (glā'-brus). Hairless, smooth.

Glacial (glā'-si-al). Resembling ice.

Gladiolus (glad-i-ō-lus). The middle piece of the sternum.

Glairy (glē'-ri). Slimy, albuminous.

Glaisher's Table. A table of figures by means of which the relative or percentage humidity of the atmosphere can be estimated from the readings of the wet and dry bulb thermometers.

Gland. An organ having the power of secreting and of abstracting certain substances from the blood and transforming them into matter of a different nature. The main kinds of glands are **Sweat G. (Sudoriferous G.),** secreting sweat. **Salivary G.,** in the region of the lower jaw; they secrete saliva. **Lymphatic G.,** these do not secrete, but are concerned with the purification of lymph. **Ductless** or **Endocrine G.,** a special group of glands whose secretion is discharged direct into the bloodstream and not through a duct. *See* **Endocrine.**

Glanders (glan'-ders). A contagious febrile disease communicable from horses to man.

Glans. The bulbous termination of the clitoris and penis.

Glauber's Salt (glaw'-ber's). Sodium sulphate; a purgative.

Glaucoma (glaw-kō'-mà). A disease of the eye characterized by swelling and hardening of the eyeball. Pain is severe, and blindness results unless the condition is relieved.

Gleet. A clear, watery discharge from the urethra, the result of chronic urethritis.

Glenoid (glē'-noid). A cavity on the scapula into which the head of the humerus fits to form the shoulder-joint.

Glioma (glī-ō'-mà). A malignant growth of the brain or cord, arising from the neuroglia.

Glisson's Capsule. The connective tissue sheath of the blood-vessels and bile ducts in the liver.

Globin (glō'-bin). A basic protein having the properties of a histone. One of the substances forming hæmoglobin.

Globulin (glob-ū-lin). One of the soluble proteins of the blood.

Globus Hystericus (glō'-bus histe'-rik-us). A feeling as if a ball forms in the throat; an hysterical manifestation.

Glomerulus (glom-e'-rū-lus). A coil of minute arterial capillaries in the capsule at the commencement of the uriniferous tubules of the kidney.

Glossal (glos'-al). Pertaining to the tongue.

Glossalgia (glos-al'-ji-à). Pain in the tongue.

Glossitis (glos'-ī-tis). Inflammation of the tongue.

Glossoplegia (glos-ō-plē-ji-à). Paralysis of the tongue, generally caused by cerebral hæmorrhage.

Glottis (glot'-is). The opening into the larynx between the arytenoid cartilages and the base of the epiglottis.

Glucose (gloo'-kōz). A monosaccharide with the chemical formula $C_6H_{12}O_6$. Synonyms, *Grape-sugar, Dextrose.* See **Carbohydrate.**

Gluteal (gloo'-tē-al). Relating to the buttock. G. Muscles, the gluteus *maximus, medius,* and *minimus.*

Gluten (gloo'-ten). The protein of cereals.

Glycerine (glis'-e-rin). The sweetish principle of oils and fats. It is odourless and colourless, and is used for many purposes in medicine.

Glycerophosphate (glis-e-rō-fos'-fāt). A salt of glycerophosphoric acid.

Glycogen (glī'-kō-jen). Animal starch found in the liver and muscles. A polysaccharide with the chemical formula $C_6H_{10}O_5$ multiplied many times.

Glycosuria (glī-kō-sū'-ri-à). The presence of sugar in the urine.

Gnathalgia (nāth-al'-ji-à). Pain in the jaw.

Gnathic (nā'-thik). Pertaining to the jaw.

Gnathoplasty (nā'-thō-plas-ti). Plastic operations on the jaw.

Goa Powder (gō'-à). Chrysarobin (*q.v.*).

Goitre (goi'-ter). Enlargement of the thyroid gland. **Cystic G.,** enlargement due to formation of cysts in the gland. **Adenomatous G.,** a general glandular enlargement occurring about the time of puberty or pregnancy. Also known as *Simple, Colloid,* or *Endemic G.* **Exophthalmic G.,** first described by Graves in 1835; the gland is enlarged and there is loss of weight, lassitude, tachycardia, tremor, dyspnœa, etc.; generally but not invariably there is *exophthalmos* or protrusion of the eyeballs. **Malignant G.**, carcinoma of the thyroid gland ; very rare.

Golden Ointment. A popular name for ointment of yellow oxide of mercury. Used in eye diseases. Synonym, *Ung. Hyd. Ox. Flav.*

Gold Treatment. Sanocrysin, used in the treatment of tuberculosis. It consists of gold sodium thio-sulphate. **G. Cure**, a method of treating alcoholism ; first, small quantities of the alkaloid daturine at 4-hourly intervals, four times per day for twelve days, is injected ; this is followed by small doses of atropine at gradually increasing intervals until only occasional doses are given ; a tonic mixture of gold chloride and cinchona bark is given in doses every 2 hours during the treatment.

Golgi Bodies (gol′-gi). A thread-like process seen in certain cells, particularly the glands ; it resembles a loosely tied knot.

Gonadectomy (gon-a-dek′-to-mi). Excision of the testes.

Gonads (gon′-ads). The organs of generation.

Gonococcus (gon-o-kok′-us). The micro-organism causing gonorrhœa.

Gonorrhœa (gon-or-rē′-à). An acute contagious inflammation of the genital tract

caused by the *gonococcus. See* **Ophthalmia Neonatorum.**

Gonorrhœal Ophthalmia. Same as *Ophthalmia Neonatorum.* **G. Arthritis**, arthritis of the joints associated with gonorrhœa. **G. Rheumatism**, the same as *G. Arthritis.*

Goodell's Law. When the cervix is as hard as one's nose, pregnancy is non-existent ; when it is as soft as one's lips, pregnancy is probable.

Gouge (gooj or gowj). A chisel with a hollow blade for cutting or boring holes in hard tissues such as bone.

Gout (gowt). A disease characterized by acute inflammation, swelling and pain of the joints, especially the big toe. The blood contains an excess of uric acid, and in time tends to form concretions around the joints. **Poor Man's G.**, a form of gout developing in poor persons, caused by insufficient food and alcoholism.

G.P.I. An abbreviation for General Paralysis of the Insane ; a progressive mental and moral deterioration, combined with paralysis, manifested in the late or quaternary stage of syphilis.

Graafian Follicles. *See* **Follicle.**

Graft. Transplantation of living tissues such as bone or skin. **Bone G.**, a piece of bone taken generally from the tibia and inserted elsewhere in the body to replace bone already lost. **Skin G.**, removal of small sections of skin to a raw, clean surface such as a large superficial burn. The whole thickness of the skin may be taken; this is known as a **Wolfe G.** When only the epidermis and a small amount of dermis is used it is a **Thiersch G. Ovarian G.**, implantation of a section of ovary into the muscles of the abdominal wall.

Grain (grān). 1/20 scruple, 1/60 drachm, 1/480 oz., etc.

Gram. The metrical unit of weight=15½ gr.; it is the weight of 1 ml. of water.

Gram's Method. A method of staining bacteria. All germs are not acted upon by this stain; those which retain it are called **G. Positive**, and those remaining unaffected are called **G. Negative**.

Granulation (gran-ū-lā'-shun). The appearance of small, rounded projections on the surface of a deep raw wound.

Granules (gran-ūlz). A small rounded body or grain; minute bodies sometimes seen in the protoplasm of tissue cells.

Granulocyte (gran'-ū-lō-sīt). Any cell containing granules, *e.g.*, a leucocyte with neutrophil, eosinophil or basophil granules in its cytoplasm.

Granuloma (gran-ū-lō'-mà). A tumour formed of granulation tissue.

Grape-sugar. Dextrose.

Gravel. A sandy deposit seen in the urine; the particles are very minute, but visible to the naked eye.

Gravid (grav'-id). Pregnant.

Gregory's Powder. A purgative powder compounded of rhubarb, ginger, and magnesia.

Grey. A colour between black and white. **G. Matter**, the cortex of the brain. **G. Oil**, an emulsion of mercury used for intramuscular injection for syphilis. **G. Powder**, a mixture of mercury and chalk 1-3, given to check infantile diarrhœa. Dose, 1-5 gr.

Grinders. The molars or double teeth.

Gripe (grīp). Acute pain caused by intestinal flatulence.

Groin. The junction of the thigh with the abdomen.

Growing-pains. Neuralgic pains in the limbs during youth, probably rheumatic in origin.

Guaiacol (gwī'-a-kol). A colourless oily liquid; much used in phthisis.

Guillotine (gil'-ō-tēn). A surgical instrument used for excision of the tonsils.

Gullet (gul'-et). The food pipe; anatomically known as the œsophagus.

Gum. (1) The edge of the jaws, including the alveolar processes. (2) Also a thick, viscid, amorphous substance obtained from certain trees. **G. Boil**, an abscess of the jaw.

Gumma (gum'-à). Pl. *gum-*

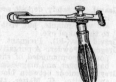

Tonsil Guillotine (or Tonsillotome).

mata. A firm tumour-like mass which constitutes the characteristic lesion of the tertiary stage of syphilis. It may occur anywhere in the body and is found most frequently in the sub-periosteal regions and in the liver and testis. It often ulcerates through the skin, the floor of the ulcer presenting a washleather appearance. It is only slightly infective as compared with the primary and secondary lesions.

Gurgling (gurg'-ling). A bubbling sound caused by the passage of air through a liquid.

Gustatory (gus-tā'-to-ri). Relating to the sense of taste. **G. Buds,** the taste-buds, *i.e.,* the specialized nerve-endings in the tongue which are concerned with the sense of taste.

Gut. The intestines.

Gutta (gut'-ä). A drop. **G.-**

percha, a juice obtained from certain trees, which, after passing through a special process, is used as a waterproof covering material.

Gutter-splint. A splint much used for fractures. It is made of tin or aluminium, and is hollowed out like a trough to fit the shape of the limb.

Gynæcologist (gī-ne-kol'-o-jist). A surgeon who specializes in gynæcology.

Gynæcology (gī-ne-kol'-o-ji). The word is derived from the Greek *gyne*, a woman, and *logus*, a discourse. It is the science which deals with diseases and disorders which are peculiar to women, having special reference to the organs of generation.

Gypsum (jip'-sum). Native calcium sulphate. The source of Plaster of Paris.

Gyrus (jī'-rus). A fold or convolution, as the convolution of the cerebral cortex.

H.

H. The symbol for hydrogen.

Habit (hab'-it). The establishment of certain actions, or the development of mental processes by constant repetition. Such actions are often carried out involuntarily, and are only acquired during the lifetime of the individual.

Habitat (hab'-it-at). The local-

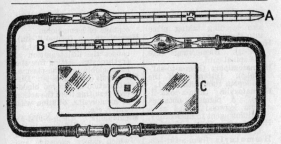

Hæmocytometer.

A, Pipette for white corpuscles count.
B, Pipette for red corpuscles count.
C, Counting chamber and cover glass.

ity where an animal or plant normally exists in the wild state ; a breeding-place or birth-place.

Hæmatemesis (hēm-a-tem′-e-sis). The vomiting of blood from the stomach. The blood is often stale, and therefore contains coagulated particles resembling coffee-grains. It is mixed with stomach contents, and shows an acid reaction if tested with litmus.

Hæmatin (hēm′-a-tin). An iron-containing constituent of hæmoglobin.

Hæmatite-miner's Lung (hēm′-a-tīt). Fibrosis of the lung, which is also rendered a brick-red colour as the result of the inhalation of red iron-ore dust. Like silicosis it predisposes to tuberculosis.

Hæmatocele (hē-mat′-ō-sēl). A swelling filled with blood.

Hæmatocyte (hē-mat′-ō-sīt). A blood-corpuscle.

Hæmatocytometer (hēm-a-tō-sī-tom′-e-ter). An apparatus designed for counting the number of blood-cells in a stated amount of blood.

Hæmatolysis (hēm-a-tol′-i-sis). The disintegration or destruction of the blood-cells.

Hæmatoma (hēm-a-tō′-mà). A tumour filled with blood.

Hæmatometra (hēm-a-tō-mē′-

trà). The retention of menstrual fluid within the uterus ; also bleeding taking place into the uterus.

Hæmatorrhachis (hēm-a-tō-răk′-is). Hæmorrhage into the spinal cord.

Hæmatosalpinx (hēm-a-tō-sal′-pinks). Distension of the Fallopian tube with blood.

Hæmatoxylin (hēm-a-toks′-il-in). A pigment obtained from logwood, used as a staining agent in microscopy.

Hæmatozoa (hēm-a-tō-zō′-á). Living parasites in the blood.

H æ m a t u r i a (hēm-a-tūr-i-á). The presence of blood in the urine.

Hæmidrosis (hēm-i-drō′-sis). Bloody sweat.

Hæmochromatosis (hēm-ō-krōm-a-tō′-sis). A rare disease in which brown pigmentation of the skin is associated with cirrhosis of the liver, diabetes, and the deposition of much iron pigment in the organs. Also known as "Bronzed Diabetes."

Hæmocytometer (hēm-ō-sī-tom′-et-er). An instrument for counting the number of blood corpuscles.

Hæmoglobin (hēm-ō-glō′-bin). The colouring matter contained in the red blood-corpuscles. It is composed of an iron-containing substance called hæmatin combined with globin.

Hæmoglobinometer (hēm-ō-glō-bin-om′-et-er). An instrument for estimating the percentage of hæmoglobin.

Hæmolysin (hēm-ō-lī′-sin). An organic substance which causes the disintegration of erythrocytes, setting free the hæmoglobin into the plasma.

Hæmolysis (hē-mol′-is-is). Disintegration of the red blood-cells resulting from the action of hæmolysins, dilution with water, etc.

Hæmophilia (hēm-ō-fil′-i-á). A congenital deficiency in the coagulability of the blood which causes excessive and protracted hæmorrhage from even minor injuries. It is hereditary, being "carried" by the female who is not the sufferer and is transmitted to the male who may suffer. It is probably due to lack of prothrombin in the blood.

Hæmopoiesis (hēm-ō-poi-ē′-sis). The production of blood, usually in the marrow. **Extra-medullary H.,** the production of blood from collections of red marrow cells outside of the bones.

Hæmopoietin (hēm-ō-poi-ē′-tin). The active principle in liver which is essential for the normal production of red blood corpuscles.

Hæmoptysis (hē-mop′-tis-is). Bleeding from the lungs. The blood is alkaline in reaction, frothy, and bright red.

Hæmorrhage (hem′-or-āj). The

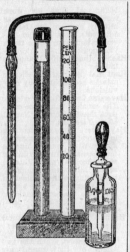

Hæmoglobinometer (Gower's).

escape of blood from a blood-vessel. **Arterial H.,** bleeding from an artery ; the blood is bright red and spurts out. **Venous H.,** the blood is a dark bluish colour and flows out. **Capillary H.,** the blood may be either bright or dark, and oozes rather than flows. **Primary H.,** that which occurs at the time of the injury. **Reactionary H.** occurs within 24 hours. **Secondary H.** occurs after 24 hours, usually between 7th and 10th day ; is always due to sepsis. The main symptoms of hæmorrhage are an *increasingly* rapid and feeble pulse, cold sweat, extreme pallor and restlessness, sighing respiration (air-hunger), thirst, nausea, failing vision.

Hæmorrhoids (hem'-or-roidz). Varicosity of the veins around the anus ; piles.

Hæmostasis (hēm-ō-stā'-sis). The arrest of hæmorrhage.

Hæmostatics (hēm-ō-stat'-iks). Agents which bring about hæmostasis. *See* **Styptic.**

Hæmothorax (hēm-ō-thawr'-aks). The presence of blood in the pleural cavity.

Hallucination (hal-oo-sin-ā'-shun). A false belief in sensations which have no actual foundation in fact ; generally associated with abnormal mental states. Such sensory disturbances may be either auditory, visual, tactile, etc.

Hallux (hal'-uks). The big toe. **H. Valgus,** displacement of the big toe away from the median line, *i.e.*, towards the other toes. **H. Varus,** displacement towards the median line.

Halogen (hal'-ō-jen). A group

171

of electro-negative chemical elements whose salts resemble those of the sea, *e.g.*, *bromine*, *chlorine*, *fluorine*, and *iodine*.

Ham. That part of the leg lying between the hip and knee-joint. **H.-strings**, the tendons of the muscles on the posterior aspect of the thigh.

Hamamelis (ham-a-mel'-is). A drug used as an astringent and styptic ; witch hazel.

Hammer Toe. A deformity in which there is dorsiflexion of the first phalanx, and plantar flexion of the second and third phalanges.

Hanot's Disease (han'-ō). Cirrhotic enlargement of the liver, associated with jaundice.

Haptophore (hap'-tō-fawr). That part of a toxin by which it is fixed and united to an antitoxin, and is thereby rendered inert. *See* Ehrlich's Theory.

Hard chancre. The primary sore of syphilis ; also known as the true Hunterian chancre.

Hare Lip. A congenital defect in the lip, a fissure extending from the margin of the lip to the nostril ; may be single or double, and is often associated with cleft palate.

Harlequin Fœtus. A fœtus born with ichthyosis.

Hartshorn. Aqua ammonia.

Harvey, William (1578-1657), of Folkestone ; discovered the circulation of the blood, and published his discovery in 1628. At first his work received scant notice and was bitterly opposed by Galen's adherents, but further investigation soon made truth victorious.

Hashish (hash'-ish). Cannabis indica.

Haut Mal (hō'-mal). Epileptic attacks accompanied by convulsions.

Haversian Canals (ha-ver'-si-an). The canals found in the compact tissue of bone. Named after *Haversius*.

Hay Fever. Coryza occurring in allergic persons possessing a sensitive nasal mucous membrane. Any irritating substance may precipitate an attack, but it most commonly occurs during the pollination of hay grasses. The symptoms are headache, malaise, and a streaming nasal catarrh.

Healing (hēl-ing). The natural repair of injured tissues ; occurs in two ways. (1) By *first intention*, when the two edges of the wound are exactly approximated and sutured. This method of healing leaves only a thin, clean scar without deformity ; is the type of healing aimed at by all surgeons, but is only possible when the strictest aseptic precautions are taken. (2) By *second intention* ; this occurs mostly in deep lacerated wounds which are already septic. Healing is by means of granulations.

Health. The normal state; freedom from disease.

Hearing. One of the special senses. Sound is interpreted by the brain, after receiving the sensation through the auditory nerve from the ear.

Heart. The hollow, muscular organ which pumps the blood through the body. Weighs 8-10 oz. in the female, and 10-12 oz. in males. **H.-block,** interference with the rhythm of contraction between the auricles and ventricles due to a lesion of the A.V. bundle; the block may be partial or complete. In the latter state, the ventricles beat independently of the auricles, with a rate of 15-30 beats per minute. **H.-burn,** a form of dyspepsia associated with a burning sensation in the stomach, and a rush of fluid with a sour, acid taste into the mouth. **H. Disease,** any abnormal state of the heart.

Heat (hēt). (1) The sensation of warmth. (2) A state of matter caused by molecular movement. The more rapid the motion, the hotter the body becomes, and these degrees of hotness are measured in terms of temperature. **Latent H.,** the amount of heat absorbed by a body,

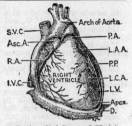

Pericardial Sac and Heart.

S.V.C., Superior vena cava.
Asc.A., Ascending aorta.
R.A., Right auricle.
I.V.C., Inferior vena cava.
P.A., Pulmonary artery.
L.A.A., Left auricular appendix.
P.P., Parietal pericardium (cut edge).
L.C.A., Left coronary artery (descending branch).
L.V., Left ventricle.
D., Diaphragm.

while changing its state from solid to liquid or liquid to gas, without showing any rise in temperature, e.g., during the conversion of ice into water, heat is used up, but the temperature does not rise until the whole of the ice has become converted into water. **Specific H.,** the relative amount of heat necessary to raise a given weight of a substance through 1° C., and the heat necessary to raise the same weight of water through 1° C. **H. Unit,** a calorie (*q.v.*).

Heb'erden's Disease. Angina pectoris. **H. Nodes,** rheumatic nodules of the small joints in arthritis deformans.

Hectic Fever. The typical fever of phthisis. The temperature rises at night and falls in the morning. **H. Flush,** the malar flush often seen in persons suffering from phthisis, and in some other diseases.

Hectogram (hek'-tō-gram). A hundred grams.

Hectolitre (hek'-tō-lē-ter). A hundred litres.

Hectometre (hek'-tō-mē-ter). A hundred metres.

Hedonism (hēd'-on-izm). A determined and exclusive pursuit of pleasure and the avoidance of pain.

Hegar's Sign. Compressibility of the soft uterine cervix noticed during bimanual examination. It is due partly to the softening of the cervix, and partly to the fact that the lower uterine segment is not filled by the embryo during the first two or three months of pregnancy.

Heliotherapy (hē-li-ō-the'-ra-pi). The treatment of disease by means of sunlight.

Heliotropism (hē-li-ō-trōp'-izm). The specific reaction of an organism towards the light,

e.g., the turning of a flower towards light. This is known as *heliotropistic action.*

Helix (hē'-liks). The outer rim of the pinna of the ear.

Heller's Test. A test for the presence of albumin in urine. *See* Appendix : Urine-testing.

Helminth (hel'-minth). A worm infesting the intestine.

Helminthagogue (hel-minth'-a-gog). Drugs which destroy intestinal worms.

Hemaralopia (hem-ar-al-ō'-pi-à). Night blindness.

Hemianopia (hem-i-an-ō'-pi-à). Blindness in one-half of the visual field.

Hemiatrophy (hem-i-at'-ro-fi). Atrophy of the tissues of one side of the body.

Hemicrania (hem-i-krān'-i-à). Unilateral headache. Imperfect development of half of the skull.

Hemidiaphoresis (hem-i-dī-a-for-ē'-sis). Unilateral sweating of the body.

Hemiplegia (hem-i-plē'-ji-à). Paralysis of one side of the body only.

Hemisphere (hem'-i-sfier). The half of a sphere. **Cerebral H.,** half of the cerebrum.

Hemlock (hem'-lok). *See* Conium.

Henbane (hen'-bān). *See* Hyoscyamus.

Henoch's Purpura (hē'-noks). A disease mainly affecting

children and paroxysmal in type. The main symptoms are a purpuric rash and bleeding from the mucous membranes associated with severe abdominal pain.

Hepar (hĕ'-pá(r)). The liver.

Hepatic (he-pat'-ik). Pertaining to the liver.

Hepatitis (hep-a-tī'-tis). Inflammation of the liver.

Hepatization (hep-a-tī-zā'-shun). Pathological changes in the tissues which cause them to resemble the liver. Thus the lung tissue in pneumonia passes first through the stage of red hepatization and later through grey hepatization.

Herbivorous (her-biv'-o-rus). Feeding only on plants and vegetables.

Heredity (he-red'-i-ti). The transmission of certain traits and characteristics from parents to their offspring. *See* **Chromosomes.**

Hermaphrodite (her-maf'-rō-dīt). An individual possessing the reproductive organs of both sexes. Although they may approximate either to the male or female type they are usually sterile through imperfect development of their gonads.

Hermetically (her-met'-ik-al-i). A term used in chemistry when sealing a tube, etc., to render it air-tight.

Hernia (her'-ni-á). The protrusion of any viscus from its normal surrounding structures. This generally occurs through a weakened spot, as the result of strain or injury such as a blow. **Cerebral H.,** protrusion of a portion of the brain through injury to the cranium. **Chronic H.,** one that has persisted for a long time without giving rise to acute symptoms. **Congenital**

Hernia Director.

H., a hernia which has existed before birth. **Crural H.,** *see* **Femoral H. Diaphragmatic H.,** the protrusion of an abdominal organ through the diaphragm ; usually the stomach or intestine. **Inguinal H.,** the passage of a loop of intestine through the inguinal canal. **Femoral H.,** a hernia descending below Poupart's ligament and through the femoral ring. **Incomplete Inguinal H.,** one in which the sac does not pass beyond the external abdominal ring. **Irreducible H.,** a hernia which cannot be reduced by manipulation. **Thoracic H.,** *see* **Diaphragmatic H. Strangulated H.,** a hernia which is tightly constricted at its neck so that

175

its circulation is interfered with and gangrene results if the condition is not relieved by operation. **Ventral H.,** hernia of a loop of intestine through a weakened part of the abdominal wall, such as a scar.

Herniotome (her'-ni-o-tŏm). A special knife with a blunt tip used for hernia operations.

Herniotomy (her-ni-ot'-o-mi). The operation for the division of the constricting band of a strangulated hernia, so that it can be reduced.

Heroic (he-rō'-ik). Venturesome, risky, drastic; applied to severe measures which may cure the condition, or on the contrary may terminate fatally.

Heroin (he'-rō-in). A derivative of morphine; depresses the respiratory centre and so allays cough. Dose, 1/25-1/8 gr.

Herpes (her'-pēz). Vesicular eruptions due to a virus infection. H. Febrilis, H. Labialis, inflammatory vesicles on lips, nose, or mouth which occur in febrile conditions such as the common cold or pneumonia. H. Zoster, *shingles*; herpes along the course of a nerve, usually the intercostals. Pain is severe and of the neuralgic type. Crops of vesicles occur which may be discrete or may coalesce. It is generally

unilateral, but may be bilateral.

Herpetic (her-pet'-ik). Relating to herpes.

Herpetiform (her-pet'-i-fawm). Resembling herpes.

Heterogeneous (het-e-rō-jē'-ni-us). Differing in type or nature; of a miscellaneous character.

Heterogenesis (het-e-rō-jen'-e-sis). The production of a living organism which bears no resemblance to its parents.

Heterophoria (het-e-rō-faw'-ri-à). Defective parallelism between the two lines of vision, caused by fatigue of the ocular muscles.

Hexagon (heks'-a-gon). Having six sides and six angles; a six-sided figure.

Hexamethylenetetramine (heks'-a-meth-e-lēn-tet'-ra-mēn). A colourless, crystalline drug commercially sold as *urotropine*. It is a urinary and spinal fluid antiseptic. Other names for it are *cystamine*, *hexamine*, and *hexamethylenamine*.

Hexose (heks'-ōz). A class of simple sugars belonging to the monosaccharide group. They contain six carbon atoms to their molecules.

Hibernation (hī-ber-nā'-shun). The process of sleeping through the cold winter months, a mode of behaviour followed by many animals.

Hiccup (hi'-kup). An involuntary spasm of the respiratory organs consisting in a quick inspiratory movement of the diaphragm ending in a sudden closure of the glottis with the production of a characteristic sound.

Hidrosis (hid-rō'-sis). Sweat secretion.

Hilum (hi'-lum). A depression on the inner or under surface of an organ where vessels, ducts, etc., enter and leave.

Hip. The upper part of the thigh. *Hip joint*—the joint formed by the articulation of the head of the femur with the acetabulum in the innominate bone.

Hippocrates (hi-pok'-ra-tēz). Famous Greek doctor and philosopher who worked in the school at Cos. Born 460 B.C. Is known as the "Father of Medicine."

Hippuria (hi-pūr'-i-à). An excess of hippuric acid in the urine.

Hirsute (her'-sūt). Hairy or shaggy.

Hirudin (hī-roo'-din). A substance secreted in the head of a leech which prevents the coagulation of blood.

Hirudo (hī-roo'-dō). The leech.

His, Bundle of. A bundle of specialized tissue passing from the right auricle to the ventricles of the heart. Also called (1) the auriculo-

ventricular tract, or the A.V. bundle ; (2) Kent's bridge.

Histology (his-tol'-o-ji). The science dealing with the microscopic study of tissues.

Histolysis (his-tol'-is-is). The disintegration of organic tissue.

Hobnail Liver. *See* **Cirrhosis of Liver.** Also known as gin-drinker's liver.

Hodgkin's Disease (hoj'-kinz). A disease characterized by multiple lymphatic enlargements. Synonyms, *Lymphadenoma* and *Pseudoleukæmia*.

Homatropine (hŏm-at'-rō-pēn). An alkaloid obtained from tropine and allied to atropine; used in 1% solution of its hydrobromide it causes dilatation of the pupil.

Homeopathy (hŏm-i-op'-ath-i). A method of treating disease by prescribing minute doses of drugs, which in maximum dose would produce the symptoms of the disease. First adopted by Hahnemann.

Home-sickness. Nostalgia, longing for home.

Homicidal (hom-i-sī'-dal). (1) The state of being a homicide. (2) Pertaining to or having a tendency to homicide.

Homicide (hom'-i-sīd). Manslaughter, murder ; a murderer.

Homogeneous (hom-ō-jē'-ni-us). Having a like nature.

Homosexuality (hom-ō-seks-ū-al'-it-i). Attraction between persons of the same sex.

Hook-worm. *See* **Ankylostoma Duodenale.**

Hordeolum (haw-dē'-ō-lum). A stye ; a furuncle on the eyelid.

Hormone (haw(r)'-mōn). The internal secretion of a gland which, when passed into the blood-stream, excites activity in some distant organ or gland, *e.g.*, *pituitrin, thyroxin, adrenalin.*

Hormopoietic System (haw(r)-mō-poi-et'-ik). The glands and tissues which are concerned in the elaboration of hormones.

Horseshoe Kidney. A congenital malformation in which the two kidneys are joined by a bridge at their lower poles ; is generally situated nearer the median line than is normal.

Host (hōst). The organic structure upon which parasites thrive.

Hour-glass Contraction. Excessive and irregular contraction of the parturient uterus during the third stage of labour. The placenta is imprisoned in the upper part of the uterus by a tightly constricting band between the upper and lower uterine segments. **H. Stomach,** a condition in which the stomach is divided by a fibrous con-

178

striction ; generally associated with gastric ulcer.

Housemaid's Knee. Inflammation of the bursa over the patella ; pre-patellar bursitis.

Houston's Folds. Three oblique folds in the mucous lining of the rectum.

Humerus (hū'-me-rus). The bone of the upper arm ; that

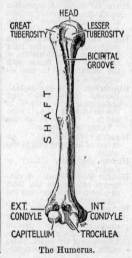

The Humerus.

which lies between the elbow and shoulder-joint.

Humid (hū'-mid). Moist.

Humidity (hū-mid'-it-i). (1) Moisture. (2) The amount of moisture in the atmosphere. This is measured by the " wet and dry bulb " thermometer. (To estimate the relative humidity, *see* **Glaisher's Table**.)

Humor (hū'-mer). Any fluid of the body. **Aqueous H.,** the fluid in the anterior chamber of the eye, between the iris and the cornea. **Vitreous H.,** the jelly-like substance filling the interior of the eyeball.

Humoral (hū-mor-ral). Pertaining to the body fluids. **H. Pathology,** the teaching which ascribes all disease to alterations in the fluids of the body.

Hunterian Chancre. The hard chancre or primary syphilitic sore.

Hutchinson's Teeth. A deformity of the teeth, particularly the upper central incisors, which are short, narrow, peg-shaped, and notched at their cutting edge; said to be a sign of congenital syphilis; peg-top teeth.

Hyaline (hī'-a-lin). Like glass; transparent. **H. Cartilage,** a variety of cartilage having a glass-like appearance.

Hyaloid (hī'-a-loid). Resembling hyaline, *e.g.,* the hyaloid

membrane which encloses the vitreous humor of the eye.

Hydatid (hī-dat'-id). A cystic tumour, caused by infestation with the larvæ of the *Tœnia echinococcus,* a species of tapeworm. The cysts are commonest in the liver and lungs. *See* **Tapeworm**. **H. of Morgagni,** a small cystic embryonic remnant attached to the Fallopian tube or epididymis.

Hydatidiform (hī-da-tid'-i-fawm). Pertaining to or resembling a hydatid. **H. Mole,** *see* **Mole**.

Hydnocarpus Oil (hīd-nō-kå(r)'-pus). The oil expressed from the seeds of trees (*Hydnocarpus wightiana,* and *h. anthelmintica,* etc.) belonging to the botanical family *Bixaceæ,* to which also belongs the Chaulmoogra tree. It is used principally in the treatment of leprosy.

Hydræmia (hī-drē'-mi-å). A watery condition of the blood.

Hydragogue (hī-drå-gog). A purgative which causes excessively watery evacuations of the intestines, *e.g.,* colocynth, croton oil, and jalap.

Hydramnios (hī-dram'-ni-os). An excessive amount of amniotic fluid.

Hydrargyrate (hī-drå(r)'-ji-råt). Relating to or containing mercury.

Hydrargyria (hī-drå(r)-jī'-ri-å). Mercurial poisoning.

Hydrargyrum (hī-drá(r)'-ji-rum). Mercury or quicksilver. *See* **Mercury.**

Hydrastis (hī-dras'-tis). A drug obtained from the dried root of *Hydrastis canadensis* or *golden seal plant.* Its action is stomachic and nerve stimulant, and is also used locally as an astringent in rectal and uterine hæmorrhage. Dose: Liq. extract, 5-15 minims; tincture, 30-60 minims.

Hydrate (hī-drāt). The combination of a chemical substance with water; hydroxide.

Hydration (hī-drā'-shun). The process by which a chemical substance combines with water.

Hydraulics (hī-draw'-liks). The science which deals with the behaviour of fluids while in motion.

Hydro (hī'-drō). A prefix signifying the presence of hydrogen or water.

Hydrocarbon (hī-drō-ká(r)'-bon). A chemical compound consisting of hydrogen and carbon.

Hydrocele (hī'-drō-sēl). An encysted serous effusion in the tunica vaginalis of the testis, or in connection with the spermatic cord.

Hydrocephalus (hī-drō-kef'-a-lus). An excess of cerebrospinal fluid inside the skull. The common and important type is the internal hydro-

cephalus in which one or more of the ventricles is dilated. It may be due to excessive production but is most frequently due to obstruction to the normal circulation of the fluid by tumours, etc., which thus interferes with the reabsorption of the fluid into the venous system.

Hydrochloric Acid (hī-drō-klor'-ik) (HCl). A normal constituent of the gastric juice; is formed in the oxyntic cells of the stomach and (1) acidifies the stomach contents; (2) activates pepsinogen, converting it into pepsin; (3) stops the action of saliva on sugar by rendering ptyalin inert; (4) relaxes the pyloric sphincter; (5) is slightly antiseptic. *See* **Achlorhydria** and **Hyperchlorhydria.**

Hydrocyanic Acid (hī-drō-sī-an'-ik). *See* **Prussic Acid.**

Hydrogen (hī'-drō-jen). A colourless, odourless gas; the lightest of all known chemical elements, having an atomic weight of 1. **H. Peroxide** (H_2O_2), a valuable antiseptic fluid; it acts by liberating an atom of oxygen, and effervesces in the presence of pus.

Hydrolysis (hī-drol'-is-is). The decomposition of water in which the two constituents (H and OH) are separated and fixed in distinct compounds ; the conversion of starch into sugar during digestion is brought about through hydrolysis.

Hydrolytic (hī-drŏ-lit'-ik). Relating to hydrolysis.

Hydrolyze (hī'-drŏ-līz). To cause a chemical change through hydrolysis.

Hydroma (hī-drŏ'-má). A cystic tumour filled with watery fluid.

Hydrometer (hī-drom'-e-ter). An instrument for determining the density of fluids.

Hydrometra (hī-drŏ-mēt'-rá). A collection of watery fluid within the uterus.

Hydrometry (hī-drom'-et-ri). The method of determining the specific gravity of fluids by means of a hydrometer.

Hydronephrosis (hī-drŏ-ne-frŏ'-sis). Distension of the pelvis and calyces of the kidney with urine.

Hydropathy (hī-drop'-ath-i). The treatment of diseases by means of water, e.g., cold baths, etc.

Hydropericardium (hī-drŏ-pe-ri-kár'-di-um). A collection of fluid in the pericardium.

Hydroperitoneum (hī-drŏ-pe-ri-to-nē'-um). The presence of fluid within the peritoneal cavity.

Hydrophobia (hī-drŏ-fŏ'-bi-á). An acute infectious disease caused by the bite of mad animals such as dogs or

wolves. The disease is transmitted by the saliva, and the virus enters the subcutaneous tissues of the bitten victim. The symptoms are increased salivation, spasm of the throat and respiratory muscles, extreme fear and mental disturbance, aversion to fluids, and the patient may try to bite other persons. Synonym, *Rabies*.

Hydrops (hī'-drops). Dropsy.

Hydrosalpinx (hī-drŏ-sal'-pinks). Distension of the Fallopian tube with watery fluid.

Hydrostatics (hī-drŏ-stat'-iks). The science which deals with the physics of liquid while in a state of rest. **H. Test**, floating the lungs of a dead infant in water as proof that it once lived.

Hydrothorax (hī-drŏ-thaw'-raks). The presence of fluid in the pleural cavity.

Hydrous (hī'-drus). Containing water.

Hydruria (hī-drū'-ri-á). The passage of a profuse quantity of watery urine with a low specific gravity.

Hygiene (hī'-jēn). The science which deals with the prevention of disease and the best means of maintaining health, by drinking pure water, obtaining suitable food and clothing, and living in sanitary surroundings, etc.

Named after *Hygieia*, the Goddess of Health.

Hygienic (hī-jĕ'-nik). Pertaining to hygiene; sanitary.

Hygroma (hī-grō'-mà). A cystic tumour containing fluid.

Hygrometer (hī-grom'-et-er). An apparatus for measuring the amount of humidity in the atmosphere. *See* **Humidity**.

Hygroscope (hī'-grō-skōp). An instrument which indicates without actually measuring the degree of humidity of the atmosphere.

Hygroscopic (hī-grō-skop'-ik). Having the property of absorbing moisture, *e.g.*, glycerine is hygroscopic when injected into the bowel in the form of an enema.

Hymen (hī'-men). A membranous structure which stretches across the entrance to the vagina. It has an opening through which the menstrual fluid can escape, and this outlet may be crescentic or round; or there may be a number of small holes, and it is then called a **Pepper-pot H.** The membrane may be absent at birth, or torn by injury or accident. Normally it is ruptured during coitus.

Hyoid (hī'-oid). The name given to a V-shaped bone at the root of the tongue.

Hyoscine (hī'-ŏ-sēn). An alkaloid of hyoscamus. A powerful cerebral sedative.

A useful narcotic in cases of acute mania. Also used as a means of lessening pain during labour. Synonym, *Scopolamine*. Dose: Hyos. Hyd., gr. 1/200-1/100.

Hyoscyamus (hī-ŏ-sī'-a-mus). A drug obtained from the leaves and flowers of *Hyoscyamus niger*. The chief alkaloids are (1) *hyoscyamine*; (2) *hyoscine*. Its action is mydriatic, and sedative in irritability of the bladder.

Hyper. The opposite of *hypo*; excessive; above or increased.

Hyperacidity (hī-per-ra-sid-it-i). Excessive acid secretion in the stomach, especially in conditions associated with gastric and duodenal ulcers. *See* **Hyperchlorhydria**.

Hyperæmia (hī-per-rē'-mi-à). Engorgement of the tissues with blood. **Active H.**, caused by an excessive flow of blood *to* a part. **Passive H.**, restriction of the flow of blood *from* a part. *See also* Bier's **Hyperæmia**.

Hyperæsthesia (hī-per-res-thēz'-i-à). Excessive sensitiveness of a part.

Hypercapnia (hī-per-kap'-ni-à). An excessive amount of CO_2 in the blood.

Hyperchlorhydria (hī-per-klor-hī'-dri-à). The presence of an excessive amount of hydrochloric acid in the gastric juice.

Hyperemesis Gravidarum (hī-per-re-mḗ-sis grav-id-ar´-um). The toxic vomiting of pregnancy; is characterized by rapid pulse, furred tongue, incessant vomiting, emaciation, rise in temperature, and albuminuria.

Hyperextension (hī-per-reks-ten´-shun). Extreme extension

Hyperglycæmia (hī-per-glī-sē´-mi-à). An excessive amount of sugar in the blood. Normally the blood sugar varies between the limits of 0·1-0·15 grams per 100 c.c.

Hyperhidrosis (hī-per-hī-drō´-sis). Excessive perspiration. Also **Hyperidrosis**.

Hyperinvolution (hī-per-rin-vo-loo´-shun). An excessive degree of uterine involution.

Hyperlactation (hī-per-lak-tā´-shun). Lactation continued after the ninth month.

Hypermetropia (hī-per-me-trō´-pi-à). Long-sightedness caused by faulty accommodation of the eye, with the result that the light rays are focused beyond instead of on the retina.

Hypernormal (hī-per-naw´-mal). Above normal.

Hyperonychia (hī-per-ro-nik´-i-à). Excessive growth of the nails.

Hyperphoria (hī-per-faw´-ri-à). A condition in which the visual axis of one eye is raised above that of the other.

Hyperpiesis (hī-per-pī-ē´-sis). An elevation of the normal blood-pressure.

Hyperpituitarism (hī-per-pit-ū´-it-ar-izm). An increased activity of the pituitary gland resulting in **Gigantism** or **Acromegaly** (*q.v.*).

Hyperplasia (hī-per-plā´-zi-à). Overgrowth of the tissues, by an increase in the number of cells.

Hyperpnœa (hī-per-(p)nē´-à). Abnormally rapid, deep, or loud breathing; panting or gasping.

Hyperpyretic (hī-per-pī-ret´-ik). Relating to hyperpyrexia.

Hyperpyrexia (hī-per-pī-reks´-i-à). Excessively high fever, characterized by a body temperature of 105° F. or over.

Hypersecretion (hī-per-se-krē´-shun). Excessive glandular secretion.

Hypertension (hī-per-ten´-shun). Increased tension of a part, particularly with reference to fluids, such as blood or cerebrospinal fluid, when these exert increased pressure upon their membranous structures.

Hyperthyroidism (hī-per-thī´-roid-izm). An abnormal condition resulting from an oversecretion of the thyroid gland.

Hypertonia (hī-per-tōn´-i-à). Increased tone in a muscular structure; great tonicity or tenseness.

Hypertonic (hī-per-ton´-ik). (1) Relating to hypertonia. (2)

Pertaining to saline : containing a greater concentration of salts than normal physiological fluid, thereby exerting a greater osmotic pressure than that of blood or lymph.

Hypertrophy (hī-per-trof'-ĭ). Abnormal increase in the size of tissues or structures, by an increase in the size of each individual cell element. **Cardiac H.,** an increased thickness of the myocardial walls, due to increased work following disease of the valves or of the arterial system. *See* **Compensation.**

Hypnosis (hip-nō'-sĭs). The state of being hypnotized ; abnormal sleep.

Hypnotic (hip-not'-ĭk). (1) Pertaining to hypnotism. (2) A drug having the action of inducing sleep.

Hypnotism (hip'-nō-tizm). An abnormal mental state in which a condition resembling sleep is produced either *voluntarily*, by gazing fixedly at a bright object, etc., or *artificially*, by means of suggestion. A method of dealing with psychoneurosis, much advocated by Charcot, and later adopted by Freud, who afterwards discarded it for psycho-analysis. *See* **Braidism.**

Hypo (hī'-pō). A Latin prefix signifying beneath or below.

Hypochlorhydria (hī-pō-klor-hī'-

dri-ȧ). Deficiency of hydrochloric acid in the gastric juice.

Hypochondriac (hī-pō-kon'-dri-ak). (1) A person suffering from hypochondriasis. (2) The region of the abdomen on either side of the epigastric region, *i.e.,* the area immediately covered by the lower ribs.

Hypochondriasis (hī-pō-kon-drī'-a-sĭs). An abnormal mental state in which there is extreme anxiety about the state of the health, minor symptoms being magnified to serious diseases in the mind of the patient.

Hypodermic (hī-pō-der'-mĭk). Beneath the dermis. The

Hypodermic Syringe.

subcutaneous injection of a drug by means of a small special syringe.

Hypodermoclysis (hī-pō-der-mō-klĭ'-sĭs). The introduction of normal saline solution into the subcutaneous tissues by means of needles inserted under the skin. The fluid is injected continuously at the rate of 60 drops per minute, and at a temperature of 120° F.

Hypogastric (hī-pō-gas'-trĭk).

Pertaining to the hypogastrium.

Hypogastrium (hī-pō-gas´-tri-um). That area of the anterior abdomen which lies immediately below the umbilical region. It is flanked on either side by the iliac fossæ.

Hypoglossal (hī-pō-glos´-al). Situated beneath the tongue.

Hypoglycæmia (hī-pō-glī-sē´-mi-à). Deficiency of blood sugar.

Hypophoria (hī-pō-faw´-ri-à). A state in which the visual axis of one eye is lower than the other.

Hypophosphite (hī-pō-fos´-fīt). Any salt of hypophosphorous acid. Sometimes combined with quinine and strychnine and dissolved in syrup, and is then known as **Syrup of H.**

Hypophysis Cerebri (hī-pof´-is-is). The small oval-shaped gland lying in the sella turcica of the sphenoid bone, and connected to the undersurface of the brain by a stalk. Same as the *Pituitary Gland.*

Hypopiesis (hī-pō-pī-ē´-sis). Lowered arterial tension.

Hypopituitarism (hī-pō-pit-ū´-it-ar-izm). An abnormal state caused by insufficient secretion of the pituitary gland.

Hypopyon (hī-pō´-pi-on). A collection of pus in the anterior chamber of the eye, *i.e.*, in the space between the iris and cornea.

Hypospadias (hī-pō-spā´-di-as). A congenital malformation of the male urethra, whereby the external opening is on the under-surface of the penis.

Hypostasis (hī-pō-stā-sis). (1) A deposit or sediment. (2) Passive congestion of a part, *e.g.*, *hypostatic pneumonia* occurs in the dependent part of the lung in weakly or elderly patients, and is often the cause of death after accidents or injuries, due to prolonged lying in the dorsal position.

Hypothenar Eminence (hī-pō-thē-nà(r)). The eminence on the ulnar side of the palm below the little finger.

Hypothyroidism (hī-pō-thī´-roid-izm). A group of symptoms caused by insufficient thyroid secretion. *See* Cretinism and Myxœdema.

Hypotonia (hī-pō-tōn´-i-à). Deficiency or lowering of muscular tone.

Hypotonic (hī-pō-ton´-ik). Having a low osmotic pressure or a low tension. *See* Hypertonic.

Hysterectomy (his-ter-rek´-to-mi). The operation of removal of the uterus. Commonly employed for cancer, but also indicated for large fibroid growths, etc. Two main methods of removal:

(1) **Abdominal H.**, the more usual route, *via* a lower abdominal incision. (2) **Vaginal H.**, through the vault of the vagina. **Pan H.**, *see* Total H. **Sub-total H.**, removal of the body of the uterus but leaving the cervix in the vaginal vault. **Total H.**, complete removal of the body and cervix of the uterus. **Wertheim's H.**, total removal of the uterus, the adjacent lymphatic vessels and glands, and also a cuff of the vagina ; an extremely serious operation, and only performed for cancer.

Hysteria (his-tēr´-i-à). An abnormal nervous condition associated with lack of self-control and convulsive attacks. It is due to a psychoneurosis which may manifest itself in many different ways. Thus it may simulate almost any disease, and aphonia and paralyses are common symptoms.

Hysterics (his-te´-riks). Attacks of hysteria. The term is usually applied to noisy screaming fits in persons who lack control of their emotions.

Hystero-oophorectomy (his-te-rŏ-ō-ō-for-ek´-to-mi). Removal of the uterus and ovaries.

Hysteropexy (his-te-rŏ-peks´-i). Fixation or suturing of the uterus to the anterior abdominal wall in order to prevent prolapse.

Hysterotomy (his-te-rot´-o-mi). Making an incision into the uterus.

I.

I. Chemical symbol for *iodine*.

Ice. Frozen water. **I.-bag** or **I.-cap**, a rubber bag with a metal screw-top. The bag is filled three-quarters full of small pieces of ice ; salt is added to lower the melting-point of the ice. After expelling the air, the metal cap is firmly screwed on. When applying, the bag is suspended from the top of the bed or from a cradle, so that the full weight does not rest upon the affected part. A piece of lint is inserted between the cap and skin to prevent frost-bite. **I. Compress**, a piece of linen or lint wrung out of ice-water and renewed frequently. **I. Poultice**, a piece of gutta-percha tissue double the size required is chosen. On one half is placed a layer of linseed, and on top of this a layer of small pieces of ice ; salt is now sprinkled over. The remaining half of the tissue is folded over the top, and the edges are sealed with turpentine or chloroform. The poultice, being light in weight, rests on the skin, with a protecting piece of lint between. **I. Cradle**, a perforated zinc tray suspended above the body of the patient by a cradle. A thick layer of flannel is placed at the bottom of the tray, and on this the ice rests; salt is again sprinkled liberally. **I. Coils**, see Leiter's Coils.

Ichor (ï'-kor). The thin fœtid discharge from ulcers.

Ichthyol (ik'-thi-ol). An oily brown fluid prepared by distilling bitumen containing the fossil remains of fish; used externally as a sedative and antiseptic in various inflammatory states.

Ichthyosis (ik-thi-ō'-sis). A disease mainly characterized by dryness, scaliness, and thickening of the epidermis; is non-infectious. Also called *fish-skin disease*.

Icterus (ik'-te-rus). Jaundice. **I. Gravis**, jaundice characterized by marked cerebral disturbance and by extensive necrosis of the liver.

Icterus Index. A measure of the degree of jaundice by a comparison of the depth of yellowness of the serum with a fixed standard.

Icterus Neonatorum (ik'-te-rus nē-ō-na-taw'-rum). The jaundice occurring in the newly born child. It is unimportant, and clears up in a few days. Occasionally, however, a severe and fatal type develops, due either to sepsis or syphilis or to a congenital abnormality of the bile ducts or of the blood.

Idea (I-dē'-à). A mental image; a conception.

Ideation (I-di-ā'-shun). The process of forming an idea.

Idée Fixe (ē-dā fēks). Having a fixed idea upon some particular point; an obsession.

Ideo-motor (I-di-ō-mō'-tor). The association of movement with ideation.

Identification (I-dent-i-fi-kā'-shun). Psychologically this is a variety of day-dream in which the individual identifies himself with the hero of a play, book, or film.

Idiocy (id'-i-ō-si). Severe form of mental deficiency. *See* **Insanity**.

Idiopathic (id-i-ō-path'-ik). Of unknown cause; primary; spontaneous. **I. Anæmia**, pernicious anæmia.

Idiosyncrasy (id-i-ō-sin'-kra-sï). A peculiarity of constitution which renders an individual susceptible to a specific drug or mode of treatment, while others are not affected.

Idiot (id'-i-ot). A person with a lowered mental intelligence; an imbecile.

Ignipuncture (ig-ni-pungkt-ūer or -sher). A method of treat-

187

ment consisting of puncturing the tissues with a hot needle.

Ileitis (īl-ē-ī'-tis). Inflammation of the ileum.

Ileum (īl'-ē-um). The lower three-fifths of the small intestine lying between the jejunum and the cæcum.

Ileus (īl'-ē-us). Intestinal obstruction accompanied by severe pain, vomiting, and other symptoms.

Iliac (il'-i-ak). Pertaining to the ilium.

Ilium (il'-i-um). The upper part of the innominate bone.

Illusion (il-loo'-zhun). A false perception, *i.e.*, a wrong interpretation placed upon a sensation, *e.g.*, a person might scream with fear on touching a cold, raw potato in the dark, mistaking it for a snake.

Image (im'-āj). A picture of an event or object as perceived by the eye or mind.

Imagery (im'-a-je-ri). Imagination ; calling up events or mental pictures. Mental imagery may be of various types, viz. : **Auditory I.,** when sounds can be recalled to mind, *e.g.*, the dash of waves on the seashore, the roar of a train, the rush of the wind, etc. **Motor I.,** when movement only is recalled, *e.g.*, the curling crests of the waves as they break on the shore ; in this case no sound is heard. **Taste I.** and **Smell**

I. are often very weak. **Tactile I.,** when the feel of an object can be readily recalled. **Visual I.,** this is probably the commonest type of imagery, and a vivid mental picture is obtained. Different persons vary greatly in their mental imagery, and generally do not possess all the types, but rather one is more fully developed than the others.

Imago (i-mā'-gō). The full-fledged mature insect when its metamorphosis is completed.

Imbecile (im'-be-sēl). Mentally feeble.

Imbibition (im-bib-ish'-un). The absorption of fluids.

Immobility (im-mō-bil'-it-i). The state of being fixed.

Immobilization (im-mō-bil-ī-zā'-shun). The process of procuring immobility.

Immunity (im-mūn'-i-ti). The state of being free from the risk of infection. **Active I.,** immunity produced by the introduction of the virus, bacteria, or toxin into the blood which is thus enabled to form its own antitoxin. **Acquired I.,** immunity gained from having once had an attack of the disease or by the processes of active or passive immunisation. **Natural I.,** the resistance to disease with which the individual is born. **Passive I.,**

188

immunity conferred by the injection of serum from an animal (or man) previously actively immunized, *i.e.*, the antitoxic or antibacterial bodies are introduced ready made.

Immunization (im-mū-ni-zā'-shun). The act of rendering immune.

Impaction (im-pak'-shun). The process of being wedged or pressed together.

Impalpable (im-pal-pa-bl). Not capable of being felt.

Imperforate (im-perf'-or-āt). Without an opening; not pervious. I. Hymen, one which has no natural outlet for the menstrual fluid. I. Anus, absence of an opening into the rectum.

Impetigo (im-pe-tī'-gō). An acute inflammatory skin affection characterized by pustules and scab formation. I. Contagiosa, a contagious form of impetigo.

Implantation (im-plan-tā'-shun). The act of putting in or grafting of tissues such as skin, tendon, or nerves; also the introduction of various drugs into the subcutaneous tissues.

Impotence (im'-pō-tens). Lack of power or desire for sex intercourse.

Impregnate (im-preg'-nāt). To render fertile; to fertilize an ovum with a spermatozoa; to make pregnant.

Inanimate (in-an'-im-āt). Dead not alive.

Inanition (in-an-ish'-un). Wasting and exhaustion from insufficient nourishment.

Inarticulate (in-ár-tik'-ū-lāt). (1) Unable to express one's ideas in words. (2) Without joints.

In Articulo Mortis. At the point of death.

Inassimilable (in-as-sim'-il-a-bl). Not capable of absorption.

Incarcerated (in-kár'-se-rā-ted). Imprisoned, *e.g.*, I. Uterus, when the gravid uterus is imprisoned beneath the promontory of the sacrum, so that it cannot rise into the abdomen.

Incest (in'-sest). Sexual intercourse between persons who are closely related.

Incipient (in-sip'-i-ent). Beginning.

Incision (in-sizh'-un). The act of cutting with a sharp instrument such as a scalpel.

Incisors (in-sī'-sorz). The eight front cutting teeth, four in the upper jaw and four in the lower jaw.

Inclusion (in-kloo'-zhun). The condition of being confined or enclosed.

Incoherent (in-kō-hier'-rent). Not connected or clear; confused.

Incompatible (in-kom-pat'-ibl). Immiscible; said of certain drugs which neutralize or decompose each other.

189

Incompetence (in-kom′-pe-tens). Inefficiency in the performance of some function.

Incompressible (in-kom-pres′-i-b'l). Not easily compressed. **I. Pulse**, a full pulse, difficult to compress.

Incontinence (in-kon′-tin-ens). Involuntary evacuation. **Double I.**, involuntary passage of both fæces and urine. **Sexual I.**, excessive indulgence in sexual intercourse.

Inco-ordination (in-kō-awr-din-ā′-shun). Inability to produce smooth harmonious muscular movements.

Incrustation (in-krus-tā′-shun). The formation of scabs or crusts.

Incubation Period (in-kū-bā′-shun). The period which elapses from the time the infecting agent enters the body to the time when the first symptoms appear. This period varies with the different infections.

Incubator (in′-kū-bā-tor). An apparatus in which the temperature is regulated so that it can be used for rearing premature or delicate babies, or for cultivating bacteria, etc.

Incurable (in-kūr-a-b'l). Not capable of being cured or healed by medical treatment.

Incus (ing-kus). The central ossicle of the middle ear; takes its name from the shape, *i.e.*, resembling an anvil.

Indentation (in-den-tā′-shun). A dent or depression.

Index (in′-deks). (1) The forefinger. (2) The ratio between the measurement of a given substance compared with that of a fixed standard. **Colour I.**, the proportion of hæmoglobin to each blood-corpuscle, the normal being regarded as 1. **Opsonic I.**, the ratio of the number of bacteria which are ingested by leucocytes contained in the patient's own serum, compared with the number ingested by leucocytes in a normal blood serum. **I. Finger**, the first finger. Pl. *indices.*

Indian Hemp. Same as *Cannabis indica (q.v.).*

Indican (in′-di-kan). Potassium indoxyl sulphate, derived from indol. Also the name given to the active principle of the indigo plant from which indigo blue is obtained.

Indicanuria (in-di-kan-ū′-ri-à). A state in which indican appears in the urine; it is present in healthy urine only in small quantities. *See* Indol.

Indication (in-di-kā′-shun). Sign that a certain line of treatment should be adopted.

Indigenous (in-dij′-e-nus). Native to a certain locality or country.

Indigestible (in-di-jest'-i-bl). Incapable of being digested.

Indigestion (in-di-jes'-chun). Imperfect digestion; dyspepsia.

Indigo (in'-dig-ō). A blue dye obtained from a plant. **I. Carmine,** a dye used for estimating the functional activity of the kidney.

Indol (in'-dol). A constituent of fæces, formed by the putrefaction of proteins.

Indolent (in'-dō-lent). A term applied to a sluggish ulcer which is generally painless but slow to heal.

Induced Current. An electrical current developed in a conductor which is in close proximity to a primary current. **I. Labour,** labour brought on by artificial means, *e.g.,* by the use of Champetiere de Ribes bag, the introduction of bougies, etc.

Induration (in-dū-rā'-shun). The process of hardening; sometimes seen in the early stages of inflammation.

Inebriation (in-ē-bri-a'-shun). A state of drunkenness.

Inelastic (in-e-las'-tik). Not elastic; rigid.

Inertia (in-er-shi-à). Inactivity; a static condition. **Uterine I.,** weakness or absence of uterine contractions due to an atonic condition of the uterine muscle, or to exhaustion

brought on by repeated but ineffective contractions.

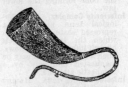

Champetier de Ribes Bag
for induction of labour.

In Extremis (in eks-trē'-mis). At the point of death.

Infant (in'-fant). A baby or a child of less than two years.

Infanticide (in-fant'-i-sīd). Murder of an infant.

Infantile Paralysis. *See* Poliomyelitis, Acute Anterior.

Infantilism (in-fant'-il-izm). The persistence of childish characteristics in adult life.

Infarct (in'-fàkt). A wedge-shaped area of dead tissue which is deprived of blood by the sudden blocking of a terminal or end artery.

Infection (in-fek'-shun). An abnormal process caused by the introduction and subsequent multiplication of living pathogenic organisms into the body.

Inferior (in-fier'-ri-or). Lower; beneath. **I. Vena Cava,** the main vein returning blood to the heart from the trunk and lower extremities. **I. Maxilla,** the bone forming the lower jaw.

Inferiority Complex. A psychological term indicating a repressed state of mind in which the individual feels himself inferior to his fellows. Such a group of ideas may be manifested indirectly by a bombastic attitude.

Infested (in-fes'-ted). Having parasites such as fleas, lice, bugs, etc.

Infiltration (in-fil-trā'-shun). Penetration of the surrounding tissues; the oozing or leakage of fluid into the tissues.

Infirm (in-ferm'). Old or weak.

Infirmary (in-ferm'-a-ri). A hospital where the sick and infirm are cared for.

Inflammation (in-flam-mā'-shun). A series of vascular and cellular changes occurring in living tissues, being the reaction of the tissues to injury.

Inflexible (in-fleks'-i-b'l). Incapable of being bent.

Influenza (in-floo-en'-ză). An acute, infectious epidemic disease caused by a filter-passing virus. There are several different manifestations of the disease, each accompanied by its own group of symptoms and sequelæ. Synonym, *La Grippe.*

Infraclavicular (in-frà-kla-vik'-ū-là(r)). Below the clavicle.

Infraorbital (in-frà-aw(r)'-bit-al). Below the orbital cavity.

Infra-red. The invisible rays beyond the red part of the spectrum. These are long waves and are not visible but produce heat.

Infraspinous (in-frà-spī'-nus). The area below the spine of the scapula.

Infundibulin. Infundin. An extract of the posterior lobe of the pituitary gland.

Infundibulum (in-fun-dib'-ū-lum). Any funnel-shaped passage; particularly applied to the terminations of the bronchioles in the lung.

Infusion (in-fū'-zhun). (1) The introduction of a liquid, such as normal saline, into the subcutaneous tissues. (2) An aqueous solution containing the active principle of a drug; made by pouring boiling water on the crude drug, and then straining after it has stood for a time.

Ingesta (in-jes'-tà). Food received into the body through the mouth.

Ingestion (in-jes'-chun). The act of introducing food into the body.

Ingredient (in-grē'-di-ent). A unit of a more complex substance; any part of a compound.

Ingrowing Toe-nail. A condition in which the toe-nail

tends to grow into the tissue of the toe, causing inflammation and pain.

Inguinal (in'-gwin-al or ing'-gwin-al). Pertaining to the groin. **I. Hernia,** one occurring through the internal abdominal ring of the inguinal canal. **I. Canal,** a tubular opening measuring 1¼ in. in length. It lies in the groin and opens from the abdomen. In the male it contains the spermatic cord; while in the female it contains the uterine round ligaments.

Inhalation (in-hal-ā'-shun). The breathing in of air or vapour.

Inhaler (in-hā'-ler). The appar-

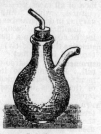

Inhaler.

atus used for the inhalation of medicinal vapours.

Inherent (in-he'-rent or in-hier'-rent). Innate; inborn.

Inherited (in-he'-rit-ed). Derived from one's forebears.

Inhibition (in-hib-ish'-un). The repression of an organic function or process by the action of the nerves or of the natural desires by the will.

Initial (in-ish'-al). Commencing.

Inject (in-jekt'). To throw in; to pour into; to introduce through a hollow needle or tube.

Injected (in-jekt'-ed). Congested, with full vessels.

Injection (in-jek'-shun). The introduction of fluid into the body or the fluid so introduced.

Innervation (in-ner-vā'-shun). (1) The nerve supply of some particular organ or structure. (2) The discharge of nerve impulses to a structure.

Innocent (in'-nŏ-sent). Not malignant; benign.

Innominate (in-nom'-in-āt). Nameless. **I. Artery,** the largest branch of the aortic arch; it divides into the right common carotid and the right subclavian arteries. **I. Bone,** one of the bones forming the pelvis; it is composed of the ilium, ischium, and pubis; also called *os innominatum.* **I. Veins,** two veins situated on either side of the root of the neck and upper part of the thorax; they are formed by the union of the subclavian and internal jugular veins. *See also* **Vena Cava Superior.**

Innoxious (in-noks'-shus). Non-injurious.

Inoculation (in-ok-ū-lā'-shun). The introduction of a specific virus or germ into the body.

Inorganic (in-or-gan'-ik). Devoid of or not derived from animal or vegetable life. I. **Chemistry,** that section of chemical science dealing specially with inorganic compounds.

Inquest (in'-kwest). Act of inquiring. A judicial inquiry before a jury, especially when death is caused by violence or injury.

Insane (in-sān'). Mad; mentally diseased.

Insanitary (in-san'-it-a-ri). Unwholesome ; not healthy.

Insanity (in-san'-i-ti). Disordered mentality. The state of being insane.

Insatiable (in-sā-shi-a-b'l). Not easily satisfied.

Insecticide (in-sek'-ti-sīd). A substance capable of destroying insects.

Insensible (in-sens'-i-b'l). Without sensation.

Insertion (in-ser'-shun). The attachment of a muscle to the bone it moves.

Insidious (in-sid'-i-us). Having an imperceptible commencement, stealthy or secret.

In Situ (in sīt'-ū). In the correct position.

Insoluble (in-sol'-ū-bl). That which cannot be dissolved.

Insomnia (in-som'-ni-á). Sleeplessness.

Inspiration (in-spi-rā'-shun). The drawing of air into the lungs.

Inspissated (in'-spis-ā'-ted). Thickened, as by evaporation or by the withdrawal of water ; dried.

Instep (in'-step). The arched top of the foot.

Instillation (in-stil-ā'-shun). The pouring in of a fluid drop by drop.

Instinct (in'-stingkt). An innate and immediate response to environment, common to men of all races, creeds, and cultures, which, although varying in degree and capable of modification, cannot be lost or acquired in a lifetime.

Instinctive (in-stingk'-tiv). Determined by instinct.

Instrumental (in-stroo-men'-tal). Pertaining to instruments. I. **Delivery,** delivery of the foetus by means of forceps.

Instruments. Appliances ; the term commonly applied to the scalpels, forceps, etc., used in surgery.

Insufflation (in-suf-flā'-shun). The blowing of powder into a cavity (obsolete). *See also* **Artificial Respiration.**

Insulation (in-sū-lā'-shun). The surrounding of an electrical appliance, such as wire, with a non-conducting material.

Insulin (in'-sū-lin). The internal secretion of the pancreas obtained from the islets of Langerhans. Its function is to control the level of the blood sugar by aiding its oxidation and utilization by the tissues.

Integument (in-teg'-ū-ment). The skin.

Intellect (in'-tel-lekt). The mind.

Intelligence (in-tel'-i-jens). The ability to understand and to profit by past experiences.

Intemperance (in-tem'-perrans). Excessive indulgence in anything, particularly food, drink, or sex functions.

Intense (in-tens'). Severe in degree ; emotional.

Intensive (in-ten'-siv). Increasing in force ; drastic ; persistent.

Intention (in-ten'-shun). Purpose ; design. *See under* **Healing**. I. **Tremor**, trembling of the limbs in voluntary movement.

Inter. A Latin prefix signifying between.

Interarticular (in-ter-ȧ(r)-tik-ū-lȧ(r)). Situated between the joints.

Intercellular (in-ter-sel'-ū-lȧ(r)). Situated between the cells of a structure.

Interclavicular (in-ter-kla-vik'-ū-lȧ(r)). Between the clavicles.

Intercondylar (in-ter-kon'-di-lȧ(r)). Between the condyles, *e.g.*, the intercondylar notch at the lower posterior end of the femur.

Intercostal . (in-ter-kos'-tal). Between the ribs.

Intercourse (in'-ter-kaw(r)s). Communication ; coitus.

Intercristal (in-ter-kris'-tal). Between the crests of two structures, *e.g.*, of the innominate bones of the pelvis. The I. **Distance** is taken between the crests or upper thickened edge of each ilium, and normally measures 11 in.

Interlobular (in-ter-lob-u-lȧ(r)). Between the lobules.

Intermittent (in-ter-mit'-ent). Occurring at intervals. I. **Pulse**, one in which a beat is dropped at intervals ; often a sign of cardiac exhaustion : it is a serious symptom in pneumonia. I. **Fever**, a fever with apyrexial periods.

Internal (in-ter'-nal). Inside. I. **Ear**, that part of the ear which comprises the *vestibule, semicircular canals,* and *cochlea.* I. **Secretions**, hormones ; the secretions produced by the ductless or endocrine glands and passed directly into the blood-stream, *e.g., thyroxin.*

Interosseous (in-ter-ros-i-us). Between bones.

Interstices (in-ter′-sti-sēz). Spaces.

Interstitial (in-ter-stish′-al). Situated between; distributed through the connective structures.

Intertrigo (in-ter-trī′-go). Erythema and eczema of the skin caused by friction or excessive sweating.

Intertrochanteric Line (in-ter-trō-kan-ter′-ik). The ridge passing between the greater and lesser trochanters of the femur on the posterior aspect of the bone.

Intestines (in-tes′-tinz). The bowels; part of the alimentary canal from the stomach to the anus. Small I., measures 20 ft. in length, commencing from the stomach, and is divided into three sections: (1) *duodenum*; (2) *jejunum*; (3) *ileum*. Large I., the colon; measures 6 ft. in length, but is of larger diameter than the small intestine.

Intima (in′-tim-à). The internal coat of a blood-vessel.

Intolerance (in-tol′-e-rans). (1) Inability to bear pain or discomfort. (2) Idiosyncrasy to certain drugs or methods of treatment.

Intra-abdominal (in-trà-abdom′-in-al). Inside the abdomen. I. Pressure, pressure within the abdomen.

Intracapsular (in-trà-kap′-sū-lár). Within the capsule. I.

Fracture, a fracture occurring within the capsule of a joint.

Intracellular (in-trà-sel′-ū-là(r)). Within a cell.

Intralobular (in-trà-lob′-ū-là(r)). Within the lobule.

Intramuscular (in-trà-mus′-kū-là(r)). Inside a muscle. I. **Injections**, drugs introduced deep into the muscle structure by means of a hypodermic needle.

Intraperitoneal (in-trà-pe-ri-ton-ē′-al). Within the cavity of the peritoneum.

Intratracheal (in-trà-trak-ē′-al). Introduced into the trachea. I. **Anæsthesia**, the administration of an anæsthetic through a catheter passed down the trachea.

Intrauterine (in-trà-ū′-te-rīn). Within the uterus. I. **Douche**, washing out the interior of the uterus.

Intravenous (in-trà-vē′-nus). Within a vein. I. **Saline**, the introduction of normal saline solution into a vein.

Intrinsic (in-trin′-sik). Inherent or inside. From within; real; natural.

Introitus (in-trō′-it-us or in-troi′-it-us). Any opening in the body; an entrance to a cavity.

Introspection (in-trō-spek′-shun). A turning inward. Psychologically, the observance of one's own thoughts and feelings; self-examination.

Introversion (in-trō-ver'-shun). A turning inward. *See* **Introspection.**

Intubation (in-tū-bā'-shun). The act of passing a tube into the larynx in order to aid respiration; may be used instead of tracheotomy in cases of diphtheria.

Intumescence (in-tū-mes'-ens). Enlargement, swelling.

Intussusception (in-tus-sus-sep'-shun). A condition in which one part of the bowel slips into the lower part; most commonly occurs in infants, and in males more often than in females.

Inunction (in-ungk'-shun). The act of rubbing oily substances or ointments into the skin.

Invagination (in-vaj-in-ā'-shun). *See* **Intussusception.**

Inversion (of Uterus) (in-ver'-shun). Turning inside out.

Involution (in-vō-loo'-shun). The normal shrinkage of an organ after activity; applied particularly to the return of the uterus to its normal size after parturition.

Iodine (ī'-ō-dēn). A poisonous non-metallic solid element with a metallic lustre. When heated it vaporizes as purple fumes without melting. Iodimitis, a weak (2½%) solution of iodine in alcohol used as an antiseptic.

Iodism (ī'-ō-dizm). Poisoning with iodides; the symptoms are those of a common cold and the appearance of a rash, frontal headache, pharyngitis, etc.

Iodoform (ī-ō'-dō-fawm). A yellow crystalline or powdered organic compound containing iodine. It has a very strong odour, and is both deodorant and antiseptic, and is largely used for suppurating cavities. Wool, lint, or gauze may be impregnated with it. Iodoform is one of the constituents of B.I.P.P. (*q.v.*).

Ion (ī'-on). Atoms or molecules which are freed by the process of electrolysis and which carry an electrical charge. If the charge is positive, the ion is known as a *cation*; but if negative, it is called an *anion*.

Ionic (ī-on'-ik). Relating to an ion.

Ionization (ī-on-i-zā'-shun). The passage of drugs in the form of ions into the body by means of electricity.

Ipecacuanha (ip-i-kak-ū-an'-à). A drug obtained from the root of a plant; contains an active principle called "emetine." In small doses it is expectorant, but in larger doses is emetic. Dose: Ipecac. Pulv., expectorant, ½-2 gr.; emetic, 15-30 gr.

Iridectomy (ir-i-dek'-to-mi). Excision of a part of the iris,

197

thus forming an artificial pupil to the eye.

Iridocyclitis (ĭr-ĭ-dō-sī-klī′-tis). Inflammation of the iris and ciliary body.

Iris (ī′-ris). The circular coloured membrane in the front of the eye. It is perforated in the centre by an opening named the pupil. The colour of the iris depends upon the amount of pigment contained in it.

Iritis (I-rī′-tis). Inflammation of the iris.

Iron. A metallic element; it forms one of the constituents of hæmoglobin, which is carried in the red blood-cells; is used in many forms medicinally; causes black stools. When taken as a tonic it should be administered half an hour after food; any signs of dyspepsia should be reported to the doctor.

Irreducible (ir-rē-dū′-si-b′l). Incapable of being reduced by manipulation.

Irregular (i-reg′-ū-là(r)). Not rhythmic or uniform. **I. Pulse,** one which does not beat regularly and steadily.

Irrigation (i-ri-gā′-shun). The act of letting water fall upon a surface, either in volume or in drops. When wounds are washed in this way a douchecan fitted with a nozzle is generally used. From 2-3 pints of saline or antiseptic lotion are prepared at a temperature of 103° F. For a slower but continuous form of irrigation *see* **Carrel-Dakin Treatment.**

Irrigator (i′-ri-gā-tor). The apparatus used for irrigation.

Irritability (ir-it-a-bil′-it-i). Capable of being excited to activity; responding easily to stimuli.

Irritant (ir′-it-ant). Any substance which causes irritability or irritation.

Ischæmia (is-kē′-mi-á). Local anæmia due to defective blood supply to the part.

Ischidrosis (is-ki-drō′-sis). Suppression of perspiration.

Ischium (is′-ki-um). The lower part of the innominate bone of the pelvis.

Isomers (I′-sō-merz). Chemical substances which have the same molecular weight and are composed of the same elements in the same proportions, but vary in the arrangement of the atoms in the molecule.

Isometric (I-sō-met′-rik). Of equal measurement.

Isotonic (I-sō-ton′-ik). Having the same osmotic pressure (as blood plasma). **I. Saline,** the same as *Normal Saline, i.e.*, 0·9% saline solution.

Isthmus (isth′-mus). A narrow band of tissue joining two larger portions.

Itch. *See* **Scabies.**

Iter (I'-ter). A passage-way in the body.

J.

Jaborandi (jab-ō-ran'-di). A drug derived from a Brazilian plant, *Pilocarpus jaborandi.* The alkaloids yielded are jaborine and pilocarpine (*q.v.*). Jaborandi increases salivation and perspiration.

Jacket (jak'-et). A small coat. **J. Poultice,** linseed poultice applied to the back and chest. **Plaster of Paris J.,** a jacket made of plaster of paris and moulded to the body to keep it rigid ; a flannel vest is worn next to the skin, and great care must be taken to prevent pressure on bony points ; the jacket is so adjusted that it can be removed for washing the body, etc. **Straight-J.,** a restraining apparatus used for dangerous maniacs.

Jacksonian Epilepsy. A form of epilepsy due to injury or lesion of the cerebral cortex. When the cause is removed, the symptoms disappear.

Jacob's Membrane (jā'-kob's). The layer of rods and cones in the retina. **J. Ulcer,** rodent ulcer.

Jacobson's Organ. A vestigial structure situated at the front part of the base of the nose. It is more developed in animals, and is said to be concerned with the association between the special senses of taste and smell. Named after *Ludwig Levin Jacobson,* a Danish anatomist.

Jacquemier's Sign (zhak'-mier's). A blue discoloration of the mucous membrane of the vagina ; a sign of pregnancy.

Jacquet's Disease. Alopecia due to reflex irritation from septic teeth.

Jactitation (jak-ti-tā'-shun). Extreme restlessness. Throwing the limbs about in an aimless manner.

Jaksch's, (Rudolph) von, Anæmia. Pseudoleukæmic anæmia of infants, due to disease of the spleen and lymphatic glands. Also called *Von J. Disease.*

Jalap (jal'-ap). A drug obtained from the dried root of a Mexican plant. A hydragogue purgative with rapid action ; used extensively in dropsy. **Pulvis Jalapæ Co.,** a powder containing jalap, acid tartrate of potassium, ginger. Dose, 5-20 gr.

Jaundice (jawn'-dis). A yellow discoloration of the conjunctivæ and skin caused by the presence of an excess of bilirubin in the blood ; is commonly caused by obstruction of the common bile duct. **J. of the New Born,** *see* **Icterus Neonatorum.**

Catarrhal J., that caused by catarrhal inflammation of the mucosa of the bile ducts in the liver. **Malignant J.,** same as acute yellow atrophy of the liver.

Jaw-bone. Either the superior or inferior maxilla.

Jejunal (je-joo'-nal). Pertaining to the jejunum.

Jejunostomy (je-joo-nos'-to-mi). The operation of making an artificial opening into the jejunum.

Jejunum (je-joo'-num). That part of the small intestine immediately following the duodenum. It constitutes two-fifths of the remaining small intestine.

Jennerian. Relating to Jenner or to the theory of vaccination.

Joint (joint). The articulation of two or more bones. **Charcot's J.,** a disease of the joints occurring in advanced syphilis ; there is great wasting of the muscles above and below the joint. **Tuberculous J.,** one which is affected with tuberculosis. **Fixed J.,** a joint which has become rigid through injury or disease, i.e., an ankylosed joint.

Jugular (jug'-ū-lā(r)). Pertaining to the throat. **J. Notch,** the notch between the jugular process and the basilar process of the occipital bone. **J. Veins,** two veins passing down either side of the neck. The internal jugular vein unites with the subclavian vein to form the innominate vein.

Juice (joos). Any of the secretions of the body, e.g., gastric or pancreatic juice.

Jumping Disease. Neurosis marked by jumping movements.

Juniper (joo'-nip-er). A drug obtained by distillation from the unripe fruit of the Juniperus communis ; used mainly as a diuretic in conditions of dropsy.

Junket (jung'-ket). Curds and whey. Prepared by warming 1 pint of milk to 100° F., and adding 1 teaspoonful of rennet. Add sugar to taste. Nutmeg can be grated over the top if desired. Leave to set in a cool place.

Jurisprudence, Medical (joo-ris-proo'-dens, or jooer-ris-proo'-dens). The inter-relation of legal and medical science.

Juxtaposition (juks-tā-pō-zish'-un). Close proximity.

K.

K. Chemical symbol for potassium.

Kala-azar (kal-à-az-á(r)'). A tropical disease caused by the Leishman-Donovan bodies.

Kaolin Poultice (kā'-ō-lin). A poultice consisting of a substance resembling antiphlogistine, though differing in composition. Kaolin provides a cleanly and antiseptic substitute for linseed poultice. Kaolin=silicate of magnesium.

Karyokinesis (kar-i-ō-kī-nē′-sis). Mitosis; the indirect process of nuclear division; a series of changes in the nuclei of cells when these divide so that one cell becomes two, two become four, etc.

Katabolism (ka-tab′-ō-lizm). The process of the breaking down of the tissue cells in the body.

Katatonia (kat-a-tōn′-i-ȧ). A form of dementia præcox insanity.

Keloid (kē′-loid). Abnormal overgrowth of scar tissue.

Keratin (ke′-ra-tin). The essential substance of horny material; used medicinally to coat pills which are required to act in the intestine, since the gastric juice does not affect it.

Keratitis (ke-ra-tī′-tis). Inflammation of the cornea.

Keratome (ke′-ra-tōm). A special surgical knife used for incising the cornea.

Keratosis (ke-ra-tō′-sis). A skin disease characterized by a thickening of the skin.

Kerectomi (ke′-rek-to-mi). An incision into the cornea.

Kerion (kē′-ri-on). A form of pustular ringworm.

Kernig's Sign. Inability to extend the leg when the patient is in the dorsal position, with the hip-joint flexed at right angles to the trunk of the body; is observed in meningitis.

Ketol (kē′-tol). A decomposition product of fæces.

Ketone (kē′-tōn). A compound consisting of the radicle CO and two univalent hydrocarbon groups. Acetone is one of the commonest examples.

Ketosis (kē-tō′-sis). _See_ Acidosis.

Kidney (kid′-ni). The organ which secretes urine. **Floating K.,** one which is displaced from its normal position and relatively unfixed. **Granular K.,** the contracted kidney with finely nodular surface seen in chronic nephritis and arteriosclerosis of the kidney. **Horseshoe K.,** abnormal and imperfect development of the kidneys which are fused into one resembling a horseshoe in shape; often situated in the midline. **Large White K.,** the large pale kidney of parenchymatous nephritis. **Surgical K.,** the same as pyelonephritis (_q.v._). **Pedicle of K.,** the renal artery and vein and the ureter situated at the hilum of the kidney.

Killian's Operation. An operation for drainage of the frontal sinus.

Kinæsthetic Sense (kĭn-es-thet´-ik). The sense by which muscular movement is appreciated.

Kinetic (kĭn-et´-ik). Capable of producing motion. **K. Energy,** the energy of a moving body.

Klebs-Lœffler Bacillus. The bacillus which produces diphtheria.

Kleptomania (klep-tō-mā´-ni-ă). An uncontrollable pathological desire to steal.

Knee (nē). The joint formed by the articulation of the lower end of the femur and the head of the tibia. **K. Cap.,** the patella. **K. Jerk,** the reflex extension of the leg due to the sudden contraction of the quadriceps extensor femoris which results when the patellar tendon is sharply rapped while the limb is held limply in flexion, e.g., in the sitting position with the knees crossed. **Knock - K,** leg distorted outwards so that knee lies inside normal line ; same as genu valgum.

Knot (not). The ends of cords or ropes twisted and interlaced and made secure by drawing tightly.

Knuckles (nuk´-ls). (1) The joints of the phalanges. (2) Loops of intestine.

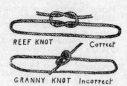

REEF KNOT   Correct

GRANNY KNOT Incorrect

Koilonychia (koil-o-nik´-i-ă). Spoon-shaped nails seen in some forms of anæmia.

Koplik's Spots (kop´-lik). Small whitish-grey spots seen on the buccal mucosa during the early stages of measles. A valuable diagnostic sign.

Koumiss (koo´-mis). Fermented mare's milk ; said to be very nutritious.

Krameria (kra-mē´-ri-ă). Rhatany.

Kraurosis Vulvæ (kraw-rō´-sis). A dry, glistening condition of the mucous membrane of the vulva, characterized by intense itching and constitutional disturbance from loss of sleep.

Kupffer's Cells (koop´-ferz). Phagocytic endothelial cells in the walls of the sinusoids of the liver.

Kyphosis (kĭ-fō´-sis). Humpback; an exaggeration of the dorsal curve of the spine.

K.Y. A lubricant substance used for the nozzles of enema syringes, etc.

L.

Kymograph (kī'-mō-graf). An instrument for recording various movements in the form of waves.

L.

Labia (lā'-bi-à). Lips. **L. Majora,** two large lip-like folds extending from below the mons veneris to the edge of the vagina; they are muscular folds, lined with skin, and covered externally with skin and hair. **L. Minora,** a pair of smaller folds covered on both sides with mucous membrane; they lie between the labia majora. Also known as *Nymphæ.* Singular =Labium.

Labial (lā'-bi-al). Pertaining to the lips.

Labioglossolaryngeal (lā-bi-ō-glos-ō-lar-in-ji'-al). Relating to the lips, tongue, and larynx. **L. Paralysis,** a nervous disease characterized by progressive paralysis of the lips, tongue, and larynx.

Labioglossopharyngeal (lā-bi-ō-glos-ō-far-in-ji'-al). Relating to the lips, tongue, and pharynx.

Laboratory (lab'-or-a-tor-i, also la-bor'-a-tor-i). A place set apart for experimental and scientific research work.

Labour (lā'-ber). The act of giving birth to a child; parturition.

Labyrinth (lab'-i-rinth). The tortuous cavities of the internal ear. **Bony L.,** that part which is directly hollowed out of the temporal bone. **Membranous L.,** the membrane which loosely lines the bony labyrinth.

Labyrinthine (lab-ir-in'-thīn). Pertaining to the labyrinth.

Labyrinthitis (lab-ir-in-thī'-tis). Inflammation of the labyrinth).

Lac. Milk. Any fluid resembling milk.

Lacerated (las'-e-rā-ted). Torn; having jagged, uneven edges.

Lachrymal (lak'-ri-mal). Relating to tears. **L. Bone,** the bone at the inner side of the orbital cavity. **L. Duct,** the duct passing from the lachrymal gland. **L. Apparatus,** the lachrymal gland, ducts, and nasal duct. **L. Secretion,** tears.

Lachrymation (lak-ri-mā'-shun). A copious outflow of tears; weeping.

Lachrymose (lak'-ri-mōs). Tearful.

Lactagogue (lak'-ta-gog). A drug which increases milk secretion.

Lactalbumin (lakt'-al-bū-min). The chief protein of milk.

Lactation (lak-tā'-shun). (1) The period during which a mother suckles her child. (2) The act of suckling.

Lacteal (lak'-ti-al). A minute tubule situated in a villus and containing chyle, which is thus passed from the intestines into the lymphatic vessels.

Lactic Acid (lak'-tik as'-id). An acid formed by the fermentation of lactose. The souring of milk is due to the presence of this acid.

Lactose (lak'-tōs). Sugar of milk.

Lactosuria (lak-tō-sū'-ri-à). The presence of lactose in the urine.

Lacuna (la-kū'-nà). A minute space or depression, *e.g.*, the canaliculi of the Haversian system terminate in the lacunæ, which lie between the lamellæ.

Lævulose (lē'-vū-lōs). Fruit sugar. Same as *Fructose*.

La Grippe. *See* Influenza.

Laking of Blood. Destruction of the erythrocytes of the blood so that the hæmoglobin is set free into the blood plasma. *See* Hæmolysis.

Lallation (la-lā'-shun). Constant usage of the letter *l* instead of *r* in speaking.

Lambda (lam'-dà). The point of union between the sagittal and lambdoidal sutures.

Lambdoidal Suture (lam-doid'-al). The union between the serrated edges of the occipital and parietal bones.

Lamella (la-mel'-à). A thin plate-like scale or partition. Pl. *lamellæ*.

204

Lamina (lam'-in-à). A thin plate of bone.

Laminaria Tents (lam-in-è'-ri-à). A species of seaweed which is compressed into rods about 2 in. in length,

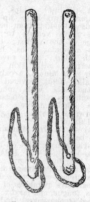

Laminaria Tents.

and with a hole at one end through which a thread can be passed. The tents swell slowly but forcibly in the presence of moisture, and therefore are sometimes used for dilating the cervix uteri in gynæcological and obstetrical procedures. When not in use they must be kept in a dry place. The use of laminaria tents is now largely superseded by other methods.

Laminectomy (lam-in-ek'-to-mi). The operation of removing the lamina of a vertebra.

Lana (lá'-ná). Wool. *See* Adeps Lanæ.

Lancet (lan'-set). A small two-edged surgical knife.

Lancinating (lan'-sin-ă-ting). Piercing or darting : used in connection with pain.

Landry's Disease (lán'-dri). An acute ascending paralysis of unknown origin. Death results when the respiratory muscles are affected.

Langerhans, Islets of (lang'-er-hans). Groups of polyhedral cells in the substance of the pancreas. They secrete a hormone called insulin, which controls the amount of blood sugar. *See* Insulin.

Lange's Colloidal Gold Curves (lang'-gi). A sensitive test for syphilitic and meningitic changes in the cerebro-spinal fluid depending on colour changes in the gold sol produced by variations in the albumin-globulin ratio in the fluid.

Lanoline (lan'-ō-lēn). Adeps lanæ. Purified wool-fat.

Lanugo (lan-ū'-gō). The soft downy hair often present on the body of new-born infants,

especially when they are premature.

Laparotomy (lap-ar-ot'-o-mi). A surgical incision into the abdomen for exploratory purposes.

Lapis (lap'-is). A stone.

Lard. The melted fat of the hog.

Lardaceous (lár-dā'-shus). Waxy, fatty. L. Disease, amyloid degeneration. The organs affected present a solid waxy appearance due to the deposit of a firm translucent substance called lardacein or amyloid. This substance when treated with iodine produces a dark mahogany-brown colour.

Laryngeal (lar-in-ji'-al). Pertaining to the larynx.

Laryngectomy (lar-in-jek'-to-mi). Excision of the larynx.

Laryngismus Stridulus (lar-in-jis'-mus strid'-ū-lus). Spasm of the glottis ; occurs in children between the ages of six months and two years ; may be associated with rickets.

Laryngitis (lar-in-ji'-tis). Inflammation of the larynx.

Laryngologist (lar-ing-gol'-o-jist). A doctor who specializes in the treatment of laryngeal diseases.

Laryngology (lar-ing-gol'-o-ji). The science dealing with the larynx and its diseases.

Laryngophthisis (lar-ing-gō-thī'-sis). Tuberculosis of the larynx.

Laryngoplasty (lar-ing-gō-plas'-ti). Plastic surgery of the larynx.

Laryngoscope (lar-ing'-gō-skōp). A reflector for examining the larynx.

Laryngoscopy (lar-ing-gos'-ko-pi). The use of the laryngoscope.

Laryngotomy (lar-ing-got'-o-mi). Surgical incision into the larynx.

Larynx (lar'-ingks). The organ of voice situated below and in front of the pharynx, and at the upper end of the trachea.

Lassar's Paste (laz'-àr). A paste much used in various cutaneous eruptions. It consists of zinc oxide, starch, vaseline, and 1% salicylic acid. It is mildly antiseptic but non-irritating.

Lassitude (las'-i-tūd). Weakness or tiredness; lack of energy.

Latent Heat. The heat which is required to convert a solid into a liquid or a liquid into gas at the same temperature. **L. H. of Fusion,** the heat which is required to convert 1 grm. of a solid into liquid at the same temperature, e.g., when 1 grm. of ice at 0° C. is converted into water at 0° C.; this process requires 80 calories, and until it is completed there will be no rise in temperature. **L. H. of Vaporization,** the heat required to change 1 grm. of a liquid at its boiling-point to vapour at the same temperature. The latent heat of steam is 540 calories, therefore when steam cools to liquid, each gram gives out 540 calories; this explains why a scald from steam is much more severe than one caused by boiling water.

Lateral (lat'-e-ral). Pertaining to the side.

Laudanum (lawd'-'num). Tincture of opium. Dose, 5-30 minims.

Laughing-gas. Nitrous oxide gas. An anæsthetic used for teeth extractions, etc.

Lavage (lav'-àzh). Washing out, e.g., of the stomach.

Lavender (lav'-en-der). An aromatic oil distilled from the *Lavandula vera.* Other preparations of the oil are *spirit* and *tincture.* The latter forms a reddish colouring matter for lotions and mixtures, e.g., lotio rubra. Lavender is generally used as a refreshing perfume.

Lax. (1) Loose. (2) Careless.

Laxative (laks'-a-tiv). A mild aperient.

Lead (led). Symbol, Pb. A metallic element. A soft, malleable, bluish substance, with a melting-point of 327° C. **L. Acetate,** a compound formed of lead and acetic acid. **Black L.**, graphite. **L. Lotion**, a solution of subacetate of lead ; is applied externally as an evaporating lotion for sprains, strains, etc. **L. Plaster**, a plaster containing oxide of lead. **L. Poisoning**, lead is readily absorbed into the blood and given out freely to the tissues, but is eliminated from the body very slowly ; this gives rise to a series of symptoms due to the retention of lead, known as *plumbism*, and include colic, tremor, pallor, wasting, and the appearance of a blue line on the margin of the gums. Paralysis of the extensor muscles of the hand results in drop wrist.

Leather-bottle Stomach. Contraction of the stomach with thickening of its walls ; usually due to diffuse infiltrating cancer.

Lecithin (les'-ith-in). A nitrogenous substance which is derived from palmitic or oleic acids and is extracted from the tissues containing fatty acids by alcohol or ether. It is widely distributed in nature, forming a constituent of white nervous tissue, bile, egg-yolk, and many plant tissues.

Leech (lēch). A blood-sucking worm obtained from the river or sea. The bleeding which results from its bite is sometimes difficult to check, because the leech secretes a substance, known as *hirudin*, from the salivary gland when biting. This prevents the coagulation of blood. Leeches should be kept in a wide jar covered with gauze. The jar is half-filled with cold clean water once a week. A little clean sand is kept at the bottom of the jar.

Leg. That part of the lower extremity below the knee.

Legitimacy (le-jit'-i-ma-si). The condition of being born in wedlock.

Legumen (leg-ŭ'-men). A nitrogenous substance obtained from certain leguminous plants, such as peas, beans, and lentils.

Leiomyofibroma (lī-ō-mī-ō-fī-brō'mà). A benign tumour composed of fibrous tissue and unstriped muscle. The common uterine fibroid is such a tumour.

Leiomyoma (lī-ō-mī-ō'-mà). A benign tumour composed of unstriped muscle fibres.

Leishman - Donovan Bodies (lēsh-man). The parasites which cause kala-azar. They are found in the spleen, liver, and other organs of the body.

Leishmaniasis (lēsh-man-ī'-a-sis). A group of diseases caused by the Leishmania-Donovani, *e.g.*, kala-azar, Oriental sore, and espundia.

Leiter's Coils (lī'-ter). Coiled flexible metal tubing through which water at any temperature may be run by syphon action.

Lenhartz Diet. *See* **Dietary Table.**

Lens (lenz). The small biconvex crystalline body which is supported in the suspensory ligament immediately behind the iris of the eye. On account of its elasticity, the lens can alter in shape, enabling the light-rays to focus exactly on the retina.

Lentigo (len-tī'-gō). Freckles and other spots on the skin.

Lentil (len'-til). A cheap and nutritious legumin containing a large amount of protein.

Leontiasis Ossea (lē-on-tī'-a-sis os'-i-á). A condition characterized by enlargement and distortion of the facial bones, giving the face a lion-like appearance. The disease is slow in progress, and not fatal.

Leper (lep'-er). A person afflicted with leprosy.

Leprosy (lep'-ro-sĭ). A chronic contagious disease caused by the *B. lepræ*; the incubation period is variable. The skin is attacked first, but later the disease penetrates the tissues, producing ulcerative changes in the bone and nerve structures, which result in terrible mutilation. There are two main types of the disease: (1) the nodular form or

lepra tuberosa; (2) blotched and anæsthetic form (*lepra maculosa*). The best results are obtained by the use of chaulmoogra oil by (*a*) in unction, (*b*) orally, (*c*) intramuscular injection.

Leptomeningitis (lep-tō-men-in-jī-tis). An infection of the pia and arachnoid membranes primarily with the meningococcus or other pathogenic organism. The main symptoms are acute headache, pain in the back, spinal rigidity, irritability, and drowsiness terminating in coma.

Leptospira (lep-tō-spī'-rá). One of the subdivisions of the spirochætes. L. Icterohæmorrhagiæ, the spirochæte which causes Weil's disease.

Leptothrix (lep'-tō-thriks). A class of branching bacteria.

Lesion (lē-zhun). An alteration in the structure of living tissues by injury or disease. Primary L., the initial local manifestations of a disease. Secondary L., one which develops some time after the primary lesion has appeared. Gross L., a lesion which can be recognized with the unaided eye. Psychic L., mental trauma, *e.g.*, as manifested by hysteria.

Lethal (lē'-thal). Pertaining to death; fatal.

Lethargy (leth'-ár-jĭ). (1) A state of lassitude. (2) Deep sleep from which the sufferer is aroused with difficulty: not true coma.

Leucin (lū´-sēn). A white crystalline substance formed by the hydrolysis of proteins during digestion.

Leucocytes (lū´-kŏ-sīts). The white corpuscles of the blood. In the blood-stream they are spherical, colourless, nucleated masses, and some are motile and phagocytic.

Leucocythæmia (lū-kŏ-sī-thē´-mĭ-ă). An abnormal increase in the number of leucocytes in the blood, usually accompanied by glandular and splenic enlargement.

Leucocytosis (lū-kŏ-sī-tō´-sis). A transient increase in the number of leucocytes in the blood.

Leusoderma (lū-kŏ-der´-mă). An abnormal state of the skin in which there are circumscribed patches showing loss of pigmentation. Normal sensation and sweat secretion in these pale areas remain unimpaired.

Leusoma (lū-kŏ´-mă). A white dense scar formation in the cornea following deep-seated ulceration of the cornea. Interference with normal sight depends upon the site of the opacity.

Leucopenia (lū-kŏ-pē´-ni-ă). A transient diminution in the number of white corpuscles in the blood.

Leucorrhœa (lū-kŏ-rē´-ă). A sticky, whitish discharge from the vagina.

Leucosis (lū-kŏ´-sis). A lymphatic disease characterized by great pallor of the skin.

Leukæmia (lū-kē´-mi-ă). A blood disease characterized by the presence in the blood of a persistent increase in the number of white corpuscles, a large proportion of which are primitive. There are different varieties depending upon the type of leucocyte affected but all of which may be acute or chronic. All are associated with anæmia which is often severe. Lymphatic L., the variety in which mature and primitive lymphocytes are present in great numbers in the blood, and accompanied by enlargement of the lymph nodes and spleen. Monocytic L., a rare variety affecting the monocytes of the blood. Myeloid or Spleno-medullary L., the variety affecting the marrow and resulting in a great increase of the polymorphonuclear leucocytes and of myelocytes and myeloblasts in the blood ; the spleen is very greatly enlarged but not the lymph nodes.

Leukoplakia (lū-kŏ-plā´-ki-ă). A condition characterized by whitening and thickening of the skin or mucous mem-

branes which are also in-
flamed, cracked, and fissured.
It may terminate in malignancy and affects chiefly the
tongue, cheeks, and vulva.

Levator (le-vā´-taw(r)). A
muscle which acts by raising
a part. **L. Ani**, the muscle
concerned with defæcation,
and which helps to keep the
pelvic organs in position. **L.
Costarum**, the muscles
which elevate the ribs. **L.
Palpebræ Superioris**, the
muscle which raises the upper
eyelid.

Leysin. A village in the Swiss
mountains near Lake
Geneva ; is world-famous for
its sun treatment of tuberculosis, first introduced in
1903 by *Dr A. Rollier*.

Lichen (lī´-ken). A designation
common to many chronic,
papular skin diseases, accompanied by inflammation.

Lichenoid (lī´-ken-oid). Resembling lichen.

Lieberkuhn's Crypts (lē´-ber-
koon). Simple tubular glands
in the mucous membrane of
the small intestine.

Liebig's Condenser, an apparatus used for condensing
water which has been heated
to steam ; the steam in the
central tube is condensed by
the stream of cold water
flowing round it. *See
Diagram* on p. 118.

Lien (lē´-en or lī´-en). The
spleen.

Lienculus (lī-eng´-kū-lus). A
small accessory spleen.

Lienitis (lī-en-ī´-tis). Same as
splenitis.

Lienteric Diarrhœa (lī-en-te´-
rik). A form of diarrhœa
associated with the passage
of undigested food.

Ligament (lig´-a-ment). Strong,
tough bands of fibrous tissue
containing elastic fibres ;
they serve to connect bones
together.

Ligation (lī-gā´-shun). The
application of a ligature.

Ligature (lig´-a-tüer). The
material used for tying the
blood-vessels or sewing the
tissues. Silk, horse-hair, catgut, kangaroo tendon, silver
wire, and fascia are used.

Lightning Pains. Darting,
piercing pains which com-
monly characterize the disease
of tabes dorsalis.

Lignum (lig´-num). Wood.

Lime (līm). (1) Calcium oxide
(CaO). An important con-
stituent of bone. (2) A
species of citrus fruit of
the natural order Rutaceæ.
L. Juice, a drink made from
the sour lime fruit *Citrus
acida*. **L. Water,** the clear
fluid which is syphoned off
after calcium hydroxide
has been shaken up with
distilled water ; used mainly
for counteracting acidity.

Linctus (lingk´-tus). A thick
syrupy preparation which
has a soothing effect in

cough. Generally given in small doses.

Linea (lin-ĭ-ȧ). A line. **L. Alba,** the white line in the centre of the abdomen, stretching from the ensiform cartilage to the pubis. **L. Albicans,** the small whitish scars found on the breasts, thighs, and abdomen of pregnant and multiparous women. **L. Aspera,** the roughened area on the posterior surface of the femur.

Ling Exercises. A system of physical culture which originated in Sweden ; first introduced by Henrik Ling.

Lingua (ling'-gwȧ). The tongue.

Lingual (ling'-gwal). Pertaining to the tongue.

Liniment (lin'-i-ment). A lotion used for rubbing on the skin, for external use only.

Linitis (lĭn-ī'-tis). Inflammation of the stomach. **L. Plastica,** inflammatory or neoplastic thickening of the wall of the stomach ; same as leather-bottle stomach.

Linseed (lin'-sēd). The seeds of the common flax. **L. Poultice,** one made from crushed linseed ; must be lightly made, and the heat tested with the back of the hand before applying. **L. Tea,** a soothing drink for common colds. One tablespoonful of linseed is added to 1 pint of water ; ¼ oz. of liquorice and ¼ oz. of candy are added together with the juice of half a lemon. The whole is then simmered in a saucepan for half an hour, strained, and served hot.

Lint. Material prepared by scraping linen. *See also* **Charpie.** Surgeon's **L.,** plain white lint ; used in a double thickness with the cotton surface outside. **Boric L.,** lint which is impregnated with boracic acid ; coloured pink as a distinguishing mark.

Lipæmia (lĭ-pē'-mi-ȧ). The presence of fat in the blood.

Liparous (lip'-ar-us). Fat, obese.

Lipase (lĭ'-pāz). A fat-splitting enzyme ; found mainly in the pancreas, but also in other tissues. Same as *Steapsin.*

Lipiodol (lip-ĭ'-ō-dol). An iodized vegetable oil obtained by fixation of iodine in poppy-seed oil. It is tasteless, has a faint odour and an amber-yellow colour. It contains 40% by weight of pure iodine and by reason of its high specific gravity (1·350 at 15° C.) each cubic centimetre of the preparation contains 54 cg. of metalloid. It may be administered by the mouth or by intramuscular injections : when taken orally it is split into iodized fatty acids and glycerine, and absorbed by

211

the villi and re-synthesized, and finally passed into the blood via the lymphatic system. Since the drug is opaque to X-rays, it is a valuable aid to the radiological diagnosis of diseases in or of the body cavities. When used for this purpose it is introduced directly into the cavity to be examined, *e.g.*, by catheter, etc., into the trachea for outlining by X-ray the bronchial tree. It does not cause iodism, and is perfectly eliminated.

Lipochrome (lĭp'-ō-krōm). A fatty pigment found in animal tissues.

Lipoid (lip'-oid). Resembling fat.

Lipoma (lĭ-pō'-má). A benign tumour arising from and composed of fat.

Lipuria (lĭ-pū'-ri-á). The presence of fat in the urine.

Liquefaction (lĭ-kwi-fak'-shun). Conversion of a solid to its liquid state.

Liquor (lĭ'-kwaw(r)). A solution. L. Amnii, the fluid contained in the amniotic sac. L. Sanguinis, the blood.

Lister (lis'-ter). Lord Lister; introduced antiseptic surgery in 1880.

Listerian (lis-tĕr'-i-an). Applied to the system of antiseptic surgery.

Listerine (lis'-ter-rēn). A proprietary antiseptic lotion

used as a mouthwash and gargle.

Listerism (lis'-ter-rizm). The principles of antiseptic surgery originated by Lord Lister in 1880.

Lithæmia (lith-ē'-mi-á). An increase in the amount of uric acid in the blood.

Lithagogue (lĭth'-a-gog). An agent which will dissolve or expel calculi.

Litharge (lĭth-árj'). Yellow oxide of lead.

Lithiasis (lĭth-ī'-a-sis). The condition in which calculi form in the body.

Lithium (lĭth'-i-um). A metallic element, the salts of which are used medicinally because of their alkalinity.

Lithopædion (lĭth-ŏ-pē'-di-on). A calcified fœtus usually found in the abdominal cavity but sometimes in the uterus.

Lithotomy (lĭth-ot'-o-mi). The operation of opening the bladder in order to remove stone. L. Position, the patient lies in the dorsal position, with the thighs and legs flexed and the knees widely abducted.

Lithuria (lĭth-ū'-ri-á). The passage of gravel or crystals of uric acid in the urine.

Litmus Paper (lit'-mus). Paper impregnated with a blue vegetable pigment which turns red when in contact with an acid. Similarly, red litmus turns blue when dipped into an alkaline substance.

Litre (lē'-ter). A fluid measure; the capacity of a cubic decimetre or 1,000 c.c.; equals 35 oz. or 1¾ pints.

Little's Disease. Congenital spastic diplegia, probably due to under-development of the brain; gives rise to the "scissor" gait. Also known as *Congenital Cerebral Diplegia.*

Liver (liv'-er). The largest gland in the body. It secretes bile, and has several other important functions. Amyloid L., waxy degeneration of the liver. Cirrhotic L., hardening of the liver due to an increase of the connective tissue, with atrophy of the parenchyma. Fatty L., fatty degeneration of the liver tissues. Hobnail L., one having an irregular knobbly surface; a form of cirrhosis. Nutmeg L., liver showing both passive congestion and fatty change.

Livid (liv'-id). Blue discoloration due to bruising, congestion, or insufficient oxygenation.

Lividity (liv-id'-it-i). A state of being livid.

Lixiviation (liks-iv-i-ā'-shun). The separation of soluble from insoluble substances by the processes of washing and filtration.

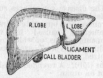

A, The Liver
(upper surface).

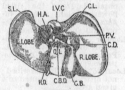

B, The Liver
(inferior surface).

S.L.,　Spigelius's lobe.
H.A.,　Hepatic artery.
I.V.C.,　Inferior vena cava.
Q.L.,　Caudate lobe.
P.V.,　Portal vein.
C.D.,　Cystic duct.
G.B.,　Gall-bladder.
C.B.D.,　Common bile duct.
Q.L.,　Quadrate lobe.
H.D.,　Hepatic duct.

Lobar (lō'-bá(r)). Pertaining to a lobe. L. Pneumonia, inflammation of one or more of the lobes of the lung.

The disease commences suddenly with a rigor, and runs a short but acute course; generally caused by the pneumococcus, of which over thirty "types" are recognized.

Lobe (lōb). A rounded division of an organ.

Lobectomy (lōb-ek'-to-mi). The surgical excision of a lobe of a lung.

Lobelia (lō-bē'-li-à). A drug obtained from the dried flowering plant *Lobelia inflata*; is a respiratory depressant and antispasmodic.

Lobular (lob'-ū-là(r)). Composed of small lobes. **L. Pneumonia**, same as *Bronchopneumonia*.

Local (lō'-kal). Circumscribed; not distributed; limited to a given area.

Localization (lō-kal-i-zā'-shun). The determining of the exact site of a disease process.

Lochia (lō'-ki-à). The vaginal discharge which occurs during the puerperium. At first pure blood, it later becomes paler, diminishes in quantity, and finally disappears altogether.

Lock Hospital. A special hospital for treating venereal diseases.

Lock-jaw. *See* **Tetanus**.

Locomotion (lō-kō-mō'-shun). Movement.

Locomotor Ataxy. *See* **Ataxia**.

Loculated (lok'-ū-lā-ted). Divided into numerous cavities.

Logwood. Same as hæmotoxylin (*q.v.*).

Loin. The lower part of the back; the area immediately above the buttocks.

Longevity (lon-jev'-it-i). Long life.

Long-sightedness. *See* **Hypermetropia**.

Lordosis (law(r)-dō'-sis). An exaggeration of the forward lumbar curve of the spinal column.

Loreta's Operation (lor-ē'-tà). The operation of opening the stomach in order forcibly to dilate the pylorus.

Lotio Rubra. Red lotion; a stimulating lotion used to promote the growth of granulation tissue. It must not be allowed to come into contact with skin, since it tends to destroy it. The solution contains 2 gr. of sulphate of zinc in 1 oz. water, and is coloured red with compound tincture of lavender.

Lotion (lō'-shun). A fluid with healing or antiseptic properties for external use.

Loupe (loop). A magnifying lens used in ophthalmology.

Louse (lows). A small parasitic insect, of which there are three varieties affecting man. *See* **Pediculus**.

Lozenge (loz'-enzh). A medicinal tablet which is slowly

sucked in cases of sore throat, etc.

Ludwig's Angina. *See* Angina.

Lues (lū'-ēz). Syphilis.

Luetin Test (lū-ē'-tin). A test for syphilis. A solution prepared from pure cultures of the spirochæte is injected beneath the skin. The reaction appears on the second day as a red area with a central papule, increasing in size and lasting several days.

Lugol's Solution (loo'-gol). A 5% solution of iodine in a 10% solution of potassium iodide in water.

Lumbago (lum-bā'-gō). Inflammation of the muscles and ligaments in the lumbar region of the back; pain in the loins.

Lumbar (lum-bá(r). Pertaining to the loins. **L. Puncture**, the introduction of a special needle into the subarachnoid space in the lumbar region of the spinal cord. Performed for (1) the relief of pressure of cerebro-spinal fluid; (2) diagnostic purposes; (3) the introduction of anæsthetic or other substances.

Lumbricoid (lum'-brik-oid). Resembling an earthworm.

Lumen (loo'-men). The interior of a tubular structure.

Luminal (loo'-min-al). A sedative drug commonly used in the treatment of epilepsy. The sodium salt is generally used on account of its solubility; $\frac{1}{2}$-2 gr. is given dissolved in water, 1 oz., night and morning.

Lunar Caustic (loo'-ná(r) kaws'-tik). Nitrate of silver; a caustic substance used for cauterizing an overgrowth of granulation tissue. The stick of lunar caustic should be held in a special holder, or in a piece of dry cotton wool, since, if it comes into contact with the fingers, it stains the skin a dark brown.

Lunatic (loo'-nat-ik). One affected with insanity.

Lungs. The two main organs of respiration which occupy the thoracic cavity; they weigh together about 42 oz., and are concerned with the oxygenation of the blood and the elimination of CO_2.

Lunula (loo'-nū-lá). The semilunar pale area seen at the root of the nail.

Lupulus (loo'-pū-lus). *Humulus lupulus* is the common English hop.

Lupus (loo'-pus). A form of tuberculosis affecting the cutaneous tissues; the common variety is known as L. Vulgaris. Another type is **L. Erythematosus**, characterized by a constant thickening and reddening of the skin on the face. This disease is not tuberculous in origin, and there is probably no relationship between the two types of lupus.

Lutein (loo'-ti-in or lū-). A bright yellow substance found in egg-yolk and in the corpora lutea of ovaries.

Luteum (loo-ti-um or lū-). Yellow. The *corpora lutea* are the yellow cellular masses which form in position of the ruptured Graafian follicles in the ovary. They persist and enlarge if pregnancy supervenes.

Luxation (luks-ā'-shun). Complete dislocation of a joint. *See* Dislocation.

Lycanthropy (lī-kan'-throp-i). A form of insanity in which the person imagines himself to be a wild beast.

Lymph (limf). The alkaline fluid contained in the lymph vessels.

Lymphadenitis (limf-ad-en-ī'-tis). Inflammation of a lymphatic gland.

Lymphadenoma (limf-ad-en-ō'-mä). Enlargement of the lymphatic glands, associated with splenic enlargement and progressive anæmia. Synonym, *Hodgkin's Disease.*

Lymphangiectasis (limf-an-ji-ek'-ta-sis). Dilation of the lymph vessels.

Lymphangioma (limf-an-ji-ō'-mä). A tumour of lymphatic vessels.

Lymphangitis (limf-an-jī'-tis). Inflammation of the lymph vessels.

Lymphatics (lim-fat'-iks). Small vessels containing lymph and distributed throughout the tissues.

Lymphocyte (limf'-ō-sīt). A variety of leucocyte formed in the lymphatic glands.

Lymphoid (limf'-oid). Pertaining to lymph.

Lymphosarcoma (limf-ō-sä(r)-kō'-mä). A form of sarcoma originating in the lymphatic tissues and composed of lymphocytes.

Lysine (lī'-sēn). (1) An amino-acid formed by the breaking down of proteins during digestion. (2) An antibody which will dissolve cells.

Lysis (lī'-sis). (1) A term which denotes a gradual fall of a high temperature to normal, *i.e.,* one taking longer than 24 hours to fall. *See* Crisis. (2) A gradual solution or disintegration of bacteria or cells as the result of the action of a lysin.

Lysol (lī'-sol). A preparation of cresol miscible with water, with a strong antiseptic and germicidal action.

M.

"M. and B. 693." Sulphapyridine; one of the sulphanilamide compounds which is particularly efficacious against pneumococcal infections.

Maceration (mas-e-rā'-shun) Softening by soaking in fluid.

Macrocephalous (mak-rō-kef'-a-lus). Having a large head.

Macrocheilia (mak-rō-kīl'-i-à). Excessive enlargement of the lips.

Macrocyte (mak-rō-sīt). A very large blood-corpuscle found in the blood of persons suffering from pernicious anæmia.

Macrocythæmia (mak-rō-sī-thēm'-i-à). The appearance of macrocytes in the blood.

Macrodactyly (mak-rō-dak'-til-i). Congenital overgrowth of the fingers.

Macroglossia (mak-rō-glos'-i-à). Overgrowth of the tongue.

Macromastia (mak-rō-mast'-i-à). Abnormal over development of the breasts.

Macronucleus (mak-rō-nū'-kli-us). A large nucleus.

Macrophage (mak'-rō-fāj). A large phagocytic cell. These cells play an important part in organization and repair.

Macroscopic (mak-rō-skop'-ik). Visible to the naked eye.

Macula (mak'-ū-là). A spot. **M. Lutea**, the yellow spot on the retina. **M. Solaris**, a sunspot ; a freckle.

Mad. Insane.

Madura Foot (ma-dū'-rà). Synonymous with *Mycetoma*.

Magendie (ma-zhon'-di). A French physiologist, born 1783, died 1855. **M. Foramen**, an opening in the roof of the fourth ventricle of the brain whereby the cerebrospinal fluid passes out into the subarachnoid space.

Maggot Treatment. A method of treating septic wounds, first introduced by Dr Baer of U.S.A. Ordinary meat maggots are introduced into a sloughing septic wound, and these ingest the necrotic material, leaving the wound with a clean granulating surface. The maggots are then removed and destroyed. The treatment is still in the experimental stage.

Magnesium Sulphate. Epsom salts ($MgSO_4 7H_2O$). A bitter, soluble salt which acts as an antacid and saline purgative, and also acts as an antidote in poisoning from lead and barium. Purgative dose, 30-240 grs. **M. Enema**, 1-2 oz. of the salts added to 6 oz. of warm water.

Magnet (mag'-net). Iron or steel which will attract other similar bodies. **M. Operation**, the removal of a piece of metal from the eye by means of a magnet.

Magnum (mag'-num). Large or great.

Maim (mām). To disable ; to injure.

Main en Griffe (man-on-gref'). Claw hand.

Mal. Sickness. **M. de Mer**, sea-sickness. **Grand M.**, major epilepsy. **Petit M.**, minor epilepsy.

Malaise (mal'-āz). A feeling of illness and discomfort.

Malar (māl'-ár). Relating to the cheek-bones. **M. Bone**, the bone forming the prominence of the cheek.

Malaria (mal-ér'-i-á). A periodic disease due to infection of the blood by protozoal parasites which are transmitted to healthy persons by a species of mosquito, the female *anopheles*. *See* Ague.

Malaxation (mal-aks-ā'-shun). The kneading movement in massage.

Male. Belonging to the masculine sex ; a man.

Male Fern. *See* Filix Mas.

Malformation (mal-faw(r)-mā'-shun). Abnormal shape or structure.

Malignant (mal-ig'-nant). Virulent and dangerous ; that which is likely to have a fatal termination. **M. Growth** or **M. Tumour**, cancer. **M. Pustule**, a form of anthrax (*q.v.*).

Malingerer (mal-ing'-ger-rer). One who feigns illness ; a sham.

Mallein (mal'-ē-in). A liquid extract of the glanders bacillus used in treatment of this infection.

Malleolus (mal-lē'-ō-lus). The protuberance at the lower end of the ankle bones. **Internal M.**, situated at the lower end

of the tibia. **External M.**, at the lower end of the fibula.

Malleus (mal'-i-us). The hammer-shaped ossicle of the middle ear. The head is in contact with the *membrana tympani*, and the handle with the *incus*.

Malnutrition (mal-nū-trish'-un). The state of being poorly nourished.

Malpighian Bodies (mal-pig'-i-an). (1) The renal glomeruli with Bowman's capsules enclosing them. (2) Small glandular patches distributed throughout the spleen.

Malposition (mal-pō-zi'-shun). Any abnormal position of a part or an organ.

Malpractice (mal-prak'-tis). Unethical, improper, or injurious treatment.

Malpresentation (mal-pres-en-tā'-shun). Any unusual presentation of the fœtus at the pelvic outlet.

Malt. Grain, usually barley, which after sprouting is fermented and dried. It contains a ferment known as diastase, which converts the starch into dextrin and maltose.

Malta Fever. An acute infectious disease occurring along the shores of the Mediterranean, and therefore also known as *Mediterranean Fever*.

Maltase (mol'-tāz). An enzyme which converts maltose to

dextrose. It is one of the enzymes of the intestinal juice.

Maltose (mol′-tōz). A form of sugar produced by the hydrolysis of starch during digestion.

Malunion (mal-ūn′-i-on). Imperfect or faulty union, *e.g.*, defective apposition of the ends of a fractured bone.

Mammæ (mam′-i). The breasts.

Mammary (mam′-a-ri). Relating to the breasts.

Mammilla (mam-il′-å). The nipple ; a small papilla.

Mandible (man′-dib-l). The lower jaw.

Mandibular (man-dib′-ū-lå(r)). Relating to the lower jaw.

Manganese (mang′-gan-ēz). A metallic element ; symbol Mn.

Mange (mǎnj). A parasitic skin disease affecting animals.

Mania (mǎn′-i-å). Insanity. **Alocholic M.**, mania caused by excess drinking of alcohol. **M. a Potu,** *see* Delirium Tremens. **Puerperal M.**, a form of insanity occurring after child-birth, generally during the puerperium. **Religious M.**, mania brought on by excessive religious fervour.

Maniac (mǎ′-ni-ak). An insane person.

Manipulation (man-ip-ū-lā′-shun). Treatment by handling.

Manometer (man-om′-et-er). An instrument for measuring

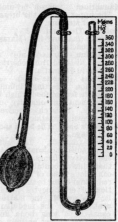

Manometer or Baumanometer. (General principles.)

the pressures exerted by liquids and gases.

Mantoux Reaction (man′-too). A test for tuberculosis depending upon an inflammatory reaction produced by the *intradermal* injection of a small quantity of dilute tuberculin.

Manual (man′-ū-al). Pertaining to or performed by the hands.

219

Manubrium (man-ū'-bri-um). The upper part of the breast bone or sternum.

Manus. The hand.

Marantic (mar-ant'-ik). Marasmic, emaciating.

Maraschino (mar-as-ki'-nō). A liquor distilled from cherries grown in Dalmatia.

Marasmus (mar-az'-mus). A condition affecting infants who are fed on food which is insufficient in quantity or quality. It is characterized by excessive wasting.

Mariotte's Spot. The blind spot of the eye.

Marrow (mar'-ō). The soft pulpy substance contained in the cavity of bones. **Red M.,** that which is contained in the cancellous tissue of bone; its red colour is due to the formation of erythrocytes within it. **Yellow M.,** the marrow contained in the medullary canal of a long bone and consisting almost entirely of fat.

Mask. A covering for the face. **Surgeon's M.,** a face-mask made of gauze or fine linen, worn by surgeons and nurses in the operating theatre. **Parkinson's M.,** an immobile appearance of the face, which develops as a result of *encephalitis lethargica*; the skin is smoothed out, with a loss of wrinkles, and the face is absolutely expressionless.

Masochism (maz'-o-kizm). A form of sexual perversion in which the pervert takes a delight in inflicting pain and degradation upon himself or in being so treated by his associate.

Massage (mas'-àzh). Treatment of various bodily disorders by scientific rubbing, kneading, stroking, and tapping by the hands of a person who is specially trained for the purpose.

Masseter (mas-ē'-ter). The chief muscle of mastication; situated at the side of the face, with its origin on the zygomatic arch, and insertion in the ramus of the inferior maxilla.

Masseur (mas-ooer). A male who practises massage.

Masseuse (mas-ooerz'). A female who practises massage.

Mastication (mas-tik-ā'-shun). The act of chewing or breaking up the food with the teeth.

Mastitis (mas-tī'-tis). Inflammation of the breast.

Mastoid (mas'-toid). The prominence on the temporal bone just behind the ear. **M. Antrum,** the air-space within the mastoid process. **M. Disease,** inflammation of the mastoid process, associated with suppuration in the antrum.

Masturbation (mas-tur-bā'-shun). The abnormal excitation of a sexual organ by manual friction or by rubbing the thighs together.

Materia Medica (mat-ier'-ri-à med'-i-kà). The science dealing with the origin, action, and dosage of drugs.

Maternal (mat-er'-nal). Pertaining to the mother.

Matrix (mā'-triks). The foundation substance in which the tissue cells are embedded.

Matter (mat'-er). (1) In physics, anything which possesses size and weight and occupies space. (2) In medicine, same as *Pus.*

Maturation (mat-ū-rā'-shun). A ripening, as of a cataract or a Graafian follicle.

Mature (mat-ūer). To ripen; to develop fully.

Maturity (mat-ū'-rit-i). Having reached full growth or development.

Matutinal (mat-ū'-tin-al). Occurring in the morning, *e.g.,* morning sickness.

Maxilla (maks-il'-à). The upper or lower jaw.

Maxillary (maks'-il-a-ri). Pertaining to the maxilla.

Maximum (maks'-i-mum). The highest degree or point attainable ; the summit.

Mazodynia (māz-ō-din-i-à). Pain in the breast ; same as mastalgia.

Measles (mēz'-'lz). An acute infectious disease characterized by coryza, rise in temperature, and the development of a blotchy rash on

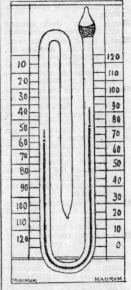

Maximum and Minimum Thermometer. A thermometer for recording and registering the maximum and minimum temperature of a room.

221

the fourth day ; the causative organism is probably a virus.

Measly Pork. Pork infected with the *Cysticercus cellulosæ*.

Meatus (mē-ā′-tus). An opening or mouth. **Auditory M.,** the opening from the pinna into the auditory canal of the ear. **Urinary M.,** the external opening of the urethra.

Mechanism (mek′-an-izm). The mechanical movements involved in carrying out a certain function, *e.g.,* **M. of Digestion,** the movements concerned with the passage of food through the alimentary canal, and which include *mastication, deglutition, peristalsis,* and *defæcation* (*q.v.*). **M. of labour,** the movements through which the fœtus passes on its way through the genital tract.

Meckel's Diverticulum (mek′-el's dī-ver-tik′-ū-lum). A blind pouch-like sac sometimes attached to the small intestine.

Meconium (mi-kōn′-i-um). The dark, sticky, greenish-black fæces expelled by an infant during the first few days after birth ; the colour gradually changes to the characteristic light brown towards the end of the first week.

Median (mēd′-i-an). The middle. **M. Line,** an imaginary line passing through the centre of the body, from a

point between the eyes to between the closed feet.

Mediastinum (mēd-i-as-tī′-num). The space between the lungs.

Medicament (med-ik′-a-ment). Any medicinal preparation.

Medicated (med′-i-kāt-ed). Impregnated with a drug or medicine.

Medico-chirurgical (med-i-kō-kī-rur-ji-kal). Pertaining to both medicine and surgery.

Medinal (med′-in-al). A hypnotic drug. Dose, 5-10 gr.

Mediterranean Fever. *See* **Malta Fever.**

Medulla (me-dul′-à). (1) The marrow in the centre of a long bone. (2) The soft internal portion of glands, *e.g.,* kidney, adrenals, thymus, lymph-nodes, etc. **M. Oblongata,** the fifth lobe of the brain ; the enlargement of the spinal cord above the foramen magnum of the occipital bone.

Megakaryocyte (meg-a-kar′-i-ō-sīt). Large multinucleated cells of the marrow which produce the blood platelets.

Megaloblast (meg′-a-lō-blàst). A large type of primitive nucleated red cell, seen especially in pernicious anæmia.

Megalomania (meg-a-lō-mān′-i-à). Delusions of grandeur, symptomatic of early G.P.I.

Meibomian Cyst (mī-bōm′-i-an). A small tumour of the eyelid caused by blockage of the duct of a meibomian gland ; when suppuration occurs it is known as a sty.

Meissner's Corpuscles (mīs'-ner). Ovoid, laminated corpuscles to which are attached nerve fibres ; they are found at the tips of the fingers and toes.

Meissner's Plexus. A nerve plexus situated in the submucosa of the small intestine. It is derived from the myenteric plexus. *See* Auerbach's Plexus.

Melæna (mel-ē'-nà). Black, tar-like stools. **M. Neonatorum,** bleeding from the bowel and other mucous surfaces in the new-born fœtus.

Melancholia (mel-an-kōl'-i-à). A morbidly depressed mental state. The individual who is strongly introspective may suffer from delusions or suicidal tendencies.

Melanin (mel'-an-in). A black pigment found in the choroid of the eye, hair, and skin, and abnormally is present in certain forms of cancer, producing the so-called malignant melanoma.

Melanoma (mel-an-ō'-mà). A tumour containing black pigment and having a great tendency towards malignancy.

Melanotic (mel-an-ot'-ik). Pertaining to melanin ; of a blackish colour.

Melanuria (mel-an-ūr'-i-à). The passage of very dark-coloured urine.

Melting-point. The temperature at which a solid will melt, *e.g.*, bismuth, 267° C. (514° F.).

Membrana Tympani. The ear-drum.

Membrane (mem'-brān). A thin lining or covering substance.

Membranous (mem'-bran-us). Of the nature of membranes.

Mendel's Law. Formulated by Gregor Mendel in 1865 as the result of his famous experiments on sweet-peas. The Law states that: (1) Characteristics are not inherited in equal proportion. (2) That characteristics vary independently.

Meningeal (men-in-ji'-al). Pertaining to the meninges.

Meninges (men'-in-jēz). The surrounding membranes of the brain and spinal cord. They are three in number : (1) the dura mater ; (2) arachnoid : (3) pia mater.

Meningism (men'-in-jizm) or **Meningismus.** (1) Condition of hyperexcitability of the meninges, probably toxic in origin, productive of some of the symptoms of meningitis but not of the characteristic changes in the cerebrospinal fluid. (2) Hysteric pseudo-meningitis.

Meningitis (men-in-ji'-tis). Inflammation of the meninges.

Meningocele (men-ing'-gō-sēl). Protrusion of the meninges.

Menopause (men'-ō-pawz). The cessation of menstruation ;

223

normally occurs between the ages of forty-five and fifty ; also called the (1) *change of life*, (2) *climacteric*.

Menorrhagia (men-o-rā'-ji-á). An excessive menstrual flow.

Menorrhœa (men-o-rī'-á). The normal menstrual flow ; sometimes used for excessive menstruation.

Menses (men'-sēz). The sanguineous fluid discharged during menstruation.

Menstruation (men-stroo-ā'-shun). The flow of blood from the uterus once a month in the female. It commences about the age of thirteen and ceases about forty-five. **Vicarious M.**, menstruation occurring through some unusual channel, *e.g.*, from the nose, bowel, or breast.

Mental (men'-tal). Relating (1) to the mind, (2) to the chin.

Menthol (men'-thol). A crystalline substance obtained from the distilled oil of peppermint.

Mercurial (mer-kū'-ri-al). Pertaining to mercury.

Mercurialism (mer-kū'-ri-al-izm). Poisoning by mercury, generally due to long-continued use of mercurial medicaments. The main symptoms include diarrhœa, fœtid breath, sponginess and soreness of the gums, and looseness of the teeth.

Mercury (mer'-kū-ri). Hydrargyrum (Hg) ; a heavy metallic fluid element obtained from native mercuric sulphide ; there are many preparations ; its action is alterative and purgative. *See* Calomel, Corrosive Sublimate, and Grey Powder. The salts are a direct poison to the *Spirochæta pallida*.

Mesencephalon (mēz-en-kef'-a-lon). The mid-brain.

Mesenteric (mes-en-te'-rik). Pertaining to the mesentery.

Mesentery (mes'-en-te-ri). A large fold of peritoneum to which the intestines are attached.

Mesial (mē'-zi-al). The same as *Medial*.

Mesmerism (mes'-me-rizm). Hypnotism.

Mesocolon (mē-zō-kō'-lon).That part of the mesentery which is attached to the colon.

Mesoderm (mē'-zō-derm). The centre layer of cells which form during the early development of the embryo ; the other two layers are the *ectoderm* (*q.v.*) and the *endoderm*.

Mesosalpinx (mē-zō-sal'-pinks). The upper portion of the broad ligament.

Metabolic (met-a-bol'-ik). Relating to metabolism.

Metabolism (met-ab'-o-lizm). The intermediate process between the breaking down and rebuilding of the tissue cells. This includes the chemical changes which occur in the foodstuffs from the time absorption takes place until they are eliminated as waste matter.

Metacarpus (met-a-kä(r)'-pus). The five bones which form the hand; they lie between the wrist and the fingers.

Metamorphosis (met-a-maw'-fō-sis). The normal structural changes which occur during the life-cycle of an organism, *e.g.*, the transformation of a tadpole into a frog.

Metaphase (met'-a-fāz). That stage in cell division during which the chromatic loop divides into two.

Metaphysis (met-af'-i-sis). The growing portion of the shaft of a long bone adjoining the epiphysis.

Metaplasia (met-a-plā'-zi-á). Conversion of one type of tissue into another.

Metastasis (me-tas'-ta-sis). An alteration in the seat of a disease from one part of a body to another; a secondary growth.

Metastatic (met-a-stat'-ik). Relating to metastasis.

Metatarsalgia (met-a-tá(r)-sal'-ji-á). Pain in the metatarsus.

Metatarsus (met-a-tá(r)'-sus). The five bones of the foot between the ankle and the toes.

Metchnikoff's Theory. The theory of a Russian physiologist which teaches that bacteria are attacked and destroyed by leucocytes and other phagocytes, which accumulate in large numbers in the presence of sepsis.

Meteorism (mē'-ti-or-izm). Abdominal distension by gas.

Methæmoglobin (met-hē-mō-glō'-bin). A stable oxidation derivative of hæmoglobin.

Methæmoglobinuria (met-hē-mō-glō-bin-ūr-i-á). The presence of methæmoglobin in the urine.

Methane (mē'-thān) (CH₄). Marsh gas.

Methylated Spirit (meth'-i-lāt-ed). A mixture of methyl alcohol or wood spirit with ethyl alcohol.

Methylene Blue (meth'-i-lēn). A blue pigment sometimes injected into a vein as a test of renal efficiency; also used as a laboratory stain.

Metritis (me-trī'-tis). Inflammation of the uterus.

Metropathia (met-ro-path'-i-á). Any uterine disease.

Metrorrhagia (met-ro-rä'-ji-á). Bleeding from the uterus between the menstrual periods.

Metrostaxis (met-ro-staks'-is). Same as *Metrorrhagia*.

Miasm (mī'-azm). A foul smell.

Michel's Clips (mī'-shel). Small metal clips used for the closure of a surgical wound instead of sutures. **M. Forceps**, forceps specially designed for the manipulation of Michel's clips.

Microbe (mī'-krōb). Bacterium ; a microscopic organism of vegetable origin. **Aerobic M.,** one which requires oxygen in order to thrive. **Anaerobic M.,** one which does not require oxygen. The three main groups are: (1) bacilli ; (2) cocci ; (3) spirilli.

Microbiology (mĭ-krŏ-bī-ol'-o-ji). That section of biology which deals with minute forms of life which are invisible to the naked eye.

Microcephalus (mĭ-krŏ-kef'-a-lus). The state of having a very small head.

Micrococcus (mĭ-krŏ-kok'-us). A minute globular organism, of which there are many kinds. They may occur singly ; in pairs, *diplococci* ; in chains, *streptococci* ; in groups or clusters, *staphylococci.*

Microcyte (mĭ'-krŏ-sīt). An undersized red blood corpuscle found in anæmic blood.

Microgyria (mĭ-krŏ-jĭ'-rĭ-à). Smallness of the gyri or convolutions of the brain ; found in some types of mental defect or idiocy.

Micron (mĭ'-kron). A millionth part of a metre, represented by the letter μ, or a thousandth part of a millimetre.

Micro-organism (mĭ-krŏ-aw(r)'-gan-izm). Any minute organism, either protozoal or bacterial.

Microphage (mĭ'-krŏ-fãj). A small phagocytic cell, viz., the polymorphonuclear leucocyte.

Microphthalmia (mĭ-krof-thal'-mi-à). The state of having abnormally small eyes.

Micropsia (mĭ-krop'-si-à). An abnormality of vision in which objects appear to be smaller than they really are.

Microscope (mĭ'-kros-kōp). An optical instrument capable of great magnification, whereby minute objects, invisible to the naked eye, become clearly seen.

Microscopic (mĭ-kros-kop'-ik). Exceedingly minute ; too small to be observed without the aid of a microscope.

Microscopist (mĭ-kros'-ko-pist). One who uses a microscope.

Microsporon (mĭ-krŏ-spaw'-ron). A minute genus of fungi which may produce disease in the skin, hair, and nails of man, *e.g.,* **M.** Audouini, the species which causes the head ringworm or *Tinea tonsurans.*

Microtome (mĭ'-krŏ-tōm). An instrument for cutting extremely thin sections of structures to be examined microscopically. There are many modifications of this apparatus, of which the most commonly used is the **Rocking M.,** in which the section to be cut is passed by a lever across a stationary knife.

Micturition (mik-tū-rish'-'n).
The act of passing urine.

Mid-brain. The same as mesen-
. cephalon.

Midriff (mid'-rif). The diaphragm (*q.v.*).

Midwife (mid'-wīf). A woman
accoucheur; one who pro-
fessionally attends another
woman in her confinement.
Such persons must pass an
examination conducted by
the Central Midwives Board.

Midwifery (mid-wif'-er-ri). The
practice of obstetrics.

Migraine (mī'-grān). Recurrent
paroxysmal attacks of severe
headache, usually unilateral.
It may be accompanied by
disturbance of vision, nausea
and vomiting, and great
prostration.

Migration (mī-grā'-shun). The
passage of cells, etc., from
one position to another; this
may be *physiological*, as,
e.g., the migration of an ovum
from the ovary into the Fallopian tube, or, again, it may
be *pathological*, as the migration of the leucocytes through
the wall of a blood-vessel into
the surrounding tissues.

Mikulicz's Disease (mik'-ū-lik).
Chronic inflammatory en-
largement of the salivary and
lachrymal glands.

Miliaria (mil-i-ér'-i-à). A skin
eruption caused by the retention of sweat in the sweat
glands where they open in
the epidermis. Such block-

age results in minute discrete
vesicular spots which are not
inflamed.

Miliary (mil'-i-a-ri). Resembling
a millet seed. **M Tuberculosis,**
a form of tuberculosis in which
small tuberculous nodules
are widely disseminated
throughout the organs and
tissues of the body.

Milk. The white fluid which
is secreted in the breasts of
mammals for feeding their
young. In the human the
composition of the milk
differs a little from that of
the cow, particularly in the
proportion of its protein.
Humanized M., cow's milk
prepared in such a way as
to resemble human milk as
closely as possible. **Citrated
M.,** milk to which sodium or
potassium citrate has been
added, 5-10 gr. to the pint,
in order to render it more
digestible. **Peptonized M.,**
milk subjected to the action
of zymogen peptonizing powder for 10 minutes at 99° F.,
and then rapidly raised to
the boil in order to terminate
the digesting action of the
zymogen. By this means
the milk proteins are rendered
more digestible. **Pasteurized
M.,** milk treated by maintaining it at a temperature of
155° F. for 20 minutes and
then rapidly cooling it on ice
or in running water. Most
of the pathogenic bacteria

are destroyed by this process, but not vitamins. The warm stage is passed through as rapidly as possible, as warmth is very favourable to the growth of bacteria.

Milk-sugar. Lactose.

Milk Teeth. The temporary teeth. They first begin to appear at the age of about six months and are shed about the age of seven years. They number twenty altogether, ten in each jaw. *See also* Teeth, Permanent.

Milligram, Millilitre, Millimetre (mil.-i-gram, -lē-ter, -mē-ter). The thousandth part of a gram, litre, and metre respectively. Abbreviations used : mgm., ml., and mm. The ml. has the same volume as 1 c.c.

"Milton." A liquid antiseptic and germicide, manufactured by an electrolytic process, and containing 1 per cent. of sodium hypochlorite. It is stable, non-caustic, non-poisonous and in the appropriate dilutions innocuous to living tissues. For sterilising water dilutions of 1/5000 to 1/1000, according to degree of pollution. For irrigating wounds: initial cleansing, 1/5 dilution (light general anæsthesia is sometimes necessary); routine treatment, 1/20 dilution. For douching, 1/40. For internal use, 1/120, and for general purposes, 1/60.

Mineral (min'-er-ral). An inorganic chemical substance occurring in nature in the solid form. **M. Oil,** petroleum.

Minim (min'-im). A drop ; 1/60 drachm ; also 1/480 fl. oz.

Minot-Murphy Diet. The liver diet used in the treatment of pernicious anæmia.

Miosis (mī-ō-sis). Smallness of the pupils of the eyes due to contraction of the sphincter muscle of the iris.

Miotic (mī-ot'-ik). (1) Relating to miosis. (2) A drug having the action of producing miosis.

Mirror. A highly polished, reflecting surface. A **Head M.,** a small mirror attached

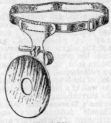

Head Mirror.

to a metal band worn on the head with the mirror on the forehead ; used for reflecting light into the eyes, nose, or throat. **M. Writing,** writing which looks like that which is read in a mirror, *i.e.,* from right to left: generally exists in persons of abnormal mentality, and is thought to be a manifestation of dual personality, since it usually occurs while the attention of the individual is otherwise occupied in conversation, etc.

Miscarriage (mis-kar´-ej). Expulsion of the fœtus from the uterus before it is viable, *i.e.,* between the third and seventh months of gestation.

Mistura (mis-tū´-rá). A mixture.

Mitchell's Treatment. *See* Weir-Mitchell.

Mite. A minute insect, *e.g.,* the itch-mite or *Acarus scabiei.*

Mitigated (mit´-i-gát-ed). Alleviated or lessened.

Mitochondria (mī-tō-kon´-dri-à). Very small proplasmic granules seen in animal cells.

Mitosis (mī-tō´-sis). Same as *Karyokinesis.*

Mitral (mī´-tral). Pertaining to the valve dividing the left auricle and ventricle of the heart; also known as the *bicuspid* valve. **M. Regurgitation,** a defect in the closure of the valve whereby blood tends to flow backward into the auricle from the ventricle. **M. Stenosis,** narrowing of the mitral orifice, usually due to recurrent attacks of rheumatism.

Mnemonics (nē-mon´-iks). Rhymes or other aids to memory.

Modus Operandi (mō´-dus op-er-ran´-di). The method of preparing for, and carrying out, any piece of work.

Molar Teeth (mō-là(r)). The double teeth or grinders. There are twelve altogether.

Mole. (1) A raised, pigmented portion of skin often containing hair. (2) A mass formed in the uterus by the death or degeneration of the ovum or fœtus. **Carneous M.,** one composed of the retained placenta, fœtal membranes, and blood after the expulsion of the fœtus, and which assumes a fleshy appearance. **Hydatidiform M.,** degeneration of the chorion in early gestation. The fœtus dies, but the mass goes on enlarging, forming cyst-like structures, varying in size; these, if not removed early, may cause rupture of the uterus or they may become malignant; sometimes the mass is expelled spontaneously from the uterus.

Molecular (mō-lek´-ū-ler). Pertaining to a molecule.

Molecule (mol´e-kŭl). The smallest particle into which matter can be divided and still retain its identity.

Mollities Ossium (mol-lish´-i-ēz os´-si-um). Softening of the bones so that they bend or break; same as *Osteomalacia.*

229

Molluscum (mol-us'-kum). A chronic skin disease showing two main forms : (1) **M. Contagiosum**, showing hard, round nodules ; (2) **M. Fibrosum**, a skin disease showing masses formed of fibro-cellular tissue.

Mongol (mong'-gol). A congenital condition characterized by obliquity of the eyes and eyebrows, protrusion of the tongue, and a low mentality usually amounting to idiocy. The cause is entirely unknown and treatment is unavailing.

Moniliform (mo-nil'-i-fawm). Having a beaded appearance ; resembling monilia—a yeast-like fungus.

Monkshood. *See* Aconite.

Monocle (mon'-o-kl). A single eyeglass.

Monocular (mon-ok'-ū-lå(r)). Possessing only one eye.

Monocyte (mon'-o-sīt). One of the forms of the leucocytes of the blood. Also known as the large hyaline mononuclear leucocyte of the blood.

Monograph (mon'-o-graf). A work written on one particular subject.

Monomania (mon-ō-mān'-i-å). Insanity on one particular point or subject.

Monoplegia (mon-o-plē'-ji-å). Paralysis of only one limb.

Monorchis (mon-aw(r)'-kis). Having one testicle.

Monsol (mon'-sol). A reliable disinfectant combining high germ-killing power with bland and non-irritant action ; does not roughen the hands, but leaves the skin soft and supple. Ideal for, and specially approved in, midwifery, as it has a selective action on the bacteria causing puerperal sepsis. Deeply penetrating, it is largely used for all skin diseases and for all antiseptic and household purposes.

Monster (mon'-ster). A fœtus born with a grossly deformed body, in which certain parts are exaggerated or missing ; they may be either single or double.

Mons Veneris (mons ven'-er-ris). The eminence formed by the pad of fat which lies over the os pubis in the female.

Moon-blindness. Dimness of vision reputed to result from exposure of the eyes to moonlight during sleep.

Mooren's Ulcer. A chronic form of ulcer which tends to spread completely round the circumference of a part, *e.g.*, the cornea ; common in old age.

Morbid (maw(r)'-bid). Relating to disease.

Morbilli (maw(r)-bil'-i). Measles.

Morbus (maw(r)'-bus). Disease. **M. Cœruleus**, congenital heart disease.

Morgue (maw(r)g). A public mortuary.

Moribund (mor'-i-bund). In a dying state.

Morning Sickness. The feeling of nausea or actual vomiting which attacks pregnant women in the morning during the first few months of pregnancy.

Morphine (maw(r)'-fēn) ($C_{17}H_{19}NO_3$). The principal alkaloid of opium; its action is sedative. Dosage: Morphine sulphate, ¼-½ gr. Morphine hydrochlor, ⅛, ¼, ½ gr.

Morphinism (maw(r)'-fin-izm). A state of poisoning resulting from a single overdose of opium or to smaller doses taken over a long period, thus forming a so-called "opium-habit."

Morphinomania (maw(r)-fin-ō-mān'-i-á). An uncontrollable and morbid craving for morphia; sufferers will go to almost any length to obtain supplies of the drug, which in time affects them not only physically, but mentally and morally as well.

Morphology (maw(r)-fol'-o-ji). The science which deals with the form and structure of living things.

Mors. Latin for death.

Mortal (maw(r)'-t'l). (1) Capable of destruction. (2) Deadly.

Mortality (maw(r)-tal'-i-ti). (1) The state of being mortal. (2) The death-rate.

Mortification (maw(r)-tif-i-kā'-shun). *See* **Gangrene.**

Mortuary (maw(r)'-tū-a-ri). A place where dead bodies are kept until burial.

Morula (mor'-ū-lá). The appearance of the ovum at a certain stage in its development in which it resembles a mulberry.

Motile (mō'-tīl). Capable of motion.

Motility (mō-til'-i-ti). The state of being motile.

Motion (mō'-shun). (1) Intestinal evacuation. (2) Movement.

Motor (mō'-ter). Relating to action. **M. Aphasia,** loss of speech through an inability to articulate caused by a cortical lesion. **M. Nerves,** the effector nerves passing from the anterior horn of the spinal cord to the muscles of the limbs, etc.

Mountain Sickness. Symptoms of sickness, tachycardia, and dyspnœa experienced by many mountaineers, and due to the low oxygen content of the rarified air at high altitudes. Also known as *Acosta's Disease.*

Mouth. (1) An opening or entrance. (2) The buccal cavity.

Mucilage (mū'-sil-áj). A solution of gum-acacia, or linseed and quince-seed.

Mucilaginous (mū-sil-aj'-in-us). Resembling mucilage; gummy.

Mucin (mū'-sin). A sticky white substance forming an important constituent of cer-

231

tain secretions, such as saliva or bile.

Mucocele (mū-kō-sēl). Cystic enlargement by distension with mucus, *e.g.*, of appendix, gall-bladder, lachrymal sac, etc.

Mucoid (mū'-koid). Resembling mucus.

Mucous Membrane. A membrane secreting mucus. Examples are the lining of the alimentary canal and the urinary tract. Such membranes have a communication with the external parts of the body in contradistinction to *serous* membranes, which have no such communication.

Mucus (mū'-kus). The viscid liquid secreted by mucous glands.

Multicellular (mul-ti-sel'-ū-lă(r)). Constructed of many cells.

Multigravida (mul-ti-grav'-id-a). A woman who has borne many children.

Multilobular (mul-ti-lob'-ū-lă(r)). Possessing many lobes.

Multilocular (mul-ti-lok'-ū-lă(r)). Possessing many smaller cysts, loculi, or pockets.

Multipara (mul-tip'-er-rà). *See* Multigravida.

Multiparous (mul-tip'-er-rus). Bearing several young at one birth.

Mumps. An acute infectious disease characterized by in-

flammation of the parotid gland. Constitutional symptoms may be severe.

Murmur (mur'-mer). An abnormal additional low sound heard during auscultation of the heart, lungs, or abdomen.

Murphy's Button. A small device for uniting the divided ends of the bowel. **M. Drip**, a method of introducing normal saline into the rectum. The solution is passed in slowly and under low pressure.

Muscle (mus'-l). The strong contractile tissue which produces movement in the body. **Cardiac M., the striated but involuntary muscle forming the heart. Skeletal M., the striated voluntary muscles which cover the bony skeleton. Visceral M.,** non-striated and involuntary muscles found in the structure of the internal organs.

Muscular (mus'-kū-lă(r)). Relating to the muscles. **M. Rheumatism.** Rheumatism affecting the muscles.

Musculocutaneous. The nerve supplying the skin and biceps muscle of the arm.

Musculospiral. The nerve supplying the triceps muscle.

Mutation (mū-tā'-shun). A difference in form resulting in a new species.

Mute. Unable to speak; dumb.

Mutilation (mūt-i-lă'-shun). Defacement; deprivation of the body of one or more of its parts.

Mutism (mūt′-izm). Dumbness.

Myalgia (mī-al′-ji-à). Pain in the muscles.

Myasthenia (mī-as-thēn′-i-à). Muscular debility.

Mycelium (mī-sēl′-i-um). The interwoven mass of filaments of certain fungi.

Mycetoma (mī-sē-tō′-mà). A tropical disease caused by infection with a parasite. Commonly infects the foot. Also known as *Madura Foot*.

Mycosis (mī-kō′-sis). Infection of the body with a parasitic fungi.

Mydriasis (mid-ri-ā′-sis). Dilatation of the pupil.

Mydriatics (mid - ri - at′ - iks). Drugs which cause dilatation of the pupil, *e.g.*, atropine.

Myelin (mī′-e-lin). The lipoid substance constituting the medullary sheath of a nerve.

Myelitis (mī-e-lī′-tis). Inflammation of the spinal cord.

Myeloblast (mī′-el-ō-blàst). The primitive non-granular precursor of all the granular leucocytes and myelocytes.

Myelocele (mī′-el-ō-sēl). A spina bifida, especially one containing a portion of spinal cord.

Myelocyte (mī′-el-ō-sīt). The large granular mononuclear cell of the marrow, derived from the myeloblast and the precursor of the granular leucocytes.

Myeloid (mī′-e-loid). Resembling marrow.

Myeloma (mī-e-lō′-mà). A tumour formed from the soft medullary centre of a long bone, *i.e.*, from marrow.

Myeloplaxes (mī-e-lō-plaks-es). Multinucleated giant cells of the normal marrow which are believed to produce blood platelets.

Myocardial (mī-ō-kà(r)′-di-al). Pertaining to the muscle of the heart.

Myocarditis (mī-ō-kà(r)-dī′-tis). Inflammation of the myocardium or heart muscle.

Myoclonus (mī-ō-klō′-nus). Clonic contractions of individual or groups of muscles.

Myoma (mī-ō′-mà). A tumour composed of muscular tissue.

Myomalacia (mī-ō-mal-ā′-si-à). Morbid softening of muscle. M. Cordis, the softening of the heart muscle resulting from cardiac infarction.

Myomectomy (mī-ō-mek′-to-mi). Surgical removal of a myoma. The term is especially applied to excision of a uterine fibroid.

Myometritis (mī-ō-me-trī′-tis). Inflammation of the uterine muscle.

Myometrium (mī-ō-mē′-tri-um). The thick muscular wall of the uterus.

Myopathy (mī-op′-ath-i). Any disease of a muscle.

Myope (mī′-ōp). A short-sighted person.

Myopia (mī-ōp'-i-à). Short-sightedness. The light-rays come to a focus in front, instead of on the retina, resulting in a blurred visual image.

Myopic. Relating to myopia.

Myositis (mī-ō-sī'-tis). Inflammation of a muscle.

Myotics (mī-ot'-iks). Drugs which cause contraction of the pupil.

Myotome (mī'-ō-tōm). An instrument for cutting a muscle.

Myotomy (mī-ot'-o-mi). The operation of cutting through a muscle.

Myotonia (mī-ō-tōn'-i-à). Tonic muscular spasm.

Myotonus (mī-ō-tō'-nus). The state of tonicity in a muscle.

Myringitis (mir-in-jī'-tis). Inflammation of the membrana tympani.

Myringotomy (mir-in-got'-o-mi). Incision into the tympanic membrane.

Myrrh (mer). A gum-resin obtained as an exudation from trees growing in Arabia and Abyssinia. It has an aromatic odour and is tonic in action.

Myxœdema (miks-ō-dēm'-à). A condition of gelatinous œdematous thickening of the skin due to deficiency of thyroid secretion.

Myxoma (miks-ō'-mà). A tumour of embryonic origin, consisting of a soft mucoid, gelatinous substance.

Myxosarcoma (miks-ō-sà(r)-kō'-mà). A tumour which is partly sarcomatous and partly contains myxomatous material.

N.

N. Chemical symbol for nitrogen.

Na. Chemical symbol for sodium.

N.A.B. Abbreviation for *nor-arsenobenzol.*

Nævoid (nē'-void). Pertaining to a nævus.

Nævus (nē'-vus). A birthmark of congenital origin, consisting of a mass of dilated capillaries. It generally forms in the skin as a bright red or purple coloured area, which is often known as a " port - wine " stain, and commonly affects the skin of the face and neck ; there are several varieties.

Nail (nāl). The horny substance covering the posterior surface of the upper terminal phalanges of the fingers and toes. **Hang N.,** a loose section of skin at the side of the nail.

Naked (nā'-ked). Uncovered ; nude. **N. Eye,** examination of an object without the aid of a microscope or magnifying glass.

Nanism (nän'-izm). Dwarfism.

Nape (nāp). The dorsal aspect of the neck.

Naphtha (naf'-thá). A distillation product from coal-tar, petroleum, etc.

Naphthalene (naf'-tha-lēn). A crystalline substance distilled from coal-tar; has antiseptic properties. (Also *Naphthol*.)

Napkin Rash. A dusky-red rash developing about the buttocks (napkin area) in infants suffering from congenital syphilis.

Narcissism (ná(r)-sis'-izm). An inordinate love and admiration for oneself. Named after Narcissus, who fell in love with his own reflection.

Narco-analysis (ná(r)-kō-an-al'-i-sis). A method of psycho-analysis in which the process is speeded up by the use of certain drugs. When injected into a vein the drug exerts a partial anæsthetic action. With the patient in a state of hypnosis the deepest secrets of the mind can be probed. Thus forgotten memories may be restored and the possibility of cure in certain mental diseases is enhanced.

Narcolepsy (ná(r)-kō-lep-sī). An uncontrolled desire for sleep occurring at intervals.

Narcomania (ná(r)-kō-mān'-í-á). A morbid and uncontrollable craving for narcotics.

Narcotic (ná(r)-kot'-ik). A drug which induces deep sleep, *e.g.*, opium.

Nares (ré'-rēs). The nostrils.

Anterior N., the cavities formed by the nostrils at the front part of the nose. **Posterior N.,** the back part of the nose.

Nasal (ná-zal). Pertaining to the nose.

Nasal Retractors.

Nascent (nās'-ent). The condition of gaseous substances at the moment of their liberation from chemical combination.

Nasopharynx (nā-zō-far'-ingks). The portion of the pharynx behind the posterior nares.

Natal (nā'-tal). (1) Pertaining to birth. (2) Pertaining to the nates.

Nates (nā'-tēz). The buttocks; the gluteal region.

Native (nā'-tiv). Belonging to a particular locality; the natural habitat of a thing.

Nauheim Treatment. *See* **Schott's Treatment.**

Nausea (naw'-si-á). A feeling of sickness without actual vomiting.

Navel (nā'-vel). The umbilicus.

Navicular (nav-ik-ū-lá(r)). Shaped like a canoe. The scaphoid bone of the tarsus and carpus.

Nebula (neb'-ū-lá). A faint greyish opacity of the cornea.

Necator Americanus. A round worm parasite found in America, similar to ankylostoma duodenale.

Neck (nek). The constricted portion immediately below the head of a structure; also refers to the narrow lower part of a hollow organ, such as the bladder and uterus. *See* Cervix and Urethra. **Anatomical N.,** the narrow constricted part of the femur between the head and the trochanters. **Wry N.,** *see* **Torticollis.**

Necropsy (ne-krop'-si). The examination of a body after death. *See* Post-mortem and Autopsy.

Necrosis (ne-krō'-sis). Cellular death and disintegration affecting small circumscribed pieces of tissue and caused by bacterial or other toxins or by loss of nutrition. *See* Sequestrum.

Necrotic (ne-krot'-ik). Having the characteristics of necrosis.

Needle (nē'-dl). A fine, sharp-pointed instrument for carrying a ligature through or under tissues. **Aneurysm N.,** one to which a handle is attached; the eye is blunt and turned up; used for passing a ligature beneath a blood-vessel preparatory to tying the vessel. **Exploring N.,** one introduced into a cavity for the purpose of ascertaining its contents.

Hypodermic N., one used for the introduction of drugs beneath the skin; it is fixed to the barrel of a

Surgical Needles.

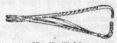

Needle Holder.

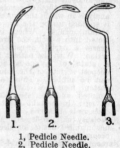

1.   2.   3.

1, Pedicle Needle.
2, Pedicle Needle.
3, Aneurysm Needle.

syringe containing the fluid. **Lumbar Puncture N.,** a special needle used for withdrawing fluid from, or introducing it into the theca of the spinal cord.

Needling (nēd'-ling). A method of treating an aneurysm in an effort to thicken and strengthen the walls of the sac. Several fine needles are introduced into the sac and left to be played upon by the blood-stream, so that the farther wall becomes scratched and irritated, thus setting up an inflammatory thickening.

Negative (neg'-a-tiv). Not positive; denial; opposition. N. Culture, one not showing the suspected organisms.

Negativism (neg'-a-tiv-izm). An abnormal psychological state in which the general attitude and ideas of an individual are in opposition to the opinions of his colleagues or to society generally.

N e m a t o d a (nē-ma-tō-dá). Round worms; among the commonest are the *Ankylostoma duodenale, Filaria,* and *Oxyuris vermicularis.*

N e m b u t a l (nem-bū'-tal). Sodium-ethyl-methyl-butyl-barbiturate; a basal hypnotic and sedative. Is administered orally, rectally, or intravenously. For pre-anæsthetic sedation 3 gr. are given orally 35-40 minutes before operation. Intravenous injection is commenced 10 minutes before operation at the rate of 1 c.c. per minute, the dose being 3-7½ gr.

Post-operative drowsiness or sleep may last from 1 to 5 hours, and vomiting is considerably lessened or entirely absent.

Neon (nē'-on), N. A gaseous element existing in fractional quantity in the ordinary atmosphere.

Neonatal (nē-ō-nā-tal). Pertaining to the new-born.

Neoplasm (nē'-ō-plazm). A new growth; one having the characteristics of a true tumour.

Neoplasty (nē-ō-plas'-ti). *See* Plastic Surgery.

Neosalvarsan (nē-ō-sal-vàr'-san). An arsenical preparation used for the treatment of syphilis, and for some other conditions in which arsenic may be of benefit.

Nepenthe (ne-pen'-thi). A narcotic drug. Dose: 5-40 minims.

Nephralgia (nef-ral'-ji-á). Pain in the kidney.

Nephrectomy (nef-rek'-to-mi). Surgical removal of the kidney. **Abdominal N.,** removal of the kidney through the abdomen. **Lumbar N.,** removal of the kidney through the dorsal lumbar region.

Nephritis (nef-rī'-tis). Non-infective inflammation of the kidney; Bright's disease; may be acute, subacute, or chronic.

Nephro- (nef'-rō). A prefix pertaining to the kidney.

237

Nephrolithiasis (nef-rŏ-lith-ī'-a-sis). The formation of calculi in the kidney.

Nephrolithotomy (nef-rŏ-lith-ot'-o-mi). The removal of a calculus from the interior of the kidney.

Nephron (nef'-ron). A single urinary unit consisting of a glomerulus and the whole length of attached tubule up to the collecting tubule.

Nephropexy (nef-rŏ-peks'-i). Keeping a displaced kidney in position by means of sutures.

Nephroptosis (nef-rop-tŏ'-sis). Prolapse of the kidney.

Nephrorrhaphy (nef-ror'-a-fi). The same as *Nephropexy*.

Nephrotomy (nef-rot'-o-mi). Surgical incision into the kidney.

Nerve. An elongated bundle of fibres which serves for the transmission of impulses between the periphery and the nerve centres. **Afferent N.,** one conveying impulses from the tissues to the nerve centres; also known as *Receptor* and *Sensory N.* **Efferent N.,** one which conveys impulses outwards from the nerve centres; also known as *Effector* or *Motor N.*; by stimulating the muscles they produce movement.

Nervous (ner'-vus). (1) Relating to nerves or nervous tissue. (2) Timid or frightened. (3) Easily stimulated. **N. System,** the structures controlling the actions and functions of the body; it comprises the brain and spinal cord and their nerves, and the ganglia forming the sympathetic system. **N. Exhaustion,** see Neurasthenia.

Nettle-rash (net'-l-rash). A transient skin rash accompanied by itching and usually by some constitutional disturbance; urticaria.

Neural (nūr-al). Pertaining to nerves. **N. Canal,** the medullary canal which passes down the whole length of the spinal cord.

Neuralgia (nū-ral'-ji-à). Severe pain along the course of a nerve fibre. The causes and varieties of neuralgia are very varied. **Trigeminal N.,** acute agonizing pain along the path of the fifth cranial nerve. The origin is unknown. Treatment consists in giving morphia to relieve the pain; injections of alcohol into the nerve have also been tried, but in intractable cases division of the Gasserian ganglion may be necessary. Also known as *Tic Douloureux.*

Neurasthenia (nūr-as-thĕ'-ni-à). A group of symptoms arising from general debility and mental and physical exhaustion. It is characterized mainly by undue fatigue on slight exertion, loss of appetite and sleep, gastro-intestinal symptoms, and mental depression.

Neurasthenic (nūr-as-then'-ik). Pertaining to neurasthenia.

Neurectomy (nū-rek'-to-mi). Excision of part of a nerve.

Neurilemma (nūr-i-lem'-á). The nucleated outer covering of a nerve fibre.

Neuritis (nū-rī'-tis). Inflammation of a nerve.

Neuroblast (nūr-ō-blást). A primitive nerve cell.

Neuroblastoma (nūr-ō-blást-ō-má). A tumour composed of primitive nerve cells; commonest in the adrenal medulla where it arises almost entirely in childhood.

Neurofibroma (nūr-ō-fī-brō'-má). A fibroma derived from the fibrous sheath of a nerve.

Neuroglia (nūr-ō-glī'-á). The supporting tissue of the brain and cord. Unlike ordinary connective tissue it is of epiblastic origin and is composed mainly of astrocytes and oligodendrocytes.

Neurology (nū-rol'-o-ji). The science and study of nerves—their structure, function, and pathology; the branch of medicine dealing with diseases of the nervous system.

Neuroma (nū-rō'-má). A tumour composed of nervous matter.

Neuron (nūr'-on). A nerve cell

and its processes. *See* Dendrites, Axis Cylinder, and Cell.

Neuronophagia (nūr-on-ō-fá'-ji-á). The destruction of nerve cells by phagocytes.

Neuropathic (nūr-ō-path'-ik). Pertaining to nervous diseases.

Neuropathology (nūr-ō-path-ol'-o-ji). The pathology of the nervous system.

Neuroplasm (nūr-ō-plazm). The protoplasm existing between the fibrils of a nerve cell.

Neurorrhaphy (nū-ror'-a-fi). Uniting the ends of a divided nerve by means of sutures.

Neurosis (nū-rō'-sis). A term used to denote any abnormal nervous condition which **ex**hibits certain functional disorders, but in which there is no manifestation of organic alteration.

Neurotic (nū-rot'-ik). (1) Pertaining to the nerves. (2) In a state of neurosis.

Neutral (nū'-tral). Neither acid nor alkaline. If tested with litmus, there is no change in colour.

Neutralize (nū'-tral-īz). To render neutral or inert.

Nicol's Prism. A prism of Iceland spar which transmits only polarized light.

Nicotine (nik'-o-tēn). A very highly poisonous alkaloid of tobacco; not used medicinally in this country.

Nicotinism (nik′-o-tin-izm). The ill-effects produced by excessive indulgence in tobacco ; nicotine poisoning.

Nictitation (nik-ti-tā′-shun). Rapid and involuntary blinking of the eyelids.

Nidus (nī′-dus). A centre or focus of infection ; a nest.

Night-blindness. An abnormal condition of the eyes in which vision is defective or absolutely lost in dim light.

Nightingale (nīt′-ing-gāl). A kind of simple bed-jacket, easily made, which can be worn by patients when in bed. It is fastened by tapes down the front, under the arms, and down the sides, and can be put on or removed with the minimum of disturbance to the patient.

Nightingale, Florence (1820-1910). A pioneer English nurse who became famous for her work in the Crimean War. She afterwards wrote several books on nursing and military topics. She may be said to be the founder of modern nursing.

Nightshade (nīt′-shād). A genus of plants, the best known being the *deadly nightshade*, a poisonous plant from which is obtained belladonna.

Night-sweat. Profuse sweating at night seen in various wasting illnesses, such as pulmonary tuberculosis and advanced rickets.

Nigrescent (nī-gres′-ent). Becoming black or dusky ; darkly pigmented.

Nipple (nip′-l). The conical eminence in the centre of each breast, through which milk is obtained during breast-feeding.

Nirvanol (ner-văn′-ol). A drug used in the treatment of chorea. It has the action of stopping the choreic movements, but has no effect on the damage already done to the heart.

Nissl's Granules. The small granular bodies in the cytoplasm of nerve cells which are darkly stained by methylene blue.

Nit. The egg of the louse, especially the *Pediculus capitis* or head louse.

Nitrate (nī′-trāt). A salt of nitric acid. N. of Silver. Lunar caustic (*q.v.*).

Nitric Acid. *See* Acid. Used in testing urine for albumin ; known as the *Cold Test* or *Heller's Test*.

Nitrite (nīt-rīt). A salt of nitrous acid.

Nitrocellulose (nīt-rō-sel-ū-lōs). Soluble gun cotton ; pyroxylin.

Nitrogen (nīt′-rō-jen). Symbol, N. A colourless, odourless, inert gaseous element contained in the atmosphere, of which it constitutes 78·09%

by volume. It serves as a diluent for oxygen. **N. Equilibrium,** the condition during a given period in which the nitrogen excreted in the urine equals the amount which is taken in by the body in the food.

Nitrogenous (nī-troj'-en-us). Containing nitrogen.

Nitroglycerin (nī-trō-glis'-e-rin). An oily liquid which is highly explosive ; medicinally it is used to lower a high blood-pressure. *Liq. Trini-trini.* Dose: ½-2 minims. Synonyms, *Trinitroglycerine, Glonoin, Trinitrin, Glyceryl Trinitras.*

Nitrous Oxide (nīt'-rus oks'-īd) (N₂O). An anæsthetic used in dentistry and minor surgery ; sometimes known as "laughing gas."

Nocturnal (nok-turn'-al). Pertaining to night. **N. Enuresis,** urinary incontinence during sleep.

Node (nōd). A small protuberance or swelling ; also a constriction. **Auriculo-ventricular N.,** the commencement of the bundle of His in the right auricle of the heart. **N. of Ranvier,** the constriction in the neurilemma of a nerve fibre.

Nodose (nō'-dōs). Characterized by the presence of nodes.

Nodule (nod'-ūl). A small node.

Noma (nō-má). *See* **Cancrum Oris. N. Pudendi** or **N.**

Vulvæ, gangrenous ulceration of the vagina in children.

Non Compos Mentis. Latin, meaning "of unsound mind."

Non-motile. Without the power of movement.

Normal (naw(r)'-mal). That which conforms to certain natural laws ; that which is typical or usual. **N. Saline Solution,** a solution of salt in water in a strength of 80 gr. of salt to 1 pint of water, *i.e.,* 0·9% solution. **N. Body Temperature,** 98·4° F. **N. Pulse:** (a) infant, 130 beats per minute ; (b) adult, 72-80 ; (c) old age, about 60 beats per minute. **N. Respiration,** breathing occurring 18-24 times per minute.

Normoblast (naw(r)'-mō-blast). A normally sized nucleated red blood-cell.

Nosocomium (nŏs-ō-kōm'-i-um). A hospital or other place where the sick are cared for.

Nosology (nŏz-ol'-o-ji). The science of diseases and particularly their classification.

Nostalgia (nos-tal'-ji-á). Homesickness.

Nostalgic (nos-tal'-jik). Relating to nostalgia.

Nostrils (nos'-trils). The anterior openings in the nose ; the anterior nares.

Nostrum (nos'-trum). A quack medicine.

Notalgia (nō-tal'-ji-á). Pain in the dorsal region.

Notifiable (nō-ti-fī'-a-bl). A

term which means that
certain diseases of an infectious nature must be
reported to the local Medical
Officer of Health.

Notochord (nŏt′-ō-kaw(r)d). A
rod-like structure, the proto-
type of the spinal column ;
it persists throughout life
in the lower vertebrates.

Novarsenobenzol (nōv-ȧrs-en-
ō-benz′-ol). An organic compound containing arsenic,
which is much used in the
treatment of syphilis ; often
abbreviated as N.A.B.

Novocain (nōv-ō-kān). A local
anæsthetic much used in
dentistry and minor surgery ;
it is much less toxic in its
action than cocaine.

Noxious (noks′-shi-us). Harmful or poisonous ; injurious.

N.P.N. Abbreviation meaning
non-protein nitrogen.

Nucha (nū′-kȧ). The nape of
the neck.

Nuclear (nūk′-li-er). Pertaining to a nucleus.

Nucleated (nūk′-li-āt-ed). Possessing one or more nuclei.

Nuclei (nūk′-li-ī). The plural
of *nucleus*.

Nucleolus (nūk-li-ō′-lus). The
small body of condensed
chromatin within the nucleus
of a cell.

Nucleus (nūk′-li-us). The inner
essential part of a tissue cell,
being necessary for the
growth, nourishment, and
reproduction of the cell.

Typically it is round in
shape and is situated near
the centre ; usually each cell
possesses one nucleus, although there may be more,
as, for example, in the giant
cells seen in tuberculous
lesions.

Nullipara (nul-lip′-a-rȧ). A
woman who has not borne a
child.

Nulliparous (nul-lip′-ar-us). The
state of never having borne
children.

Numb (num). Insensible ;
locally anæsthetic ; insensi-
tive.

N u m m u l a r (num′-ū-lȧ(r)).
Shaped like a coin. **N.
Sputum,** the appearance of
sputum in a receptacle after
it has been expectorated
from the lung, when it
assumes a flattened, circular
shape like a coin ; frequently
seen in cases of phthisis.

Nutation (nū-tā′-shun). Nod-
ding of the head.

Nutmeg Liver. *See* **Liver.**

Nutrient (nūt′-ri-ent). Nutritious ; nourishing.

N u t r i m e n t (nūt′-ri-ment).
Nourishment.

Nux Vomica (nuks vom′-ik-ȧ).
A drug obtained from the
nux vomica plant ; contains
strychnine. Dose : *Tincture,*
10-30 minims.

Nyctalopia (nik-tal-ō′-pi-ȧ).
Night-blindness.

Nymphæ (nim′-fī). The labia
minora.

242

Nymphomania (nim-fō-mān'-i-ă). Excessive sexual desire to an insane degree in women.

Nymphomaniac (nim-fō-mān'-i-ak). One who suffers with nymphomania.

Nystagmus (nis-tag'-mus). Involuntary and jerky oscillations of the eyeballs ; may be congenital, but is usually associated with mental or nervous diseases.

O.

O. The symbol for oxygen.

Obese (ō-bēs'). Extremely fat and corpulent.

Obesity (ō-bēs'-it-i). The state of being fat ; corpulency.

Obfuscation (ob-fus-kā'-shun). The condition of becoming obscured ; cloudiness.

Objective (ob-jek-tiv). (1) The object glass or lens of a microscope. (2) Pertaining to things external to one's self, *i.e.*, the opposite of subjective.

Oblique (ob-lēk'). Slanting. **O. Muscles,** two muscles of the eye ; also two in the abdomen.

Obsession (ob-sesh'-un). The dominance of the mind by some haunting idea. This state, in lesser degree, is fairly common among normal people, but becomes overpowering and excludes reasoned judgment in persons

suffering from mental derangement. The obsession may be harmless, or, on the contrary, extremely grave, leading to homicide or suicide.

Obsolete (ob'-so-lēt). No longer in use ; out of date.

Obstetrician (ob-stet-rish'-n). One who practises the science and art of obstetrics.

Obstetrics (ob-stet'-riks). The science dealing with the care of the pregnant woman during the ante-natal, parturient, and puerperal stages ; midwifery.

Obstruction (ob-struk'-shun). Blockage of a structure from any cause, so as to prevent the free outflow of its contents. **Intestinal O.,** blockage of the lumen of the intestine.

Obturator (ob'-tū-rāt-aw(r)). That which closes an aperture. **O. Foramen,** the opening in the ischium of the pelvis, which is closed by muscles and obturator fascia.

Occipital (ok-sip'-it-al). Pertaining to the occiput or back part of the head.

Occiput (ok'-si-put). The posterior region of the skull.

Occlusion (ok-kloo'-zhun). The closure of an opening.

Occult Blood (ok'-ult). Blood which is not visible to the naked eye, but the presence of which can be demonstrated by microscopical or chemical tests.

Occupation Disease. One which

is the direct consequence of the occupation of the patient.

Oeular (ok'-ū-lár) Pertaining to the eye.

Oeulist (ok'-ū-list). One who makes a special study of the defects and diseases of the eye and their treatment.

Oeulomotor (ok-ū-lō-mōt'-awr). The name given to the third cranial nerve, which moves the eye and supplies the upper eyelid.

Odontalgia (ō-don-tal'-ji-à). Toothache.

Odontoblast (ō-don-tō-blást). The cell which forms the dentine of teeth; also known as enameloblast or adamantoblast.

Odontoid (ō-don'-toid). Resembling a tooth. O. Peg, the tooth-like projection from the upper surface of the body of the second cervical vertebræ, *i.e.*, the *axis*.

Odontoma (ō-don-tō'-mà). A tumour developing from dental tissue.

Odoriferous (ō-der-rif'-e-rus). Emitting a smell; having an odour.

Odour (ō'-der). A smell.

O'Dwyer's Tubes. Tubes used for laryngeal intubation.

Œdema (ē-dēm'-à). Dropsy; an excess of fluid in the tissues, shown by swelling, pitting and translucency.

Œdipus Complex (ē'-dip-us). An extension of the normal heterosexual stage in which a boy's love for his mother rivals that of his father; may be associated with the development of mental disease later on. The condition is named after Œdipus, who, according to Greek mythology, unknowingly married his mother.

Œsophageal (ē-sof-a-jē'-al). Pertaining to the œsophagus. **Œ. Feeding,** the introduction of nourishment into the œsophagus by means of a rubber tube. **Œ. Obstruction,** constriction of the lumen of the œsophagus.

Œsophagus (ē-sof'-a-gus). The gullet or food pipe.

Œstrus (ēs'-trus). The period of sexual excitement in the female animal.

Œstrin (ēs'-trin). A proprietary preparation of the œstrus-producing hormone of the placenta.

Official (of-ish'-al). Authorized and recognized by the British Pharmacopœia.

Ohm (ōm). The unit of resistance in electricity.

Oidium (ō-id'-i-um). A parasitic fungus. **O. Albicans,** the fungus causing thrush.

Ointment (oint'-ment). A soft fatty substance possessing antiseptic or healing properties. The base of an ointment is usually lard, vaseline, or lanoline to which the medicament is added. Ointment is applied on lint or linen, and should be spread from the centre of the lint outwards, so that the edges are completely covered.

Oleaginous (ō-li-aj'-i-nus). Oily.

Oleate (ō'-li-āt). A compound of a base with oleic acid.

Olecranon (ō-lek'-ra-non). The large process at the upper end of the ulna; it forms the tip of the elbow when the arm is flexed.

Olein (ō'-lē-in). The chief constituent of fatty oils; a compound of glycerin and oleic acid.

Oleum. Latin for oil. **O. Morrhua,** cod-liver oil. **O. Ricini,** castor oil. Abbreviation is Ol. Ric.

Olfactory (ol-fak'-to-ri). Pertaining to the sense of smell. **O. Nerve,** the nerve supplying the nasal organ; the first cranial nerve. **O. Organ,** the nose.

Oligæmia (ol-i-gē-mi-ȧ). A diminution in the total quantity or volume of the blood.

Oligodendroglia (ol-i-gō-den-drō-glī'-ȧ). One constituent of the glia or supporting tissue of the brain and consisting of small cells with a few short processes.

Oliguria (ol-ig-ūr-i-ȧ). Scantiness of urine.

Olivary (ō-liv'-a-ri). Olive-shaped. **O. Bodies,** two small olive-shaped bodies situated just above the medulla oblongata.

-oma (-ō-mȧ). A suffix denoting a tumour or swelling.

Omental (ō-men'-tal). Pertaining to the omentum.

Omentum (ō-men'-tum). The large double fold of peritoneum which hangs from the lower border of the stomach and covers the front of the intestines, reaching as far as the pelvis; this is known as the *Greater O.* The Lesser O. is a smaller fold, passing between the transverse fissure of the liver and the lesser curvature of the stomach. The functions of the omentum are concerned with protection and repair and with fat storage.

Omni (om'-ni). From the Latin *omnis,* meaning all.

Omnivorous (om-niv'-or-us). Feeding on all kinds of food without discrimination.

Omphalus (om'-fal-us). The umbilicus or navel.

Onanism (ō'-nan-ism). (1) Masturbation. (2) Incomplete coitus.

Oncology (on-kol'-o-ji). The science of tumours or new growths.

Oncosphere (on'-kō-sfier). The embryonic stage in the life-cycle of tapeworms.

Onychia (ō-nik'-i-ȧ). Acute inflammation of the matrix of the nail. The suppuration may spread beneath the nail, causing it to become detached and fall off.

Onychogryphosis (on-ik-ō-grī-fō-sis). An enlarged, thickened, and deformed state of the nails, usually of the big toes and due to neglect.

Oogenesis (ō-ō-jen'-e-sis). The production and formation of ova in the ovary.

Oophorectomy (ō-ō-for-ek'-to-mi). Excision of an ovary.

Oophoritis (ō-ō-for-ī'-tis). Inflammation of an ovary.

Oophoron (ō'-ō-for-on). The ovary.

Oosperm (ō-ō-sperm). A fertilized ovum.

Opacity (ō-pas'-it-i). The state of being opaque.

Opaque (ō'-pāk). Dense; solid; not transmitting light.

Operculum (ō-perk'-ū-lum). A lid or cover; a cylindrical-shaped plug of mucus which blocks the cervix at the commencement of labour, and which is later released by the dilatation of the cervix.

Ophthalmia (of-thal'-mi-à). Inflammation of the eye. There are several varieties, the chief of which are: **Gonorrhœal O.**, due to infection of the eye with the *gonococcus*. **O. Neonatorum**, purulent infection of the eyes of an infant at birth as it passes through the genital tract; also due to infection with the gonococcus. **Sympathetic O.**, inflammation of one eye

following infection of the other.

Ophthalmic (of-thal'-mik). Relating to the eye.

Ophthalmitis (of-thal-mī'-tis). Inflammation of the eye; choroiditis.

Ophthalmocele. *See* **Exophthalmos.**

Ophthalmologist (of-thal-mol'-o-jist). One who studies ophthalmology.

Ophthalmology (of-thal-mol'-o-ji). The science which deals with the structure, function, and diseases of the eye.

Ophthalmoplegia (of-thal-mō-plē'-ji-à). Paralysis of the eye muscles.

Ophthalmoscope (of-thal'-mō-skōp). An instrument for

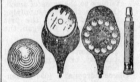

Ophthalmoscope.

examining the interior parts of the eye.

Ophthalmoscopy (of-thal-mos'-kop-i). Examination of the interior of the eye.

Opiate (ō'-pi-āt). A drug acting as an hypnotic, *e.g.*, opium.

Opisthotonos (op-is-thot′-on-os). Arched rigidity of the body brought about by violent muscular spasms ; seen in strychnine poisoning and tetanus. The spine may be so bent backwards that the body only rests on the head and the heels. *See also* **Emprosthotonos** and **Pleurothotonus.**

Opium (ō′-pi-um). A drug obtained from the unripe capsules of the white poppy, the *Papaver somniferum.* It contains many alkaloids, the chief of which are morphine, ⅛-⅓ gr., and codeine, ¼-1 gr. Common preparations of opium are :—

Tincture of opium, 5-30 minims (laudanum).
Ext. Opii Sicc., ¼-1 gr.
Tr. Opii Camph., 30-60 minims (Paregoric).

It is also embodied in pills, suppositories, liniments, and powders. Its action diminishes the gastric secretions and paralyses the peristaltic action of the intestines and relieves pain. It is sometimes given to allay cough, since it depresses the respiratory system, but in this connection must always be used with caution.

Opsonic Index (op-son′-ik). The ratio between the number of bacteria destroyed and ingested by the leucocytes in normal blood serum, as compared with the number ingested by leucocytes under the influence of the patient's own serum.

Opsonins (op′-son-ins). Substances, the exact nature of which is unknown, existing in the normal circulating blood, and which act by increasing the susceptibility of bacteria to phagocytosis. The amount of opsonin in the blood can be increased by immunization.

Optic (op′-tik). Pertaining to sight. **O. Organ,** the eye. **O. Disc,** the point where the optic nerve enters the eyeball.

Optical (op′-tik-al). Pertaining to sight.

Optics (op′-tiks). The science which deals with light-rays and their relation to sight.

Optimum (op′-tim-um). Most suitable ; best ; maximum, *e.g.,* **O. Temperature,** that temperature which is most suitable for the development of bacteria.

Ora Serrata. The fringed terminations of the ligaments of the lens and retina.

Oral (aw′-ral). Pertaining to the mouth.

Orbicular (awr-bik′-ū-lăr). Resembling a globe ; spherical or circular.

Orbicularis Oris. The name of the sphincter muscle forming the lips.

Orbit (awr′-bit). The bony

247

socket containing the eye-ball and its appendages.

Orbital (awr'-bit-al). Pertaining to the orbit.

Orchidectomy (awr-ki-dek'-to-mi). Excision of one or both testicles ; castration of the male.

Orchis (awr'-kis). The testicle.

Orchitis (awr-kī'-tis). Inflammation of the testicle.

Organ (awr'-gn). A part of the body so constructed as to exercise a special function.

Organic (awr-gan'-ik). (1) Pertaining to an organ. (2) Possessing either animal or vegetable life. O. Chemistry, the special branch of chemistry which deals with the compounds of carbon.

Organotherapy (awr-gan-ō-thĕr'-a-pi). The treatment of disease by the administration of animal organs, or certain hormones obtained from them.

Orgasm (awr'-gazm). The crisis of sexual passion.

Orientation (awr-i-en-tā'-shun). The location of an object with relation to the points of a compass and also to its environment.

Orifice (or'-i-fis). A mouth or opening.

Origin (or'-i-jin). The commencement or source of anything. O. of a Muscle, the proximal end of a muscle.

Orthodiagraph (awr-thō-dī-a-graf). The apparatus which uses X-rays to determine the size of organs, *e.g.*, the heart, within the body.

Orthodontia (awr-thō-don-shi-à). The correction of irregularities of dentition.

Orthopædics (awr-thō-pē'-diks). That branch of surgery which deals especially with the correction and cure of deformities.

Orthopædist (awr-thō-pē'-dist). One who practises orthopædics.

Orthopnœa (awr-thop-nē'-à). Difficulty in breathing when lying down and relieved by the upright position.

Os. Pl. *ossa*. Latin for bone.

Os. Pl. *ora*. A mouth.

Osazone (ō'-sa-zōn). A crystalline substance which forms when certain sugars are heated with phenylhydrazine and acetic acid. The crystals are diagnostically characteristic for different sugars. All *monosaccharides* form osazones, as also do the *disaccharides* maltose and lactose, but not cane sugar.

Oscillation (os-il-ā'-shun). A swinging or moving to and fro ; a vibration.

Osmium (oz-mi-um). One of the rare very hard metals ; symbol Os.

Osmosis (os-mō'-sis). The diffusion of fluids through permeable membranes. The liquid of lower specific gravity flows through the membrane to a fluid of higher specific gravity. When both fluids have reached an identical specific gravity, the motion ceases.

Osmotic Pressure (os-mot'-ik). The pressure exerted by a concentrated solution upon the membrane which separates the fluid from one of lesser concentration.

Osseous (os'-ē-us). Pertaining to or resembling bone.

Ossicles (os'-ik-ls). The small bones contained in the middle ear: (1) *malleus*, (2) *incus*, (3) *stapes*.

Ossiculectomy (os-ik-ū-lek'-to-mi). Removal of the ossicles by surgical means.

Ossification (os-if-i-kā'-shun). The conversion of cartilage, etc., into bone; the hardening of bone.

Osteitis (os-ti-ī'-tis). Inflammation of bone.

Osteitis Deformans (o. dē-fawr'-mans). A chronic disease affecting the bones, which at first become rarefied but later harden with resulting deformity; also known as *Paget's Disease*.

Osteitis Fibrosa (o. fī-brō'-zà) or **Fibrocystica** (fī-brō-sis-tik-à). A chronic disease of the skeleton due to over-action of the parathyroid glands, usually a simple tumourous condition of one of the glands, and characterized by softening of the bones with cystic formations, much

deformity and even spontaneous fractures. Also known as *Von Recklinghausen's disease of bones*.

Osteo-arthritis (os-ti-ō-àr-thrī'-tis). Chronic arthritis, accompanied by bony changes in the joints.

Osteo-arthropathy (os-ti-ō-àr-throp'-ath-i). Disease of any bony articulation.

Osteoblast (os'-ti-ō-blàst). The cells, especially on the under-surface of the periosteum, which are concerned in the formation of new bone.

Osteochondritis (os-ti-ō-kon-drī'-tis). Inflammation involving both bone and cartilage.

Osteochondroma (os-ti-ō-kon-drō'-mà). A benign tumour composed of bone and cartilage.

Osteoclast (os'-ti-ō-klàst). The cell which dissolves or removes unwanted bone.

Osteoclastoma (os-ti-ō-klàst-ō'-mà). A benign tumour composed of a round or oval celled matrix in which are numerous multinucleated giant cells (osteoclasts); also known as the benign giant-celled tumour of bones.

Osteogenesis (os-ti-ō-jen'-e-sis). Formation of bone.

Osteogenic Sarcoma (os-ti-ō-jen'-ik). Sarcoma arising from bone-forming tissues and usually producing bony specules within the tumour mass.

Osteoid (os'-ti-oid). Resembling bone; particularly applied to the soft uncalcified organized matrix with bony pattern which precedes the formation of true bone.

Osteoma (os-ti-ō'-mà). A bony tumour.

Osteomalacia (os-ti-ō-mal-ā'-si-à). A pathological softening of bone; it results in bending and deformity.

Osteomyelitis (os-ti-ō-mī-el-ī'-tis). Inflammation of the bone marrow.

Osteopath (os'-ti-ō-path). One who practises osteopathy.

Osteopathy (os-ti-op'-ath-i). A method of therapeutic treatment which is based on the belief that there is a close association between the structure and functions of the body; therefore abnormal states are treated by manipulation of the joints, muscles, etc.

Osteophyte (os'-ti-ō-fīt). A bony excrescence or outgrowth.

Osteosarcoma (os-ti-ō-sàr-kō'-mà). A sarcoma arising from and producing bone.

Osteosclerosis (os-ti-ō-skle-rō'-sis). The process in which bone is made harder and denser than normal.

Osteotome (os'-ti-ō-tōm). A surgical appliance used for cutting into bone.

Osteotomy (os-ti-ot'-o-mi). The operation of cutting through a bone.

Ostium (os'-ti-um). The opening or mouth of any tubular passage.

Otalgia (ō-tal'-ji-à). Earache.

Otic (ō'-tik). Relating to the ear.

Otitic (ō-tit'-ik). Pertaining to otitis.

Otitis Media (ō-tī'-tis mē'-di-à). Inflammation of the middle ear.

Otophone (ō'-tō-fōn). An eartrumpet.

Otorrhœa (ō-tō-rē'-à). An aural discharge of blood, pus, or serum.

Otosclerosis (ō-tō-skle-rō'-sis). Fibrosis and hardening of the tissues of the middle ear and labyrinth, leading to deafness.

Ova (ō'-và). Pl. of *ovum*, an egg; the female cells of generation.

Ovarian (ō-vē'-ri-an). Pertaining to an ovum or an ovary.

Ovaries (ō'-ver-rēz). Two small oval bodies situated on either side of the uterus on the posterior surface of the broad ligament. The structures in which the ova are developed.

Ovariotomy (ō-vē-ri-ot'-o-mi). Surgical removal of one or both ovaries.

Ovaritis (ō-ver-rī'-tis). Inflammation of an ovary.

Oviduct (ō'-vi-dukt). *See* **Fallopian Tubes.**

Oviparous (ō-vip-er-rus). Bearing or producing eggs.

Ovulation (ov-ū-lā'-shun). The maturation and rupture of a Graafian follicle with the discharge of an ovum.

Ovum (ō'-vum). An egg; the female cell of generation.

Oxalic Acid (oks-al'-ik as'-id). An acid derived from woodsorrel. *See* **Acid.**

Oxaluria (oks-al-ū'-ri-à). The presence of an excessive amount of calcium oxalate in the urine.

Oxidase (oks'-i-dāz). An active principle contained in the cells which are concerned in oxidative changes.

Oxidation (oks-i-dā'-shun). The process whereby oxygen is combined with any other substance, also the process by which oxygen is made to remove hydrogen from a substance as in the case of oxidizing ethyl alcohol into aldehyde, *i.e.*, $C_2H_6O + O = C_2H_4O + H_2O$.

Oxycephaly (oks-i-kef'-a-li). The condition of having a high-pointed skull.

Oxygen (oks'-i-jen). O. A colourless, odourless, gaseous element; necessary for life and combustion; used medicinally as an inhalation in respiratory diseases, etc.

Oxymel (oks'-i-mel). A mixture of vinegar and honey.

Oxyntic (oks-in'-tik). Producing acid. **O. Cells,** the cells in the gastric mucosa which produce hydrochloric acid.

Oxytocic (oks-i-tō'-sik). Hastening parturition; an agent promoting uterine contractions.

Oxyuris Vermicularis (oks-i-ū'-ris ver-mik-ū-lē'-ris). Threadworm; especially prevalent among children; they exist in large numbers in the rectum and lower bowel.

Ozæna (ō-zē'-nà). A disease characterized by nasal ulceration, accompanied by the formation of crusts and foulsmelling discharge.

Ozone (ō'-zōn). An allotropic form of oxygen existing in small quantity in pure air. Chemical symbol, O_3.

Ozonic Ether (ō-zon'-ik). A solution of hydrogen peroxide combined with ether; it is used in testing urine for the presence of blood.

P.

P. Symbol for phosphorus.

Pabulum (pab'-ū-lum). Latin for food; anything of a nourishing nature.

Pacchionian Bodies (pak-i-ōn'-i-an). Enlarged and fibrosed arachnoid villi appearing as small rounded masses attached to dural venous sinuses of the brain.

Pachy (pak'-i). A prefix denoting thick.

Pachydermia (pak-i-derm'-i-à). Excessive thickness of the skin.

Pachymeningitis (pak-i-men-in-ji'-tis). Inflammation of the dura mater.

Pacinian Corpuscles (pas-in'-i-an). Oval-shaped corpuscular terminations of the peripheral ends of the sensory nerves.

Pack. A method of treatment in which the patient is enveloped in moist wrappings, such as a blanket or sheet. **Cold P.**, one in which the patient is wrapped in a sheet wrung out of cold water; over this is placed a mackintosh and blanket. It is important to ensure that every part of the skin is in contact with the sheet, especially the axillæ and groins. The pack is continued for 30 minutes, and signs of collapse must be watched for. **Ice P.**, the method is the same as for cold pack, except that ice water is used and the sheet sprinkled with ice water when in position; alternatively towels may be used, which are frequently changed in turn. Both these packs are used to reduce the temperature, which must not be allowed too great a fall, and is therefore taken at frequent intervals. **Hot P.**, sometimes used for cases of nephritis in which there is much œdema. A blanket is immersed in hot water and then wrung out very dry, and the patient is quickly wrapped in it. This is covered by one or two large mackintoshes, and the rest of the blankets placed in position. If desired, three or four covered hot-water bottles may be placed outside the first dry blanket. The patient may be given a very hot drink to sip, as this helps to promote perspiration. An ice-cap is applied to the head to prevent congestion.

Paget's Disease. (1) Osteitis deformans. (2) An eczematous condition of the nipple and areola of the breast associated with a carcinoma within that gland. Named after Sir James Paget.

Pain (pān). Acute sensory disturbance of which the sufferer is aware; distress or suffering. **After-P.**, the pains immediately following labour which are caused by the contraction and retraction of the uterine muscle during involution. **Boring P.**, a severe piercing type of pain. **False P.**, pains occurring in the later stages of pregnancy, and which are sometimes mistaken for true labour pains. **Girdle P.**, pain resembling a constricting cord round the waist region, commonly associated with tabes. **Growing P.**, pains of rheumatic origin in the limbs of growing persons. **Mental P.**, mental distress or grief; pain having a psychic origin.

Painter's Colic. Colic due to chronic lead poisoning.

Palatal (pal-a´-tal). Pertaining to the palate.

Palate (pal´-at). The roof of the mouth. **Cleft P.**, a congenital cleft between the palatal bones, which leaves a gap in the roof of the mouth opening directly into the nose. **Hard P.**, the front part of the roof of the mouth formed by the two palatal bones. **Soft P.**, situated at the posterior end of the palate, and consisting of muscle covered by mucous membrane.

Palatine (pal´-a-tīn). Pertaining to the palate. **P. Arches**, the double pillars or arch-like folds formed by the descent of the soft palate as it meets the pharynx.

Palladium (pal-ā´-di-um). A rare metal of the platinum group; symbol Pd.

Pallæsthesia (pal-ăs-thēz´-i-ă). Vibration sense or osseous sense; the capacity for recognizing a vibration thrill when a low-pitched tuning fork is set in vibration and placed upon the skin immediately over a bone.

Palliative (pal´-i-a-tiv). An agent which relieves pain.

Pallor (pal´-er). Paleness.

Palm (păm). The anterior or flexor surface of the hand.

Palmar (păm´-er). Pertaining to the palm of the hand.

Palpate (pal´-pāt). To examine with the hand.

Palpation (pal-pā´-shun). The act of manual examination.

Palpebra (pal´-pe-bră). The eyelid.

Palpitation (pal-pi-tā´-shun). Forcible and rapid beating of the heart of which the patient is conscious.

Palsy (pawl´-zi). Paralysis.

Pampiniform (pam-pin-i-fawm). Shaped like a tendril.

Panacea (pan-a-sē´-ă). A drug or other agent which is said to possess the qualities for curing all ills.

Pancarditis (pan-kăr-dī´-tis). Inflammation of all three layers of the heart, i.e., of the peri-, myo-, and endocardium.

Pancreas (pan´-kri-as). A tongue - shaped glandular organ lying below and behind the stomach. See **Insulin**.

Pancreatectomy (pan-kri-a-tek´-to-mi). Excision of the pancreas.

Pancreatic (pan-kri-at´-ik). Relating to the pancreas.

Pancreatitis (pan-kri-a-tī´-tis). Inflammation of the pancreas.

Pandemic (pan-dem´-ik). Widely distributed everywhere; not confined to any particular

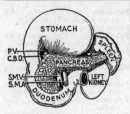

The pancreas and its relations.

P.V., Portal vein.

C.B.D., Common bile duct.

S.M.V., Superior mesenteric vein.

S.M.A., Superior mesenteric artery.

Stomach has been reflected upwards.

area or country; generally used with reference to infectious disease.

Panhysterectomy (pan-his-ter-rek'-to-mi). Complete removal of the uterus. Total hysterectomy.

Pannus (pan'-us). A generalized inflammation of the cornea causing haziness, and therefore seriously affecting the sight.

Panophobia (pan-ō-fō'-bi-à). A morbid fear of everything.

Panophthalmitis (pan-of-thal-mī'-tis). Inflammation of all the tissues of the eyeball.

Panotitis (pan-ō-tī-tis). Inflammation of the ear, especially the middle and internal ear.

Pant. To breathe hard; gasping and heaving respiration, as occurs after running or great exertion; is also produced by fear.

Papain (pap-ān). A ferment similar to pepsin, obtained from the juice of the papaw.

Papaver (pa-pā-ver or -pà-). The poppy plant which produces opium.

Papaverine (pa-páv'-er-rēn). An alkaloid of opium.

Papilla (pa-pil'-à). A minute nipple-shaped eminence. **Circumvallate P.**, the large papilli found at the base and dorsal aspect of the tongue. **Filiform P.**, the fine hair-like papilli at the tip of the tongue. **Fungiform P.**, papilli shaped like a fungus, found chiefly on the dorso-central area of the tongue.

Papillary (pa-pil'-a-ri). Pertaining to or resembling papillæ.

Papilliform (pa-pil'-i-fawm). Having the appearance or characteristics of a papilla.

Papillitis (pap-il-ī'-tis). Inflammation of the optic disc; optic neuritis.

P a p i l l o m a (pap-i-lō'-mà). A proliferative pedunculated benign tumour of the skin or mucous membranes; a wart-like growth.

254

Papular (pap'-ū-lår). Having the characteristics of or resembling a papule.

Papule (pap'-ūl). A small red raised elevation of the skin; often precedes vesicular or pustular formation.

Papyraceous (pap-ir-ā'-shus). Parchment-like. A term sometimes used to denote a fœtus which has been retained in the uterus beyond the natural term and has assumed a mummified appearance.

Paracentesis (pa-ra-sen-tē'-sis). The withdrawal of dropsical effusions by puncturing the tissues, thus permitting the fluid to drain away. **P. Abdominis,** tapping the abdomen with a trocar and cannula for the drainage of fluid. **P. Thoracis,** drainage of fluid from the chest cavity. *See also* Aspiration.

Paracolon (par-a-kō'-lon). The name given to a group of relatively harmless bacilli belonging to the coli-typhoid family.

Paracusis (par-a-kū'-sis). Disordered hearing.

Paradox (par'-a-doks). That which is contrary to generally accepted opinion.

Paræsthesia (par-ās-thēz'-i-à). Any abnormality of sensation.

Paraffin (par'-af-in). A saturated hydrocarbon. **Liquid P.,** refined paraffin, which when taken medicinally is not absorbed from the ali-mentary canal, but acts as an excellent lubricant. **P. Durum,** hard paraffin, *i.e.,* paraffin wax. *See* Ambrine. **P. Molle,** soft vaseline.

Paraldehyde (pa-ral'-de-hīd). A powerful hypnotic with a burning taste. On account of its unpleasant taste it is often administered in capsules, but may also be given as a draught, or per rectum as a pre-operative sedative. Dose, 30-120 minims.

Paralysis (par-al'-i-sis). A loss of the power of motion or muscular action which may affect any set of muscles and may be partial or complete. **P. Agitans,** *see* Parkinson's Disease. **Ascending P.,** *see* Landry's Disease. **Bulbar P.,** paralysis due to degeneration of the nerve roots in the medulla oblongata. **Crutch P.,** caused by pressure of a crutch upon the musculo-spiral nerve in the axilla. **General P. of the Insane,** *see* G.P.I. **Infantile P.,** same as *Acute Anterior Poliomyelitis.* **Hysterical P.,** paralysis resulting as a manifestation of hysteria, but without any organic lesion to account for it; according to psychological theories, it is in the nature of an unconscious defence mechanism. **Pseudohypertrophic Muscular P.,** a chronic form of paralysis affecting certain

255

muscles of the lower extremities and other parts of the body ; the main features are weakness, and often enlargement of the muscle groups affected. **Spastic P.,** a form of paralysis associated with contraction and rigidity of the muscles.

Paralytic (par-a-lit′-ĭk). Pertaining to paralysis.

Parametritis (par-a-met-rī′-tis). Inflammation of the pelvic cellular tissue.

Parametrium (par-a-mĕt′-rĭ-um). The tissues immediately surrounding the uterus.

Paranoia (par-a-noi′-á). A form of chronic but slowly progressive insanity which is characterized by delusions of persecution. The term is often used for several different forms of insanity.

Paraphimosis (par-a-fĭ-mŏ′-sis). Retraction of the prepuce, causing constriction of the glans penis.

Paraplegia (par-a-plē′-ji-á). Paralysis of both lower limbs.

Parasite (par′-a-sīt). An animal or plant existing and living upon or in some other living animal or plant. Human parasites are divided into two main groups : (1) **Internal P.,** consisting of various kinds of worm, especially *round-worms, tape-worms,* and *thread-worms.* (2) **External P.,** consisting of bugs, fleas, and lice. *See* **Pediculus.**

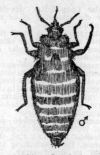

Cimex lectularis
(bed bug).

Parasitic (par-a-sit′-ik). Pertaining to parasites.

Parasiticide (par-a-sit′-i-sīd). An agent which will destroy parasites.

Parasitology (par-a-sit-ol′-o-ji). The science which studies the life-cycles and habits, etc., of parasites.

Parathormone (par-a-thaw(r)-mōn). The internal secretion of the parathyroid glands.

Parathyroid (par-a-thī′-roid). Four small endocrine glands lying close to, or embedded in, the posterior surface of the thyroid gland. They may vary in size and number, and control the calcium and phosphorus metabolism.

Parathyroidectomy (par-a-thi-roid-ek-to-mi). Excision of a parathyroid gland.

Paratyphoid Fever (par-a-tī'-foid). An infectious disease resembling typhoid fever, but caused by the *paratyphoid bacillus*, which is not identical with the *B. typhosus* of Eberth.

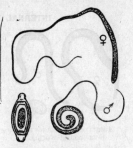

Trichocephalus Trichiurus and Ovum (whip-worm).

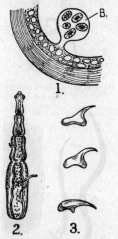

Hydatid.

1, Wall of hydatid cyst, with brood capsule B.
2, *Tænia echinococcus*.
3, Hooklets.

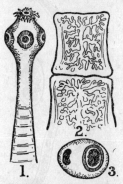

Tænia solium (tape-worm).

1, Scolex (head).
2, Strobila (segments of the body).
3, Oncosphere embryo.

I

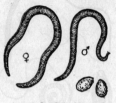

Ascaris lumbricoides and
Ova (round-worm).

Oxyuris vermicularis and Ovum
(thread-worm), not to scale.

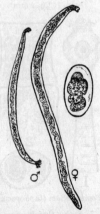

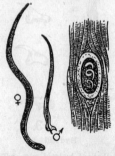

Ankylostoma duodenale and
Ovum (hook-worm).

Trichinella spiralis, with Embryo encysted in Muscle
(measly pork).

Paregoric (par-e-gor'-ik). Camphorated tincture of opium.

Parenchyma (par-en'-ki-mà). The parts of an organ which are concerned with its function in contradistinction to its interstitial tissue.

Parenteral (par-en'-ter-ral). Associated with injections either subcutaneous or intravenous, but not through the alimentary canal.

Paresis (par-ē'-sis). Partial or slight paralysis.

Paretic (par-ē'-tik). Pertaining to paresis.

Pareunia (par-ūn'-i-à). Coitus.

Parietal (par-ī'-et-al). Pertaining to a wall. **P. Bones,** the two bones which form the sides and vault of the skull.

Parietes (par-ī'-et-ēz). The walls of a cavity.

Parietofrontal (par-ī'-et-ō-fron'-tal). Pertaining to the parietal and frontal bones.

Parieto-occipital (par-ī'-et-ō-ok-sip'-it-al). Pertaining to the parietal and occipital bones.

Parkinson's Disease (pår'-kin-sons). A chronic nervous disease characterized by tremor of the head and limbs, a peculiar gait, emaciation, and muscular rigidity. Synonyms, *Paralysis Agitans,* also *Shaking Palsy.* **Parkinson's Mask,** an expressionless appearance of the face, which becomes smoothed out, all wrinkles disappearing, and with absolute immmobility of the facial muscles. This *mask* is typical of Parkinson's disease and post-encephalitic states.

Paronychia (par-ō-nik'-i-à). Inflammation about the nail of the finger. *See* **Onychia, Felon,** and **Whitlow.**

Paroophoron (par-ō-oof'-or-on). Same as *Parovarium.*

Paropsis (par-op'-sis). Disordered vision.

Parosmia (par-os-mi-à). Abnormal sense of smell, generally of an hallucinatory nature.

Parotid (par-ot'-id). (1) Near the ear. (2) The parotid salivary gland, which is situated in front of and below the ear.

Parotidectomy (par-ot-id-ek'-tō-mi). Removal of the parotid gland.

Parotitis (par-ō-tī'-tis). Inflammation of the parotid gland. **Epidemic P.,** mumps. The cause is believed to be a virus infection, but a secondary low grade bacterial parotitis may result as a complication of typhoid fever, scarlet fever, abdominal operations, and neglect of oral hygiene. **Septic P.** is rare, and is accompanied by adenitis of the adjacent lymphatic glands. The chief complications of epidemic parotitis or mumps are mastitis and ovaritis in the female, orchitis in the male.

Pancreatitis occasionally develops.

Parous (pār'-us). Fruitful; bringing forth young; parturient.

Parovarium (par-ō-vēr'-i-um). The vestigial remains of the Wolffian body in the broad ligament of the uterus.

Paroxysm (par'-oks-izm). (1) A sudden increase and exacerbation in the symptoms and gravity of a disease. (2) Fits and convulsions. (3) Sudden rapid development of any particular emotional state, such as joy, fear, or grief.

Paroxysmal (par-oks-iz'-mal). Pertaining to a paroxysm.

Parrot Disease. Psittacosis.

Parrot's Nodes. Bony excrescences or osteophytes on the frontal and parietal bones around the anterior fontanelle in congenital syphilis.

Parry's Disease. Exophthalmic goitre; also known as Graves' disease and Basedow's disease.

Pars. A part. **P. Nervosa,** the posterior lobe of the pituitary gland.

Parthenogenesis (pār-then-ō-jen'-e-sis). An asexual form of reproduction.

Parturient (pār-tūr'-i-ent). The condition of being in labour, or of giving birth to young.

Parturition (pār-tūr-i'-shun). The act of bearing a child.

Partus (pār'-tus). Latin for child-birth; labour.

Passage (pas'-azh). The laboratory process of transmitting a diseased state from one animal to another in order to prove the living nature of the causal agent, especially used in virus culture.

Passive (pas'-iv). Submissive; not active. **P. Congestion,** congestion due to defective circulation, especially venous obstruction. **P. Immunity,** see **Immunity. P. Movements,** movement of the joints of a patient by a masseuse, the patient herself remaining inactive.

Pasteur Treatment. Treatment by the inoculation of a special vaccine for the prevention and cure of hydrophobia.

Pasteurization (pas-tūr-ī-zā'-shun). A process whereby certain pathogenic organisms in milk are destroyed by heat. See **Milk.**

Patella (pat-el'-a). The knee-cap; the triangular-shaped sesamoid bone developed in the rectus femoris tendon. **Patellar Reflex,** the knee-jerk.

Patent (pā'-tent). Open; not closed.

Pathogenesis (path-ō-jen'-e-sis). The origin and development of disease.

Pathogenic (path-ō-jen'-ik). Capable of causing disease.

Pathognomonic (path-ō-nō-

Pathologic (path-ō-loj′-ik). Pertaining to pathology.

Pathologist (path-ol′-o-jist). One who studies pathology.

Pathology (path-ol′-o-ji). The science which deals with the cause and nature of disease. There are many specialized branches of this science, as *e.g., comparative, experimental, general, medical, special,* and *surgical, etc.*

Pathophobia (path-ō-fō′-bi-à). A morbid dread of disease.

Patulous (pat′-ū-lus). Opened out ; expanded.

Pavement Epithelium. Epithelial lining consisting of large irregular polygonal flattened cells.

Pawlie's Grip (paw′-liks). A method of determining how far the presenting part of a fœtus, during the onset of labour in a parturient woman, has descended into the true pelvis.

Pearl (perl). (1) A cataract. (2) A peculiar concentric arrangement of epithelial cells (epithelial pearl or cell-nest).

Pea-soup Stool. The characteristic stool of typhoid fever. It is the colour and consistency of pea-soup and is highly infective.

Pectinate (pek-tin-āt). Resembling a comb.

Pectineal (pek-tin′-i-al). Re-

lating to the pubis. **P. Ridge,** the iliopectineal line.

Pectoral (pek′-tor-al). Relating to the chest.

Pectoriloquy (pek-tor-il′-ō-kwi). Abnormal distinctness of articulate speech heard on auscultation of the chest.

Pedal (pēd′-al). Pertaining to the foot.

Pedialgia (pēd-i-al′-ji-à). Pain in the foot.

Pediatrics (pēd-i-at′-riks). That branch of medical science which specially deals with the diseases and disorders of children.

Pedicle (ped′-ik-l). A stalk ; the narrow part by which a tumour is attached to the surrounding structures.

Pediculosis (ped-ik-ū-lō′-sis). A state of being infested with lice.

Pediculus (ped-ik′-ū-lus). A louse. **P. Capitis,** the head louse. **P. Corporis,** the body louse. **P. Pubis,** the louse which infests the pubis ; the crab-louse.

Pedunculated (pe-dungk′-ū-lā-ted). Possessing a pedicle.

Peliosis (pē-li-ō′-sis). Purpura (*q.v.*).

Pellagra (pel-à′-grà). A deficiency disease due to lack of Vitamin B., characterized by skin, digestive, and nervous disturbances. *See* **Vitamins.**

Pellet (pel′-et). A little pill.

Pellicle (pel′-ik-l). A thin film

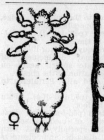

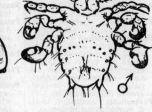

Pediculus capitis (head louse), with Ovum or Nit attached to a Hair.

Pediculus pubis (crab louse).

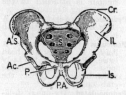

The Pelvis, Adult Male (front view).

A.S., Antero-superior spine.
Ac., Acetabulum.
P., Os Pubis.
P.A., Subpubic arch.
S., Sacrum.
Cr., Iliac crest.
Il., Ilium.
Is., Ischium.

or covering on the surface of a fluid.

Pelvic (pel'-vik). Relating to the pelvis. **P. Girdle,** a girdle formed by the innominate bones.

Pelvimeter (pel-vim'-et-er). An instrument especially devised to measure the diameters of the pelvis.

Pelvis (pel'-vis). A large bony, basin-shaped cavity formed by the innominate bones and the sacrum ; it contains and protects the bladder, generative organs, and the rectum. **False P.,** the wide expanded part of the pelvis above the brim. **Flat P.,** one in which the anteroposterior diameter is shortened. **True P.,** that part of the pelvis below the brim.

Pemphigus (pem'-fig-us). An infectious skin complaint characterized by the appearance of large bullæ. **P. Neonatorum** appears soon after birth ; also known as *Ritter's Disease*, generally due to septic infection, but is sometimes luetic. **P. Syphiliticus**, a form of the disease definitely caused by syphilis.

Pendulous (pen'-dū-lus). Hanging down.

Penicillin (pen-i-sil'-in). The extract from the saprophytic fungus penicillium, used in the treatment of a large number of bacterial infections.

Penis (pē'-nis). The male organ of copulation.

Pennyroyal. A species of mint used medicinally as a carminative.

Pentnucleotide (pent-nūk'-li-ō-tīd). A compound of nuclein and pentose, used to produce leucocytosis in agranulocytosis.

Pentose (pen-tōs). One of a group of sugars with the formula $C_5H_{10}O_5$.

Peppermint (pep'-er-mint). An aromatic carminative and stimulant.

Pepsin (pep'-sin). A proteolytic enzyme of the gastric juice, formed by the interaction of HCl on pepsinogen.

Pepsinogen (pep-sin'-ō-jen). A precursor of pepsin into which

it is changed by contact with HCl. It is formed in the peptic cells of the gastric glands.

Peptic (pep'-tik). Pertaining to pepsin and to digestion generally.

Peptone (pep'-tōn). A substance produced during the hydrolysis of protein by the action of pepsin.

Peptonize (pep'-tō-nīz). A method of enabling food to be more easily digested by previously adding pepsin, which partially digests the food before it is taken.

Peptonuria (pep-tōn-ūr'-i-à). The presence of peptones in the urine.

Per Anum (per ā-num). Through or via the anus.

Peracute (per-a-kūt'). Extremely acute.

Percaine (per'-kān). A local anæsthetic belonging to the quinoline group of drugs. Acts in extreme dilution. Produces intense and lasting anæsthesia. Employed for regional infiltration and spinal anæsthesia, and also in the form of an ointment. **Percainal.**

Perception (per-sep'-shun). The reception and recognition of external impulses as conveyed by the senses.

Perchloride of Mercury. *See* **Corrosive Sublimate.**

Percolation (per-kō-lā'-shun).

The process by which fluid slowly passes through a hard but porous substance.

Percussion (per-kush'-n). The act of striking or tapping the body sharply but lightly in order to gain information as to the position, size, and consistency of structures lying beneath; also performed to detect the presence of fluid or pus in a cavity.

Perforate (per'-for-āt). To puncture; to make holes.

Perforation (per-for-ā'-shun). The state of being perforated.

Perfusion (per-fū'-zhun). The forcing of blood through an organ by way of the blood-vessels.

Periarteritis (pe-ri-àrt-e-rī'-tis). Inflammation of the outer sheath of an artery. **P. Nodosa**, an arterial disease in which the periarteritis results in local aneurysmal swellings and thrombosis.

Periarthritis (pe-ri-àrth-rī'-tis). Inflammation around the joints.

Pericardial (pe-ri-kàrd'-i-al). Pertaining to the pericardium.

Pericarditis (pe-ri-kàr-dī'-tis). Inflammation of the pericardium.

Pericardium (pe-ri-kàrd'-i-um). The double membranous sac which envelops the heart.

Pericellular (per-i-sel-ū-làr). Surrounding cells. **P. Cirrhosis**, a pericellular fibrosis

in the liver resulting from congenital syphilis.

Perichondrium (pe-ri-kond'-ri-um). The membranous covering of cartilage.

Pericranium (pe-ri-krān'-i-um). The periosteal covering of the cranium.

Pericystitis (pe-ri-sis-tī'-tis). Inflammation of the tissues surrounding the bladder.

Perihepatitis (pe-ri-hep-a-tī'-tis). Inflammation of the peritoneal surface of the liver.

Perilymph (pe'-ri-limf). The fluid contained in the internal ear, between the bony and membranous labyrinth.

Perimeter (pe-rim'-et-er). (1) The outer edge or periphery. (2) An instrument for measuring the field of vision.

Perimetritis (pe-ri-met-rī'-tis). Inflammation of the pelvic peritoneum. It is often though not necessarily, associated with parametritis.

Perineal (pe-ri-nē'-al). Pertaining to the perineum.

Perineoplasty (pe-ri-nē-ō-plast'-i). See **Perineorrhaphy**.

Perineorrhaphy (pe-ri-nē-or'-raf-i). The operation for the repair of a torn perineum.

Perinephric (pe-ri-nef'-rik). Around the kidney. **P. Abscess**, the formation of an abscess in the perinephrium.

Perinephrium (pe-ri-nef'-ri-um). The tissues immediately surrounding the kidney.

Perineum (pe-ri-nē'-um). The

muscular structure lying between the vagina and anus.

Perineurium (per-i-nūr′-i-um). The outer sheath of a funiculus of nerve fibres.

Period (pē′-ri-od). An interval of time. **Incubation P.**, the interval which passes between the time when the germ first gains entrance into the body to the time when the first symptoms appear. This varies for most of the common infectious diseases. **Isolation P.**, the time during which those suffering from infectious diseases must be kept separate from the general population. **Quarantine P.**, the time during which " contacts " must be kept isolated. **Monthly P.**, menstruation.

Periosteal (per-i-ost′-i-al). Pertaining to the periosteum.

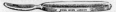

Periosteal Elevator.

Periosteum (per-i-ost′-i-um). The membrane which covers a bone. In long bones only the shaft as far as the epiphysis is covered.

Periostitis (per-i-os-tī′-tis). Inflammation of the periosteum.

Periostosis (per-i-os-tō′-sis). Hypertrophy of bone due to inflammation.

Peripheral (pe-rif′-er-ral). Relating to the periphery.

Periphery (pe-rif′-er-ri). The outer circumference of anything.

Periphlebitis (pe-ri-fle-bī′-tis). Inflammation of the outer coat of a vein.

Perirenal (pe-ri-rēn′-al). Around the kidney.

Perisplenitis (pe-ri-splen-ī′-tis). Inflammation of the capsule of the spleen.

Peristalsis (pe-ri-stal′-sis). The characteristic movement of the intestines by which the contents are moved along the lumen. It consists of a wave of contraction preceded by a wave of relaxation.

Peristaltic (pe-ri-stal′-tik). Pertaining to peristalsis.

Perithelioma (pe-ri-thēl-i-ō-má). A tumour which is supposed to arise from the perivascular lymphatics.

Peritoneal (pe-ri-tō-nē′-al). Pertaining to the peritoneum.

Peritoneum (pe-ri-tō-nē′-um). The delicate membrane which lines the abdominal and pelvic cavities, and also covers the organs contained in them.

Peritonitis (pe-ri-tō-nī′-tis). Inflammation of the peritoneum. **General P.**, general infective inflammation of the whole of the abdominal peritoneum. **Local P.**, inflammation confined to one particular area of the peri-

I*

toneum. **Pelvic P.,** infection of the peritoneal lining of the pelvic cavity. **Plastic P.,** a form in which the bowel becomes bound by the development of inflammatory adhesions. **Tuberculous P.,** inflammation caused by the presence of numerous tuberculous nodules in the peritoneum. *See Miliary Tuberculosis, also* **Ascites.**

Perityphlitis (pe-ri-tĭf-lĭ''-tis). Inflammation of the peritoneum and tissues immediately surrounding the cæcum.

Periurethral (pe-ri-ū-rē'-thral). Surrounding the urethra.

Perivascular (pe-ri-vas'-kū-làr). Around a blood vessel.

Perls' Reaction. The Prussian blue test for the excess of free iron in tissues, by immersing these in a freshly prepared mixture of solutions of weak hydrochloric acid and potassium ferrocyanide.

Permanganate (per-mang'-a-nāt). The salt of permanganic acid. **P. of Potash** (KMnO₄), dark purple crystals which, when dissolved in water, produce a rich purple fluid ; its action is antiseptic, astringent, and deodorant. A weak solution makes an excellent douche, mouth-wash, and gargle ; Condy's fluid.

Permeable (per'-mi-a-bl). Capable of being penetrated ; porous. **P. Strata,** soil which

will readily allow water to soak through it.

Pernicious (per-nish'-us). Having a tendency to end fatally. **P. Anæmia,** a blood disease of unknown etiology ; a primary form of anæmia. The number of erythrocytes becomes diminished, although the colour index remains high. Nucleated red cells are found as well as the conditions of anisocytosis, megalocytosis, polychromasia and poikilocytosis. Cachexia, glossitis, weakness, and a characteristic velvety state of the skin, which is lemon coloured, are important symptoms, and the disease shows remissions. Treatment consists of administration of the specific hæmopoietic principle in the form of fresh liver or liver extracts. Synonym, *Addison's Anæmia.* **P. Vomiting,** *see* **Hyperemesis Gravidarum.**

Pernio (per'-ni-ō). A chilblain.

Peroneal (pe-rō-nē'-al). Pertaining to the fibula.

Peroneum (pe-rō-nē'-um). The fibula.

Peroxidase Test (per-roks'-i-dāz). A chemical test on blood films by which the granules of the cells of the granulocytic series are stained black.

Peroxide of Hydrogen (H₂O₂). A substance nearly related to water chemically and differing therefrom in that its molecule contains one more atom of oxygen. When brought into contact with septic material, this extra atom of oxygen is liberated with effervescence. It owes its antiseptic properties to this capacity of acting as an oxidizing agent.

Pertussis (per-tus´-is). Whooping-cough; a contagious paroxysmal cough which is characterized by a peculiar "whoop." The causative germ is the *bacillus of Bordet and Gengou.*

Perversion (per-ver´-shun). Deviation from the normal. **Sexual P.,** abnormal manifestation of the sex instinct.

Pervious (per´-vi-us). The state of being permeable.

Pes. A foot. **P. Cavus.** *See* **Talipes.**

Pessary (pes´-a-ri). An appliance fixed in the vagina to

Hodge's Pessary.

serve as a support for a prolapsed or displaced uterus; it is usually constructed of rubber or vulcanite. There are many patterns and sizes,

the commonest being the *ring, Hodge's,* and *stem* pessaries. Also a medicated lozenge or cone of coco-butter, etc., used for vaginal antisepsis or as a contraceptive.

Pest. The plague.

Pestilence (pes´-til-ens). A virulent, deadly epidemic disease.

Pestis (pes´-tis). The name of the micro-organism causing bubonic plague.

Petechiæ (pe-tēk´-i-ē or pe-tēch´-i-ē). Small hæmorrhagic spots in the skin.

Petechial (pe-tēk´-i-al). Pertaining to petechiæ.

Petit mal (pet-ē´ mal). A mild form of epilepsy usually without convulsions.

Petri Dish (pet´-ri). A small shallow glass dish used in chemical and bacteriological laboratories.

Petrification (pet-ri-fi-kā´-shun). The process of converting matter into a hard stone-like condition.

Pétrissage (pā´-tris-äzh). A kneading movement used in massage.

Petroleum (pet-rō´-li-um). An inflammable mineral oil obtained from the earth in various parts of the world.

Petrous (pē´-trus). Resembling stone; hard. **P. Bone** or **Petrosa,** the lower portion of the temporal bone which contains the canals of the 7th and 8th cranial nerves.

Peyer's Patches. Flat patches of lymphatic tissue situated in the small intestine, but mainly in the ileum ; they are the seat of infection in typhoid fever and in tuberculosis enteritis.

Pfeiffer's Bacillus (fīf'-er). A short slender bacillus often found in cases of influenza, but not the cause of this disease. Also known as *Hæmophilus influenzæ.*

Phagedena (faj-e-dē'-nà). Rapidly spreading ulceration of the tissues, with a tendency to sloughing and gangrene.

Phagocyte (fag'-ō-sīt). A cell which exhibits the special function of ingesting and destroying bacteria and other substances foreign to the blood and other tissues.

Phagocytosis (fag-ō-sī-tō'-sis). The action of phagocytes in destroying bacteria.

Phalanges (fal-an'-jēs). The small bones of the fingers and toes. Singular, *phalanx.*

Phallic (fal'-ik). Pertaining to the penis.

Phallus (fal'-us). The penis.

Phantom Tumour. An apparent tumour due to flatus or muscular contraction, seen in hysterical patients. *See* **Pseudocyesis.**

Pharmaceutical (fàm-a-sūt'-ik-l). Pertaining to pharmacy.

Pharmacist (fàm'-a-sist). A title restricted by the Pharmacy Acts to persons possessing the qualifying certificate of the Pharmaceutical Society of Great Britain and who are registered as chemists and druggists. Persons skilled in the science and art of pharmacy. An apothecary or druggist.

Pharmacology (fàm-a-kol'-o-ji). The science of the nature and action of drugs.

Pharmacopœia (fàm-a-cop-ē'-er). A book containing a list of drugs for use in medicine, the manner of preparing and compounding them, and the weights and measures by which they are to be mixed. Information is also given concerning the characters of the substances enumerated, the test for their identity, and the dosage of the drugs suitable for internal administration. The " British Pharmacopœa " is published under the direction of the General Council of Medical Education and Registration of the United Kingdom, and it is revised and republished periodically. The term British Pharmacopœia is often abbreviated B.P. Each country has its own Pharmacopœia.

Pharmacy (fàm'-a-si). The science and art of preparing, compounding, and dispensing drugs for medicinal purposes.

Pharyngeal (far-in-jē'-al). Pertaining to the pharynx.

Pharyngismus (far-in-jis'-mus). Spasm of the pharynx.

Pharyngitis (far-in-jī'-tis). Inflammation of the pharynx.

Pharyngotomy (far-in-got'-o-mi). Incision into the pharynx.

Pharynx (far'-ingks). The cavity at the back of the mouth. It is cone-shaped, 4½ in. long, and is lined with mucous membrane; at the lower end it opens into the œsophagus.

Phenazone. Synonym antipyrin.

Phenol (fē'-nol). Carbolic acid.

Phenolphthalein (fē-nol-tha'-lē-in). A coal-tar derivative used as an indicator of alkalinity in chemistry and as a laxative in medicine.

Phimosis (fī-mŏ'-sis). Narrowing of the meatus of the prepuce such that the foreskin cannot be retracted over the glans penis.

Phlebectasis (fle-bek'-ta-sis). Local dilatation of a vein.

Phlebitis (fle-bī'-tis). Inflammation of a vein.

Phlebolith (fleb'-ō-lith). A vein stone; a calcareous concretion in a vein.

Phlebotomy (fle-bot'-o-mi), Venesection (q.v.).

Phlegm (flem). The secretion of mucus expectorated from the bronchi.

Phlegmasia Alba Dolens. White-leg; a thrombo-phlebitis which commonly follows parturition, but may also occur in some other conditions. The leg becomes white, œdematous, and painful. Careful nursing is essential in these cases, as there is a danger of a piece of the thrombus becoming detached, so forming an *embolus*. Complete rest, immobilization of the limb, and administration of sedatives are the main features of treatment.

Phlegmatic (fleg-mat'-ik). Sluggish; apathetic.

Phlegmoncus (fleg'-mon-us). Of the nature of a phlegmon which is a condition of acute suppuration of loose connective tissue.

Phloem (flō'-em). A biological term indicating the outer vascular layer of a tree stem.

Phlyctena (flik-tē'-nā). A cutaneous swelling filled with clear fluid; a blister.

Phlyctenule (flik-ten'-ūl). A minute phlyctena.

Phonation (fō-nā'-shun). The utterance of vocal sounds.

Phonetics (fō-net'-iks). The science which studies sounds produced vocally.

Phosphate (fos'-fāt). A salt of phosphoric acid.

Phosphaturia (fos-fa-tū'-ri-à). The presence of an excess of phosphates in the urine.

Phosphorated (fos'-for-ā-ted). Containing phosphorus.

Phosphorescence (fos-for-es'-ens). The property of shining in the dark without emitting heat.

Phosphorus (fos'-for-us). A non-metallic element forming an important constituent of osseous and nervous tissue.

Photometer (fō-tom'-et-er). An apparatus used for measuring the intensity of light.

Photometry (fō-tom'-et-ri). The determination of the degree of intensity of light.

Photomicrograph (fō-tō-mīk'-rō-graf). An enlarged photograph taken of a microscopic object by the combined use of a double-extension camera and a microscope.

Photophobia (fō-tō-fōb'-i-à). Inability to stand exposure of the eyes to light ; extreme sensitiveness to light.

Photosynthesis (fō-tō-sin'-the-sis). The process by which plants are able to manufacture carbohydrates from the air in the presence of light. Only plants containing chlorophyll are capable of thus producing sugars. It is obvious, therefore, that there is some association between chlorophyll and sunlight. The red and blue waves of the spectrum are absorbed by the chlorophyll, but all others are rejected. CO_2 and H_2O are also necessary factors. When grape-sugar is formed, the plant splits up CO_2, uses the carbon by photosynthesis, and liberates the oxygen. The sources of energy for this disruption are the blue and red rays which are absorbed by the plant. To make 1 grm. of synthetic sugar the plant requires 750 cub. ft. of CO_2.

Phototropism (fō-tō-trōp'-izm). *See* **Tropistic Action.**

Phren (fren). The diaphragm.

Phrenalgia (fren-al'-ji-à). Pain in the diaphragm.

Phrenic (fren'-ik). Pertaining to the diaphragm.

Phrenology (fren-ol'-o-ji). Character reading from the shape of the head.

Phthiriasis (thi-rī'-a-sis). The presence of lice and their irritating effects.

Phthisical (thīs'-ik-al). Pertaining to phthisis.

Phthisis (thīs'-is). Pulmonary tuberculosis ; a wasting disease.

Phylogeny (fī-loj'-en-i). The development of a group or species of animal life.

Phylum (fī'-lum). A primary division in biological classification.

Physic (fiz'-ik). (1) The science of healing. (2) A drug.

Physical (fiz'-ik-al). Pertaining to physics or to the body generally.

Physician (fiz-ish'-un). A doctor who specializes in medicine.

Physicist (fiz'-is-ist). One who is an expert in the knowledge and science of physics.

Physics (fiz'-iks). The science

which deals with the forces, formation, properties, and measurement of matter.

Physiognomy (fiz-i-og′-no-mi or fiz-i-on′-o-mi). (1) A study of character as revealed by the contours of the face. (2) The face.

Physiological (fiz-i-ō-loj′-ik-al). Pertaining to physiology. **P. Saline Solution**, 0·9% sodium chloride in water.

Physiology (fiz-i-ol′-o-ji). The science which deals with the manifestations of life as revealed by the functions of the body tissues. It is closely allied to such subjects as physics, chemistry, and biochemistry.

Physiotherapy (fiz-i-ō-the′-rap-i). Treatment of disease by heat, massage, hydrotherapy, light, etc.

Physique (fiz-ēk′). The general build and constitution of the body.

Physostigmine (fī-zō-stig′-min). An alkaloid of the Calabar bean; much used as a myotic. Same as *Eserine* (*q.v.*).

Phyto (fī-tō-). Prefix signifying pertaining to plants.

Pia Arachnoid (pē′-à or pī′-à a-rak′-noid). The term used to denote the pia mater and arachnoid membranes when regarded as forming one structure.

Pia or **Pia Mater** (pē′-à or pī′-à mā′-ter). The inner membrane of the meninges; the vascular membrane which lies in close contact with the substance of the brain and spinal cord.

Pial (pī′al). Pertaining to the pia mater.

Pica (pī′-kà). Desire for extraordinary articles of food.

Pick's Disease. Pseudocirrhosis of the liver combined with adhesive pericarditis and adhesive peritonitis.

Picric Acid (pik′-rik). A poisonous lemon-coloured crystalline substance, the solution of which is much used as a dressing for burns and as an antiseptic.

Picrotoxin (pik-rō-toks′-in). A drug used as a motor stimulant; it also checks the night-sweats which appear in phthisis. Dose, 1/100-1/25 gr.

Pigment (pig′-ment). Any colouring matter of the body.

Pigmentation (pig-men-tā′-shun). The deposit of pigment, especially when abnormal or excessive.

Piles. *See* Hæmorrhoids.

Pilocarpine (pī-lō-kár′-pin). The alkaloid drug obtained from jaborandi; is a cardiac depressant, increases salivation, and is a powerful diaphoretic, and is therefore extremely useful in renal disease associated with œdema. Dose, Pilocarpine nitrate, 1/20-1/5 gr.

Pilonidal (pī-lō-nī'-dal). Containing an accumulation of hairs in a cyst. **P. Sinus,** a discharging sinus near the anus resulting from infection of a congenital pilonidal cyst.

Pilula (pil'-ū-là). Latin for pill.

Pimple (pim'-pl). A raised red and pustular spot.

Pineal Body (pīn'-ē-al). A small red gland lying immediately above the superior colliculi of the mid brain ; it is thought to be a vestigial remnant of what was possibly once a functioning third eye, which still exists in certain lizards.

Pink Disease. First described in 1914 by Swift. The disease occurs in children, and is characterized by pyrexia and constitutional disturbance, œdema of the hands and feet, with erythema, which also appears on cheeks, ears, and nose. Also known as *Erythrœdema.*

Pink-eye. Popular name for acute contagious conjunctivitis.

Pinna (pin'-à). That part of the ear which is external to the head ; the ear-flap.

Pint (pīnt). A fluid measure equal in value to 20 oz., or 160 drachms, or 9,600 minims.

Pipette (pip-et'). A fine graduated glass tube for taking up fluids.

Piqûre (pi-kūr'). Puncture.

Pisiform Bone (pīz'-i-fawm). A small pea-shaped bone in the wrist.

Pithing (pith'-ing). The destruction of the central nervous system by piercing the brain and cord.

Pitting (pit'-ing). (1) Making an indentation in dropsical tissues. (2) The scars left on the skin after an attack of smallpox.

Pituitary Extract (pit-ū'-it-a-ri). The internal secretion of the pituitary gland ; it contracts plain muscle and raises the blood-pressure ; it also has a marked effect upon the gravid uterus. Also known as *Pituitrin.* **P. Gland,** the pea-shaped gland lying in the *sella turcica* of the sphenoid bone ; the hypophysis cerebri.

Pityriasis (pit-i-rī'-a-sis). A scaly skin disease.

Placebo (pla-sē'-bō). An inert drug given merely to satisfy the patient.

Placenta (pla-sen'-tà). A thick, circular, fleshy mass which is attached to the wall of the pregnant uterus. It is formed early in pregnancy, and serves as an organ of nutrition for the fœtus. It is expelled from the uterus after the birth of the child, and is therefore often known as the *afterbirth.* **Adherent P.,** one which remains adherent to the uterine wall beyond the normal period for its separation after childbirth. **Battledore P.,** one in which the cord is attached to the edge instead of the middle of the placenta. **P. Prævia,** an abnormality in which the placenta is developed in the lower uterine segment, and therefore presents before the fœtus at the onset of labour ; the condition is usually recognized by ante-partum bleeding. There are three varieties : (1) *Central,* when it lies across the opening of the cervix ; (2) *marginal,* when it lies at the margin of the cervix ; (3) *lateral,* when situated at the side of the lower uterine segment. **Retained P.,** one which is retained in the uterus as the result of uterine contraction. **P. Succenturiata,** a smaller secondary placenta.

Plague (plăg). A virulent contagious disease occurring in epidemic form. **Bubonic P.,** that variety which is caused by the *B. pestis,* and characterized by the presence of buboes. The Great Plague of London was of this type.

Planocaine (plan'-ō-kān). A white crystalline powder, odourless and stable under ordinary atmospheric conditions ; very soluble in water ; used as a local anæsthetic. For spinal anæsthesia a 5% solution combined with adrenalin is generally used ; approximately 3 c.c. are given. This may be prepared from planocaine powder and dissolved in the patient's own cerebrospinal fluid if desired, ·1-·15 grm. being dissolved in 3 c.c. of cerebrospinal fluid.

Plantar (plan-tă(r)). Pertaining to the sole of the foot. **P. Arch,** the union of the plantar and dorsalis pedis arteries in the sole of the foot.

Plaque (plăk or plak). A flat plate or surface.

Plasma (plaz'-mă). The straw-coloured fluid in which the solids of the blood float.

Plasmodium (plaz-mō'-di-um). A motile mass of protoplasm formed by the fusion of two or more amœboid bodies. **P. falciparum,** the parasite of sub-tertian or malignant malaria. **P. malariæ,** the parasite of quartan malaria. **P. vivax,** the parasite of tertian malaria.

Plaster (plăs'-ter). An adhesive material used medicinally for strapping the edges of cuts, etc., together, for supporting structures, keeping splints and dressings in position, and for the purpose of extension in case of fracture, etc. *See also* **Lead P.** and **Court P. P. of Paris,** heated calcium sulphate, which sets to a hard mass when mixed with small

273

quantities of water. **P. of P. Bandages,** the dry powder is rubbed into 6-yd. length muslin bandages and stored in air-tight tins ; before applying they are immersed in tepid water.

Plastic (plas'-tik). Capable of being moulded. **P. Surgery,** that branch of surgery which specializes in restoring and repairing physical defects.

Platelets, Blood. *See* Blood.

Platyhelminth (plat-i-hel'-minth). One of the *platyhelminthes* or flat worms which include the tape worms.

Pleomorphic (plē-ō-maw(r)'-fik). Having many distinct shapes ; multiform.

Plethora (pleth'-o-rà). Abnormal fullness of the blood-vessels. Full-bloodedness.

Pleura (plooer'-ra). A thin membrane covering the surface of the lung, and reflecting, at the root of the lung, on to the chest wall.

Pleurisy (plooer'-ri-si). Inflammation of the pleura ; pleuritis.

Pleurodynia (plooer-rō-din'-i-à). Pain in the intercostal nerves.

Pleurothotonos (plooer-rō-thot'-on-os). Bending of the body sideways in muscular spasms, *e.g.,* in tetanus and strychnine poisoning.

Plexus (pleks'-us). A network of vessels or nerves.

Plica (plī'-kà). A fold.

Plicate (plī'-kàt). Folded.

Plumbago (pium-bà-gō). Graphite or lead.

Plumbism (plum'-bizm). Lead-poisoning.

Plumbo-solvent Action. The dissolving action of soft water on lead.

Plumbum (plum'-bum). Lead.

Pneumobacillus (nū-mō-bas-i-lus). A bacillus which sometimes causes pneumonia ; Friedlander's bacillus.

Pneumococcus (nū-mō-kok'-us). A bacterium causing pneumonia. There are at least thirty different types. The microbe is encapsuled and a diplococcus.

Pneumoconiosis (nū-mō-kōn-i-ō'-sis). A fibrotic disease of the lungs caused by the inhalation of dust or grit. Also written *Pneumonokoniosis.*

Pneumogastric (nū-mō-gas'-trik). The tenth cranial nerve ; supplies the heart, lungs, and stomach. Also known as the *Vagus Nerve.*

Pneumonia (nū-mō'-ni-à). Inflammation of the lungs. **Acute Lobar P.,** inflammation of one or more lobes of the lung. **Broncho-P.,** *see* Lobular P. **Double P.,** disease affecting both lungs. **Hypostatic P.,** a type of pneumonia occurring in the aged and feeble, and attacking the most dependent part of the lung. **Septic, P.** a form resulting from inhaling septic material.

Pneumonic (nū-mon′-ik). Relating to the lungs.

Pneumonitis (nū-mon-ī′-tis). Same as *Pneumonia*.

Pneumopericardium (nū-mō-per-i-kå(r)′-di-um). The presence of air or gas in the pericardial sac.

Pneumothorax (nū-mō-thaw′-raks). The presence of gas or air in the pleural cavity.

Pock. A pustule of smallpox.

Podagra (po-dag′-rå). Gout.

Podalgia (pō-dal′-ji-å). Pain in the feet.

Podalic (pō-dal′-ik). Relating to the feet. **P. Version,** turning of the fœtus while in utero, so that the head is uppermost and the feet presenting.

Podophyllin (po-dof′-il-in). A powerful gastro - intestinal irritant, producing a bile-stained liquid motion.

Poikilocytosis (poik-il-ō-sī-tō′-sis). An alteration in the shape of the erythrocytes.

Polarimeter (pōl-a-rim′-et-er). An instrument for measuring the degree of rotation of polarized light.

Polarization of Light (pōl-ar-i-zā′-shun). The changing of light rays in such a way that vibrations take place in one plane only. The property of rotating this plane through varying but specific degrees is characteristic of sugar

solutions and other substances.

Polioencephalitis (pō-li-ō-en-kef-al-ī′-tis). Inflammation of the cortex of the brain.

Poliomyelitis (pō-li-ō-mī-el-ī′-tis). Acute inflammation of the grey matter of the spinal cord. **Acute Anterior P.,** infantile paralysis ; the main symptoms are pyrexia and paralysis of various groups of muscles.

Politzer Bag (po-lit′-zer). An apparatus consisting of a rubber bag with a rubber tube and nozzle ; the latter is introduced into a nostril,

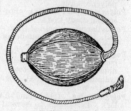

Politzer Bag.

and the patient asked to swallow. The doctor simultaneously squeezes the rubber bulb ; by this means air is forced up the Eustachian tubes into the middle ear.

Poly. A prefix meaning many.

Polyarthritis (pol-i-år-thrī′-tis).

Inflammation of several joints at the same time.

Polyblast (pol'-i-blast). The large motile phagocytic cells of newly developing connective tissue. These cells are derived from various sources and eventually exhibit different functions.

Polychromasia (pol-i-krō-māz'-i-à). The property of some cells of being stained by different types of stain; such cells show abnormal coloration in stained preparations.

Polychromatophilia (pol-i-krō-mat-ō-fil'-i-à). The same as polychromasia.

Polycystic (pol-i-sis'-tik). Possessing many cysts.

Polycythæmia (pol-i-sī-thēm'-i-à). An excessive number of red blood-corpuscles.

Polydactylism (pol-i-dak'-til-izm). Having an excessive number of fingers and toes.

Polydipsia (pol-i-dip'-si-à). Excessive thirst.

Polyglandular (pol-i-gland'-ū-làr). Pertaining to several glands.

Polygraph (pol'-i-graf). An apparatus designed for recording simultaneously the arterial and venous pulses, the apex beat, or other movements.

Polymastia (pol-i-mast'-i-à). Having one or more accessory breasts; these may be found in the axilla, thigh, or other unusual place.

Polymorphonuclear (pol-i-mawrf-ō-nūk'-li-àr). Having nuclei of many different shapes; a name given to the common and most abundant type of leucocyte in the blood, because the nucleus of the cell is lobulated and of variable shape; they constitute about 70% of the total number of leucocytes.

Polyneuritis (pol-i-nū-rī'-tis). Inflammation affecting several nerves at the same time.

Polyopia (pol-i-ōp'-i-à). Seeing many images of a single object.

Polyp or Polypus (pol'-ip(-us)). A small pedunculated tumour growing from the mucous membrane of the nose, vagina, or uterus, etc.

Polyposis (pol-i-pō'-sis). A condition, e.g., of colon, rectum, or stomach, in which there are numerous and widespread polyps.

Polysaccharide (pol-i-sak'-ar-īd) $(C_6H_{10}O_5)n$. One of the carbohydrate groups; it includes starches, glycogen, dextrin, and cellulose; chemically they consist of the saccharide group $(C_6H_{10}O_5)$ multiplied many times; they are non-crystallizable, non-reducible, and do not form osazones.

Polyserositis (pol-i-sē-rō-sī'-tis).

General inflammation of serous surfaces, *e.g.*, of pleuræ, pericardium and peritoneum.

Polyuria (pol-i-ūr'-i-à). An excessive secretion of urine.

Pompholyx (pom'-fol-iks). A skin disease affecting the hands and feet with multiple bullæ or blisters.

Pomum Adami (pōm'-um a-dăm'-i). The prominence in the front of the neck due to the thyroid cartilage in the male; commonly known as *Adam's Apple.*

Pons Varolii. The white convex mass of nerve tissue at the base of the brain which serves to connect the various lobes of the brain.

Popliteal (pop-lit-tē'-al). Pertaining to the popliteus. **P. Space,** the space in the popliteus.

Popliteus (pop-lit-tē'-us). The region behind the knee-joint.

Pore. One of the mouths of the ducts leading from the sudoriferous or sweat gland on the surface of the skin; they are controlled by fine papillary muscles, contracting and closing in the cold, and dilating in the presence of heat.

Porencephaly (por-en-kef'-al-i). The condition of the brain in which the surface is pitted by depressions; cysts might also be present in its substance.

Poroplastic Felt. Sheets of thick, tough, brown felt which are used for making supports, jackets, and splints.

Porosity (por-os'-it-i). A state of being porous.

Porous (paw'-rus). (1) Having pores. (2) Allowing the ready passage of fluid.

Portal Vein. The vein formed by the veins of the splanchnic area, and which conveys this blood into the liver.

Port-wine Stain. A purplish-red birth-mark; a nævus; often occurs on the face or neck.

Position (pō-zish'-'n). Posture; attitude. *See* **Decubitus** and **Presentation. Dorsal P.,** lying on the back. **Fowler's P.,** the sitting position, with the back and head well supported by pillows, and the knees flexed over a pillow to prevent slipping. **Genu-pectoral P.,** a position sometimes used to correct a cord presentation, etc., during delivery; the patient rests upon her knees and breasts with the head resting upon the folded arms. *See Diagram,* p. 279. **Knee-chest P.,** same as *Genu-pectoral P.* **Left Lateral P.,** the patient lies on the left side with the knees flexed, the right thigh being drawn up a little more than the left. **Sim's P.,** a position much used in gynæcology for vaginal examination; the patient assumes an

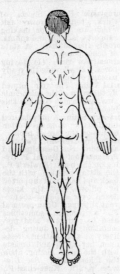 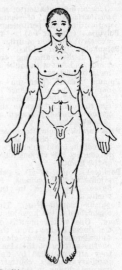

Anatomical Positions.

Posterior View.   Anterior View.

exaggerated left lateral posture with the head well flexed and resting on a pillow, the buttocks are brought well to the edge of the bed, and the left arm is placed along the back.

Posology (pŏz-ol'-o-ji). The science which deals with the dosage of drugs.

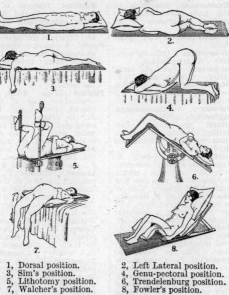

1, Dorsal position.
3, Sim's position.
5, Lithotomy position.
7, Walcher's position.

2, Left Lateral position.
4, Genu-pectoral position.
6, Trendelenburg position.
8, Fowler's position.

Posthumous (post'-ū-mus). A term applied to a child who is born after the death of the father.

Posticus (pŏs'-tĭk-us). Posterior; dorsal.

Post-mortem (pŏst-maw(r)'-tem). After death. **P.**

279

Examination, dissection of the body after death for medical purposes; an autopsy.

Post-natal (pŏst-nā'-tal). After birth.

Post-operative (pŏst-op'-e-ra-tiv). After operation.

Post-partum (pŏst-pär'-tum). After parturition. **P. Hæmorrhage,** severe bleeding occurring after labour; it may be (1) *primary* or (2) *secondary*. See **Hæmorrhage.** Abbreviation P.P.H.

Postural (pos'-tū-ral). Pertaining to position or posture.

Potash (pot'-ash). Potassium hydroxide.

Potassium (pot-as'-i-um), K. One of the chemical elements, a soft malleable metal. Several of its salts are prescribed medicinally, four of the chief being : **P. Bromide,** a nerve sedative; dose, 5-30 gr. **P. Citrate,** a powerful diuretic; dose, 15-60 gr. **Iodide of P.,** much used in the treatment of aneurysm and in syphilitic conditions; dose, 5-20 gr. **Permanganate of P.,** a useful disinfectant and deodorizer; has an astringent and antiseptic action, and is therefore prescribed for douching and gargles.

Potion (pō'-shun). A draught or drink.

Pott's Disease. Spinal caries due to tuberculosis. **P.**

Fracture, fracture of the lower end of the fibula; often accompanied by dislocation of the tarsal bones and injury to the ligaments.

Pouch. A pocket or recess. **P. of Douglas,** the cavity in the pelvis lying between the posterior wall of the uterus and the anterior surface of the rectum.

Poultice (pōl'-tis). A hot, moist application made of bread, linseed, mustard, etc. **Bread P.,** the crumb of bread is moistened by pouring boiling water over it; the water is then pressed out, and the bread mash spread between old linen and applied. **Ice P.,** see **Ice. Linseed P.,** see **Linseed. Mustard P.,** dry mustard is added to the dry linseed in proportions of 1/8 for adults, but 1/12 to 1/16 for children; the poultice is then made as for an ordinary linseed poultice. **Charcoal P.,** is used for foul septic wounds; it can either be made in the same way as a mustard poultice in the proportion of 1/3, or an ordinary linseed poultice can be made and the charcoal powdered over the top; the former method is the more usual. **Jacket P.,** a poultice made both for the chest and back; used in acute lobar pneumonia. **Starch P.,** used in eczema and other skin affections ; a thick paste of ʒii of starch is made, to which is added 1 dram of boracic acid to water, 1 pint; the mixture is boiled to burst the starch granules, and is then spread on old linen and applied to the part ; it is renewed four-hourly.

Poupart's Ligament (poo'-part's). The ligament which stretches between the anterior-superior spine of the ilium and the spine of the pubis.

Pox (poks). A contagious pustular disease ; syphilis.

Practitioner (prak-ti'-shun-er). A practising physician or doctor.

Precancerous (prē-kan'-se-rus). Occurring before cancer with special reference to non-malignant pathological changes which are nevertheless believed to lead on to or to be followed by cancer.

Precipitation (prē-sip-it-ā'-shun). The process of throwing down solids from their solutions in liquids, leaving clear fluid above.

Precordial (prē-kaw(r)'-di-al). Pertaining to the area of the chest immediately over the heart.

Predisposition (prē-dis-pō-zi'-shun). A natural susceptibility to develop or contract certain diseases.

Pregnancy (preg'-nan-si). The state of being with child.

Abdominal P., the growth and development of the embryo within the abdominal cavity. **Extra-uterine P.,** see Ectopic Gestation. **False P.,** see Pseudocyesis. **Multiple P.,** a condition in which there is more than one embryo in the uterus. **Ovarian P.,** a rare condition in which conception occurs within the ovary. **Phantom P.,** an imaginary pregnancy. See Pseudocyesis.

Pregnant (preg'-nant). Having conceived ; with child.

Prehensile (prē-hen'-sīl). Equipped for grasping.

Prehension (prē-hen'-shun). Grasping.

Premature (prē'-ma-tūr). Occurring before the proper time. **P. Labour,** expulsion of the fœtus before the 280th day of gestation.

Premolar (prē-mōl'-âr). One of the two bicuspid teeth which immediately precede the molars.

Premonition (prē-mōn-i'-shun). A warning of future events ; a feeling of impending disaster.

Prenatal (prē-nāt'-al). Prior to birth ; during the period of gestation.

Prepuce (prē'-pūs). The foreskin of the penis.

Presbyopia (pres-bi-ōp'-i-à). Long-sightedness, due to failure of accommodation in elderly persons of about the age of forty-five and onwards.

Prescription (prē-skrip'-shun). A written formula for dispensing drugs signed by a physician. A prescription consists of four main parts: (1) The **Superscription**, represented by the symbol ℞, which signifies *Recipe*, from the Latin *recipere*, meaning take. (2) The **Inscription**, containing the ingredients; this again is generally constructed of four parts; (*a*) the *basis* or principal drug; (*b*) the *adjuvant*, which assists the action of the basis; (*c*) the *corrective*, which diminishes unpleasant taste or pain or griping, etc.; (*d*) the *vehicle* to hold the drugs either in solution or suspension. (3) The **Subscription**, or directions to the dispenser as to the manner of preparation of the drugs. (4) The **Signature**; this is concerned with directions to the patient with regard to the manner of taking, dosage, etc.; finally, the physician's signature and the date must be added.

Presentation (pres-en-tā'-shun). That part of the fœtus which appears at the pelvic outlet during labour.

Pressure-point. A point very sensitive to pressure; the place where pressure should be applied to stop an arterial hæmorrhage; a point or area particularly liable to develop a pressure sore when the patient is kept in bed for long periods.

Presystole (prē-sis'-to-li). The period preceding the systole or contraction of the heart.

Priapism (prī'-ap-izm). Persistent and painful erection of the penis.

Prickly Heat. *See* Miliaria.

Primary (prīm'-a-ri). First. Also means of unknown origin, *e.g.*, in P. Anæmia. **P. Hæmorrhage**, bleeding occurring at the time of injury.

Primigravida (prīm-i-grav'-i-dà). A woman who is pregnant for the first time.

Primipara (prī-mip'-a-rà). A woman who is giving birth to her first child.

Primitive (prim'-it-iv). New or original; also means undeveloped.

Principle (prin'-sip-'l). The essence or primary quality of a body.

Privates (prī'-vets). The non-technical name for the external genitalia.

Probang (prō'-bang). A flexible rod-like instrument which is used for removing foreign bodies from the Œsophagus.

Probe (prōb). A straight, slender instrument, used (1) for examining the depth and dimensions and contents of a wound; (2) when threaded to carry gauze through a perforating wound; (3) as a director ; (4) for applying drugs to the os uteri, etc.

Procidentia (pro-si-den'-shi-à). Complete prolapse of the uterus.

Procreation (prō-krē-ā'-shun). The reproduction of the species.

Proctalgia (prok-tal'-ji-à). Pain about the area of the rectum.

Proctitis (prok-tī'-tis). Inflammation of the rectum.

Proctoclysis (prok-tō-klī'-sis). The slow introduction of a fluid, such as saline, into the rectum.

Proctoscope (prok'-tō-skōp). *See* Rectoscope.

Proctoscope.

Prodromal Rash (prō-drōm'-al). A rash which sometimes precedes the true rash of an infectious disease, *e.g.*, the " bathing-drawers " rash of smallpox.

Profeta's Law (pro-fēt'-à) states that a syphilitic mother cannot infect her own child

if it is born healthy. *See also* **Colles' Law.**

Progeny (proj'-en-i). Offspring.

Progeria (prō-jē'-ri-à). A rare condition in which premature senility supervenes upon infantilism. The skin becomes loose and wrinkled, the arteries become hardened, and baldness is a common feature. The cause is unknown.

Proglottides (prō-glot'-id-ēz). The plural of proglottis.

Proglottis (prō-glot'-is). One of the segments of the body of a tape-worm.

Prognathous (prog'-nā-thus). Having projecting jaws.

Prognosis (prog-nō'-sis). A forecast of the probable course and termination of a disease.

Prognosticate (prog-nos'-ti-kāt). To predict or prophesy ; to make a prognosis.

Projection (prō-jek'-shun). (1) The act of throwing forward ; a part extending beyond the level of the surroundings. (2) A psychological term meaning a transference of a painful emotion from its source to some other innocent object.

Prolan (prō'-lan). The hormone secreted by the anterior lobe of the pituitary which stimulates ovarian activity. Given by intramuscular injection in doses of 100-300 rat units daily.

Prolapse (prō'-laps). Descent ;

283

the falling of a structure, such as the uterus or rectum.

Proliferation (prŏ-lif-e-rā'-shun). Increase, *e.g.*, cell mitosis.

Prolific (prŏ-lif'-ik). Fruitful; multiplying abundantly.

Promontory (prom'-on-to-ri). A projection; a prominent part.

Pronation (prŏ-nā'-shun). The act of turning the ventral surface face downwards, *e.g.*, to lie on the face, or to turn the palm of the hand downwards.

Prone (prōn). Face downwards.

Pronephros (prŏ-nef-ros). The primitive tubular excretory organ from which the kidney is developed.

Prontosil. The trade name of a synthetic dye of great value in streptococcal and some other bacterial infections. The name is often applied to the whole group of sulphanilamide compounds (*q.v.*).

Prophylactic (prŏ-fil-ak'-tik). Pertaining to prophylaxis.

Prophylaxis (prŏ-fil-aks'-is). Treatment which aims at preventing disease, *e.g.*, the administration of antitetanic serum for the prevention of tetanus, etc.

Proprietary Medicine (pro-prī'-et-ar-i). A medicine which is patented, trade-marked, or secret.

Proptosis (prop-tō'-sis). Protrusion forwards.

Prosencephalon (prŏs-en-kef'-a-lon). The forebrain; the anterior part of the brain

consisting mainly of the cerebral lobes.

Prostate (pros'-tāt). A small gland surrounding the first part of the urethra in the male.

Prostatectomy (pros-ta-tek'-to-mi). Excision of the prostate gland. It is usual to use some kind of suction apparatus for keeping the

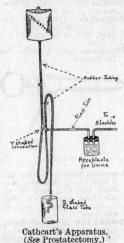

Cathcart's Apparatus.
(*See* Prostatectomy.)

bladder free of urine after the operation. A modification of Cathcart's appliance is often used for this purpose. (*See* diagram.)

Prostatic (pros-tat'-ik). Pertaining to the prostate gland.

Prostatitis (pros-ta-tī'-tis). Inflammation of the prostate gland.

Prosthetics (pros-thet'-iks). The part of surgery (and particularly dental surgery) which deals with the artificial replacement of lost parts.

Prostitution (pros-ti-tū'-shun). Indiscriminate and promiscuous sexual intercourse.

Prostration (pros-trā'-shun). Extreme mental and physical exhaustion.

Protamine Insulin (prŏt-a-mēn). A combination of insulin with an amino-acid (protamine). The value of this preparation is that after injection the insulin is only slowly liberated from the protamine into the tissues and the insulin effect is thus considerably prolonged. Zinc protamine insulin, a combination of the above with zinc. The addition of the zinc serves still further to delay the liberation of the insulin so that its effect becomes spread over 24 to 36 hours.

Protean (prŏ'-tē-an). Taking various forms ; manifesting itself in many ways ; variable ; changing.

Protective (prō-tek'-tiv). A thin waterproof material. such as gutta-percha, used for covering moist dressings.

Proteid. *See* Protein.

Protein (prŏ'-tē-in). A complex organic substance occurring in a variety of forms, a common one being egg-albumin (white of egg). The molecules of proteins contain the elements C, H, O, N, and sometimes S and P.

Proteolysis (prō-ti-ol'-is-is or prō-ti-ō-lī'-sis). The breaking down of a complex protein substance into the simpler form of peptones.

Proteolytic (prō-ti-ō-lit'-ik). Pertaining to proteolysis.

Proteose (prŏ'-ti-ōs). The first formed product found during the proteolysis of protein ; it forms an intermediate stage between protein and peptone.

Proteus (prŏ'-tē-us). A genus of bacilli, frequently found in infected urine.

Prothrombin (prō-throm'-bin). A chemical substance existing in the circulating blood, and which, through the medium of *thrombokinase*, interacts with calcium salts to produce thrombin ; also known as *Thrombogen*.

Protopathic (prō-tō-path'-ik). (1) Primary. (2) Pertaining to the earliest return of function, *e.g.*, of a nerve after injury. (3) Pertaining

285

to the diffuse poorly localized sensations of pain and extreme changes in temperature ; also used in relation to the nerves conveying such sensations.

Protoplasm (prō'-tō-plasm). A jelly-like semi-transparent substance with a complex chemical structure of which protein forms an important part ; it constitutes the main part of the tissue cells, and may be clear or granulated.

Protoplasmic (prō-tō-plas'-mik). Pertaining to protoplasm.

Protozoa (prō-tō-zō'-à). The smallest type of animal life known to exist ; unicellular organisms, of which the amœba is a well-known example.

Protozoon (prō-tō-zō'-on). The singular of protozoa.

Proud Flesh. Excessive granulation of healing tissue.

Proximal (proks'-im-al). Nearest to the head or centre.

Prurigo (proo-rī'-gō). A skin disease characterized by the appearance of papules accompanied by intense irritation.

Pruritis (proo-rī'-tis). Intense itching ; may be due to lack of cleanliness, but is also a symptom of several diseases, *e.g.*, P. Vulvæ is often an early symptom of *diabetes mellitus*.

Prussic Acid (prus'-ik). Same as *Hydrocyanic Acid* ; a violent and rapid poison.

Psammoma (sam-ō'-mà). A

brain-sand tumour. *See* **Brain-sand.**

Pseudo. A prefix meaning false.

Pseudoarthrosis (sū-dō-ar-thrō'-sis). The condition of having a false joint.

Pseudocrisis (sū-dō-krī'-sis). A false crisis.

Pseudocyesis (sū-dō-sī-ē'-sis). An abnormal psychological state of mind in which a woman who is very desirous of having children imagines herself to be pregnant. The abdomen may become distended, and other signs may be present, such as morning sickness. Under an anæsthetic the abdominal enlargement disappears and the true condition is thus obvious.

Pseudohermaphroditism (sū-dō-her-maf'-rō-dit-ism). False hermaphroditism in which gonads of one sex only are present but the external genitalia are those of the other sex.

Pseudomucin (sū-dō-mū'-sin). A gelatinous substance (not mucin) found in some ovarian cysts.

Pseudoplegia (sū-dō-plē'-ji-à). A form of paralysis due to hysteria and not to any organic defect.

Pseudopodia (sū-dō-pō'-di-à). The projectile parts of the amœba which assist it in movement : literally, false legs.

Psittacosis (sit-a-kō'-sis). A

fatal disease affecting parrots and communicable to man.

Psoriasis (so-rī'-a-sis). A chronic scaly skin disease.

Psychasthenia (sīk-as-thēn'-i-à). An abnormal mental state caused by mental fatigue.

Psychiatrist (sik-ī'-a-trist). A physician who specializes in the treatment and study of mental disorders.

Psychiatry (sik-ī'-a-tri). The treatment of mental disorders.

Psychic (sīk'-ik). Pertaining to the mind.

Psycho-analysis (sīk-ō-an-al'-i-sis). A method of investigation and treatment of persons who are suffering from neurasthenia, obsessions, hysteria, and other mental disturbance. The process is based upon the theory that such phenomena are due to repression of painful or undesirable past experiences, which, although totally forgotten, later manifest themselves in various abnormal ways. Psycho-analysis, therefore, makes an effort to bring up such forgotten memories into the conscious mind. The patient is thus enabled to view the occurrence in its true perspective, and so loses its harmful effect. The method is usually associated with the name of *Freud*, who laid much stress upon the sex instinct as a causal factor. This, however, is not accepted by all psychologists. There are two main methods : (1) dream analysis ; (2) the method of free association.

Psychology (sīk-ol'-o-ji). The science which deals with the mental processes, both normal and abnormal. There are two main approaches to the study : (1) Introspective method, *i.e.*, looking inwards, or self-examination of one's own mental processes. (2) The objective method, *i.e.*, studying the minds of others. In this latter there are four chief lines of attack : (a) The experimental method ; (b) the comparative method ; (c) the genetic method ; (d) the pathological method.

Psychopathology (sīk'-ō-path-ol'-o-ji). The science dealing with the pathology of mental diseases.

Psychosis (sīk-ō'-sis). A general term denoting any mental disorder.

Psychotherapy (sīk-ō-the'-ra-pi). The treatment of disease through the mind.

Pterygoid (te'-ri-goid). Resembling a wing.

Ptomaine (tō'-mān). Poisonous substances produced by bacteria in putrifying food.

Ptosis (tō-sis). Drooping of the upper eyelid due to paralysis of the third cranial

nerve. The term is also applied to the downward displacement of other organs.

Ptyalin (tī-a-lin). An enzyme present in saliva, which acts by converting starch into dextrin and maltose.

Ptyalism (tī'-a-lizm). An excessive flow of saliva.

Pubertas præcox (pŭ-ber'-tas prē'-koks). Precocious or premature sexual development.

Puberty (pū'-ber-ti). The age at which an individual becomes capable of reproduction.

Pubes (pū'-bēz). (1) Pubic hair. (2) The hair region over the os pubis ; the mons veneris region. (3) the os pubis.

Pubescence (pū-bes'-ens). The age of developing sexual maturity ; puberty.

Pubiotomy (pū-bi-ot'-o-mi). The operation of cutting through a pubic bone to facilitate delivery through a contracted pelvis.

Pubis (pū'-bis). The pubic bone or *Os Pubis* forming the centre bone of the front of the pelvis.

Pudendum ; plural, **pudenda** (pū-den-dum, -dà). The external genitals of the female.

Puerperal (poo-er'-pe-ral). Pertaining to child-birth. **P. Insanity,** insanity developing during the puerperium.

Puerperium (poo-er-pē'-ri-um). The period immediately following child-birth to the time when involution is completed.

Pullulation (pul-ū-lā'-shun). Germination sprouting ; reproduction.

Pulmonary (pul'-mon-a-ri). Pertaining to the lungs. **P. Consumption,** phthisis. **P. Circulation,** the flow of blood from the right cardiac ventricle through the lungs, where it is oxygenated, and back to the left auricle of the heart.

Pulmonectomy (pul-mon-ek'-to-mi). The surgical excision of a part of the lung.

Pulpitis (pulp-ī'-tis). Inflammation of the dental pulp, *i.e.,* of the soft contents of the central cavity of a tooth.

Pulsation (pul-sā'-shun). Beating or throbbing, as of the heart or arteries.

Pulse. The impulse felt in an artery when the left ventricle of the heart, by contracting, forces from 4-6 oz. of blood into the already full aorta. The normal pulse rates are : Infants at birth, 130 beats per minute ; adults, 72-80 beats per minute ; old age, 60-70 beats per minute. The pulse is taken by placing the first three fingers over the radial artery, just below the ball of the thumb. The *rhythm, rate, force,* and *volume* should be noted. An **Intermittent P.** is one which misses one or more beats, often a sign of cardiac exhaustion. An **Irregular P.** is one in which the beats occur at irregular intervals. A **Dicrotic P.** is one with an excessive recoil wave, best seen in a sphygmogram. A **Soft P.** is one which is easily compressible, while one which is not easily compressible is a **Hard P.**

Pulsus Alternans. A pulse which is alternately weak and strong although regular in time. **P. Bigeminus,** a pulse in which the beats occur in pairs so that a longer interval occurs after every two beats. **P. Paradoxus,** a pulse which becomes weaker during inspiration.

Pultaceous (pul-tā'-shi-us). Soft and mushy.

Pulvis (pul'-vis). A powder.

Pump. An apparatus for drawing or forcing fluid. **Breast P.,** one which is used to withdraw milk from the breast of a nursing mother. **Stomach P.,** a glass funnel with rubber tubing attached which is used for introducing or withdrawing fluid from the stomach.

Puncta (pungk'-tă). The plural of punctum; spots; points; pin-point hæmorrhages seen in purpura.

Punctate (pungk'-tāt). Having many points; spotted. **P. Basophilia,** the same as "basophilic stippling," the condition in which red blood corpuscles are dappled with bluish dots in stained (Leishmann) films.

Puncture (pungk'-tūr). A stab; a wound made with a sharppointed instrument.

Pupil (pū'-pil). The opening in the centre of the iris.

Pupillary (pū-pil'-a-ri). Pertaining to the pupil.

Purgative (pur'-ga-tiv). A drug which will cause an evacuation of the bowels, *e.g.,* pulv. jalapæ co., etc.

Purpura (pur'-pū-rá). The appearance of purple blotches under the skin due to hæmorrhage; a serious symptom in many diseases. **P. Hæmorrhagica** or **Thrombocytopenic P.** A grave form of blood disease with purpura and a greatly reduced platelet count. **P. Rheumatica** or **Peliosis R.** or **Schönlein's Disease.** Purpura with pyrexia and swollen joints. **P. Simplex,** a mild, apyrexial purpura. **Henoch's P.,** *see* Henoch.

Purulent (pū'-rū-lent or pur'-ū-lent). Pertaining to or resembling pus.

Pus. Matter; consists of albuminous fluid containing many bacteria and dead leucocytes; is generally yellowish-white; if red, suggests rupture of small vessels due to congestion; if blue or

K

green, indicates infection with the *B. pyocyaneus*.

Pustule (pus'-tūl). A small inflammatory swelling containing pus. **Malignant P.**, the typical boil of *anthrax*.

Putrefaction (pūt-ri-fak'-shun). The rotting or decay of animal or vegetable matter; advanced organic decomposition.

Putrefactive (pūt-ri-fak'-tiv). Pertaining to putrefaction.

Putrid (pū'-trid). Showing signs of putrefaction; rotting.

Pyæmia (pī-ēm'-i-à). A condition in which collections of pyogenic bacteria circulate in the blood at intervals, producing abscesses wherever they lodge.

Pycnosis or **Pyknosis** (pik-nō'-sis). A degenerative change whereby the nucleus of the cell is condensed so that its chromatin pattern is lost and it stains uniformly dark.

Pyelitis (pī-e-lī'-tis). Inflammation of the pelvis of the kidney.

Pyelography (pī-e-log'-ra-fi). Examination of the renal pelvis by means of the X-rays after it has been filled with some opaque substance such as *uroselectan* (*q.v.*).

Pyelonephritis (pī-e-lō-nef-rī'-tis). Inflammation of the kidney and its pelvis.

Pylephlebitis (pī-lē-fle-bī'-tis).

Inflammation of the portal vein.

Pylorectomy (pī-law-rek'-to-mi). Excision of the pylorus.

Pyloroplasty (pī-law-rō-plas'-ti). A plastic operation for widening the pylorus.

Pylorus (pī-law'-rus). The opening of the stomach into the duodenum.

Pyocolpos (pī-ō-kol'-pos). The retention of pus in the vagina.

Pyogenic (pī-ō-jen'-ik). Producing or causing pus formation.

Pyohæmothorax (pī-ō-hēm-ō-thawr'-aks). Pus and blood in the pleural sac.

Pyonephrosis (pī-o-nef-rō'-sis). The distension of the renal pelvis with pus.

Pyopneumothorax (pī-ō-nū-mō-thawr'-aks). Pus and gas or air within the pleural sac.

Pyorrhœa (pī-o-rē'-à). A flow of pus. Term is generally regarded as **P. Alveolaris**, a disease characterized by the presence of pus at the roots of the teeth. Also known as *Rigg's Disease*.

Pyosalpinx (pī-ō-sal'-pingks). The presence of pus in the Fallopian tube.

Pyramidon. *See* **Amidopyrine**.

Pyrexia (pī-reks'-i-à). A rise in temperature above normal; fever.

Pyriform (pir'-i-fawm). Pear-shaped.

Pyrosis (pī-rō′-sis). A burning sensation in the stomach due to acidity, with a return of gastric contents into the mouth. *See* **Water-brash**.

Pyuria (pī-ūr′-i-á). The presence of pus in the urine.

Q

Quack. One who pretends to medical knowledge or skill which he does not possess; also a person who sells preparations unrecognized by the medical profession.

Quadriceps (kwod′-ri-seps). The *quadriceps extensor femoris* muscle of the thigh, which possesses four heads: (1) Vastus internus; (2) vastus externus; (3) crureus; (4) rectus femoris.

Quadrilateral (kwod-ri-lat′-e-ral). Having four sides.

Qualitative (kwol′-i-tā-tiv). Pertaining to quality.

Quantitative (kwon′-ti-tā-tiv). Pertaining to quantity.

Quarantine (kwor′-an-tēn). The period during which persons who have been in contact with infectious diseases are segregated in order to prevent the spread of disease.

Quart (kwawrt). The fourth part of a gallon; 2 pints.

Quartan (kwawr′-tan). The term applied to intermittent fever with paroxysms occurring every fourth day.

Quassia (kwas-i-á or kwash- or kwosh-). A bitter tonic; the rasped wood of the quassia tree which is made into an infusion for the treatment of thread-worms in children; $\frac{1}{2}$-1 oz. of the infusion is added to 1 pint of warm water and injected per rectum.

Quickening (kwik′-en-ing). The first perceptible movement of the foetus in utero; generally felt at the end of the fourth month.

Quickenstedt's Sign. When pressure is applied to the veins of the neck, there is a rise in the pressure of cerebro-spinal fluid in healthy persons, such rise being reduced again when the pressure is released. The pressure of the fluid is unaffected if there is any obstruction in the vertebral canal.

Quick-lime (kwik līm). Calcium oxide. CaO.

Quick-silver. Mercury.

Quinidine (kwin-i-dēn). An isomer of quinine possessing similar action, but with greater incidence on the heart muscle (depression), used in auricular fibrillation for its specific effect on the muscle of the auricle; most likely to be of service when fibrillation is of recent development with no cardiac enlargement and no valvular affection. In all cases digitalisation is first carried out and the heart failure relieved. The patient must be at rest and under frequent observation. Quinidine possesses an anti-malarial action equally powerful to that of quinine, and may be employed in cases showing idiosyncrasy to quinine. Dose : Quinidine sulphate, 3-10 gr.

Quinine (kwin-ēn'). A bitter tonic obtained from the *Cinchona succirubra*, the bark of the stem and branches being used. It is antipyretic and sedative, and has a marked effect in malaria. It also stimulates the muscular contractions of the gravid uterus. Dose : Tincture, 30-60 minims ; liq. quin. ammon., 30-60 minims ; quin. bisulph., 1-10 gr. ; sulphate, 3-10 gr.

Quinism (kwin'-izm). A series of symptoms arising from an idiosyncrasy to or long-continued use of quinine, *e.g.*, headache, noises in the ears and partial deafness, disturbed vision, and nausea. Also known as *Cinchonism.*

Quinsy (kwin'-zē). The formation of an abscess in the deep structures behind the tonsil, accompanied by severe inflammation and much constitutional disturbance ; peritonsillar abscess.

Quintan (kwint'-an). Recurring every fifth day.

Quintessence (kwint-es'-ens).

The concentrated activating principle of any substance.

Quotidian (kwo-tid'-i-an). The term given to a fever which recurs every day.

R.

Rabid (rab'-id). Affected with rabies.

Rabies (rā'-bēz). *See* **Hydrophobia.**

Racemose (ras'-i-mōs). Resembling a bunch of grapes.

Rachis (rāk'-is). The vertebral column.

Rachitis (rak-ī'-tis). A synonym for *Rickets.*

Radial (rā'-di-al). Pertaining to the radius.

Radiation (rā-di-ā'-shun). Emanation from some central point ; divergence.

Radical (rad'-ik-al). Pertaining to the root of a thing. **R. Operation,** one which is meant to be not merely palliative but curative.

Radicle (rad'-ik-'l). (1) The initial fibril of a nerve. (2) The small beginning of a vein. (3) The group of atoms in a compound which react as a whole and have unsatisfied valency.

Radiculitis (rad-ik-ū-lī'-tis). Inflammation of a nerve root.

Radioactivity (rā-di-ō-ak-tiv'-it-i). The power of spontaneous emission of rays having electrical and chemical properties.

Radiography (rā-di-og′-raf-i). The art of making a radiograph or X-ray picture.

Radiology (rā-di-ol′-o-gi). The theory and science of radioactivity and particularly of its application to medicine.

Radiostoleum (rā-di-ō-stōl′-i-um). An official liquor with oil as a vehicle. The same as irradiated ergosterol, but containing also a concentrate of vitamin A. *See* **Ergosterol.**

Radiotherapy (rā-di-ō-the′-ra-pi). The treatment of disease by means of radium and radioactive rays, *e.g.*, Roentgen or X-rays.

Radium (rā′-di-um) Ra. A valuable metal obtained from pitchblende and ores containing uranium. It was discovered by Madame Curie in 1898. It is a pure white metal, becoming darker on exposure to air, and emitting three types of rays : (1) The *alpha-rays*, which are electrically charged atoms of the gas *helium* ; (2) *beta-rays*, which are electrons ; (3) *gamma-rays*, which are analogous to the X-rays. Radium is an unstable substance, and is therefore used in the form of the sulphate. These salts are inserted into fine glass capillary tubes, which for safety are then put into silver or lead containers. Fine hollow needles of platinum containing radium salts are also used. Radium emanation is used in the form of tiny tubes or seeds of *radon*. Medically, radium is used extensively in the treatment of cancer.

Radius (rā′-di-us). The bone on the outer side of the forearm.

Radix (rā′-diks). A root.

Rales (råls). Rattling or bubbling sounds on auscultation of the chest in certain pulmonary diseases, such as bronchitis, pneumonia, and phthisis.

Rami (rā′-mī). The plural of *ramus*, a branch. **R. Communicantes**, the small nerve fibres passing between the nerves of the sympathetic ganglia and the fibres which emerge from the anterior roots of the spinal cord.

Ramification (ram-i-fi-kā′-shun). Branching or subdivision of certain structures.

Ramstedt's Operation (ram′-sted's). An operation for the relief of pyloric stenosis in infants. The pyloric muscle is divided, but the mucous lining of the duodenum is left intact.

Rancid (ran′-sid). Sour or partially decomposed.

Ranula (ran′-ū-là). A cystic swelling beneath the tongue.

Rape (rāp). Forcible sexual intercourse without the consent of the woman.

Raphe (raf'-ā). A ridge or crease.

Rarefaction (rē-ri-fak'-shun). Becoming less dense, as of bones in rickets, acute inflammation, etc.

Rash. An exanthematous eruption on the skin. **Bathing-drawers R.**, the prodromal rash of smallpox, which spreads from just below the umbilicus to the upper part of the thighs. **Drug R.**, a rash caused by the use of certain drugs, *e.g.*, bromide or iodine. **Enema R.**, a rash resembling measles, caused by using too much soap in an enema. **Mulberry R.** the dusky-coloured rash of typhus fever. **Nettle R.**, *see* Urticaria. **Rose R.**, rose-coloured rash of typhoid fever.

Raspatory (ras'-pator-i). A surgical instrument used for scraping the surface of bone.

Rathke's Pouch (rath-ki). The embryological diverticulum of the pharynx from which is developed the anterior lobe of the pituitary.

Ray. A beam of light or heat. **R. Fungus**, the actinomyces causing actinomycosis (*q.v.*).

Raynaud's Disease (rā'-nō). A sym-

Raspatory.

metrical disturbance of the circulation of the extremities due to vascular spasm; in severe cases gangrene may supervene.

Reaction (rē-ak'-shun). Response to a stimulus on the part of a structure or body; also a rebound or acting in an opposite direction. **R. of Degeneration**, a loss of response to the faradic current when applied to muscular tissue; abbreviation, R.D. **R. Period**, the period of recovery after an operation or other injury. **R. Time**, in the psychological *time and reaction test*, it is the time which elapses between the giving of the stimulus word and the response to it.

Reagent (rē-ā'-jent). An agent capable of producing a chemical reaction.

Réaumur (rā'-ō-mur). A thermometric scale having 0° for the freezing-point and 80° for the boiling-point of water.

Receptaculum Chyli (rē-sep-tak'-ū-lum kī'-li). The pear-shaped enlargement at the lower end of the thoracic duct.

Recessive (rē-ses'-iv). Receding; having a tendency to disappear.

Recklinghausen's Disease. (1) A disease characterized by cutaneous pigmentation and multiple neurofibromata; (2) osteitis fibrosa; both named

294

from Friedrich Danial von Recklinghausen, a German pathologist (1833-1910).

Recrudescence (rē-kroo-des'-ens). The return of symptoms.

Rectal (rek'-tal). Pertaining to the rectum.

Rectified (rek-ti-fīd). (1) Purified. (2) Made right.

Rectocele (rek'-tō-sēl). Prolapse of the rectum.

Rectoscope (rek'-tō-skōp). A speculum used for examining the rectum. *See also* **Electric Rectoscope**.

Rectovaginal (rek-tō-va-jī'-nal). Pertaining to the rectum and vagina.

Rectovesical (rek-tō-ve-sīk'-al). Pertaining to the rectum and bladder.

Rectum (rek'-tum). The lower 5 or 6 in. of the large intestine ending in the anus.

Recumbent (rē-kum'-bent). Lying or reclining.

Recuperation (rē-kūp'-e-rā-shun). Convalescence; return to health.

Recurrent (rē-kur'-rent). Returning periodically.

Red Lotion. *See* **Lotio Rubra**.

Reduction (rē-duk'-shun). The restoration of anything to its normal state.

Reef Knot. One in which the ends lie parallel with the cord; does not slip; should always be used for tying slings, bandages, etc. *See* **Knot**.

Reflection (rē-flek'-shun). (1) The throwing back of a ray of light or heat from a smooth, polished surface. (2) The bending back or withdrawal of a part to expose underlying structures.

Reflex (rē'-fleks). An involuntary response to a stimulus. The majority of the bodily acts are reflex in type, *e.g.*, sneezing, blinking, coughing, etc. **R. Arc**, the structures which are concerned with reflex action, *i.e.*, receptor and effector nerves, and a nerve centre. **R. Action**, same as *Reflex*. **Conditioned R.**, a reflex which arises as a response to some particular situation, the reflex being aroused and modified by association with some past experience.

Refraction (rē-frak'-shun). The bending of light-rays as they pass through media of different densities. Thus light passing from a rarer to a denser medium, *e.g.*, air to water, becomes refracted towards the normal. In errors of refraction of the eye, the light-rays do not focus directly on to the retina. This prevents a clear production of the image, and must be corrected by suitable glasses.

Refractory (rē-frak'-tor-i). Resistent to treatment.

Regeneration (rē-jen-e-rā'-shun).

Restoration; renewal; repair.

Regimen (rej'-i-men). A stated or fixed rule of life or conduct; also a special method of dieting which is adhered to strictly.

Regional Ileitis. Hypertrophic granulomatous inflammation of a portion of the ileum, usually the terminal portion. The infection is non-tuberculous but often classed as pseudo-tuberculous. Also known as *Crohn's Disease.*

Regurgitation (rē-gur-ji-tā'-shun). A throwing or flowing back, as of blood returning from the ventricles into the auricle when the valves of the heart are defective.

Reinfection (rē-in-fek'-shun). Infection occurring again after recovery from the original disease.

Rejuvenation (rē-joo-ven-ā'-shun). The renewal of youth.

Relapse (rē-laps'). A sudden return of grave symptoms during the convalescent period of a disease.

Relative Humidity is the ratio of the actual amount of water-vapour in the atmosphere to the amount present if the air is saturated at the same temperature.

Remedial (rē-mēd'-i-al). Having the nature of an agent used in the treatment of disease.

Remission (rē-mi'-shun). The period of abatement of a fever or other disease.

Remittent (rē-mit'-ent). Increasing and decreasing at periodic intervals. **R. Temperature,** one in which the temperature varies two or more degrees, but does not actually touch the normal.

Ren. The kidney.

Renal (rē'-nal). Pertaining to the kidney. **R. Rickets,** thinning and deformity of bones resembling those of rickets but resulting from chronic renal disease.

Reniform (rē'-ni-fawm). Shaped like a kidney.

Renin (rē'-nin). A substance produced in the kidney to which the arterial supply is reduced and believed to be the cause of essential hypertension.

Rennet (ren'-et). An infusion of the inner coat of the stomach of the calf. A fluid containing rennin and used for making junket. *See* **Junket.**

Rennin (ren'-in). The enzyme in gastric juice which curdles milk.

Repositor (rē-poz'-i-tor). An instrument for replacing a part.

Reproduction (rē-prō-duk'-shun). The act of bringing forth young.

Resection (rē-sek'-shun). The excision of any structure.

Residual (rē-zid'-ū-al). Remaining. **R. Air,** the air remain-

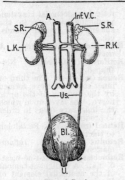

The Renal System
(posterior view).

L.K., Left kidney.
R.K., Right kidney.
S.R., Suprarenal capsules.
U., Urethra.
Us., Ureters.
Bl., Urinary bladder.
A., Aorta.
Inf. V.C., Inferior vena cava, with branches forming the renal veins.

ing in the lung after forced expiration. **R. Urine**, urine remaining in the bladder after urination.

Residuum (rē-zid'-ū-um). The balance or remainder.

Resilience (rē-zil'-i-ens). Elasticity.

Resin (rez'-in). A vegetable exudate soluble in alcohol ether and volatile oils but insoluble in water. Used for making varnishes and in pharmacy.

Resistance (rē-zis'-tens). Opposition, *e.g.*, that offered by conducting material to the passage of an electrical current.

Resolution (rez-ō-loo'-shun). A medical term denoting a disappearance of certain diseased conditions of the tissues or of an inflammatory exudate ; the return to the normal.

Resonance (rez'-o-nans). The sounds heard on auscultation of the chest during speech, or on percussion.

Respiration (res-pi-rā'-shun). The act of breathing. **Abdominal R.**, the use of the diaphragm and abdominal muscles in breathing. **Artificial R.**, the induction of breathing by artificial means.

Respirator (res'-pi-rā-tor). An apparatus worn over the face to prevent the inhalation of noxious or dangerous gases.

Restitution (res-ti-tū'-shun). (1) A return to the normal. (2) The act of making amends. (3) In midwifery practice, the turning of the fœtal head to the right or left after it has completely emerged through the vulva.

Restorative (rē-staw'-ra-tiv). A

remedy for restoring health and strength.

Resuscitation (rē-sus-i-tā'-shun). The bringing about of recovery ; restoration to life of one apparently dead ; the special method of treating cases of shock.

Retardation (rē-tå(r)-dā'-shun). Delay ; a holding back ; a slowing down.

Retch. To strain at vomiting.

Rete (rē'-tē). A network or an interlacing.

Retention (rē-ten'-shun). Holding back ; stoppage. **R. of Urine,** inability to void urine from the bladder.

Retentive Memory. The ability to store events and facts in the mind, so that they can be readily called up when required.

Reticular (rē-tik-ū-lå(r)). Resembling a network.

Reticulocyte (rē-tik'-ū-lō-sīt). A young non-nucleated red blood cell which stains with polychrome methylene blue and shows a reticulum.

Reticulo-endothelial System. A diffusely scattered series of cells mainly in the marrow, spleen, liver, and lymph glands which is concerned with the removal of foreign particles from the blood and with the making of antibodies.

Reticulosis (rē-tik-ū-lō'-sis). A diffuse overgrowth of the cellular elements of the

reticulo-endothelial system producing tumours in the spleen and lymph glands, etc.

Reticulum (rē-tik-ū-lum). A network.

Retiform (rē-ti-fawm). Net-shaped.

Retina (ret'-in-à). The third or inner coat of the eye, formed by the division of the optic nerve ; the layer upon which the light-rays focus in order to produce sight.

Retinal (ret'-in-al). Pertaining to the retina.

Retinitis (ret-in-ī-tis). Inflammation of the retina.

Retinoblastoma (ret-i-nō-blast-ō'-må). A malignant tumour of the neuroglial element of the retina. The tumour occurs exclusively in children.

Retort (rē-taw(r)t). A vessel used in distillation.

Retraction (rē-trak'-shun). The act of holding back ; receding.

Retractor (rē-trak'-tor). A surgical instrument for holding apart the cut edges of a wound.

Retro (rē'-trō). A prefix meaning backwards or behind.

Retrobulbar (rē-trō-bul'-bà(r)). At the back of the eyeball.

Retrocæcal (rē-trō-sēk'-al). Behind the cæcum, *e.g.*, a retrocæcal appendix.

Retroflexion (rē-trō-flek'-shun). Bending backwards. **R. of Uterus,** bending backwards

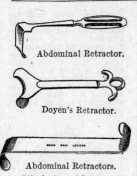

Abdominal Retractor.

Doyen's Retractor.

Abdominal Retractors.

of the body and fundus of the uterus.

Retroperitoneal (rĕ-trŏ-pe-ri-ton-ē'-al). Behind the peritoneum.

Retropharyngeal (rĕ-trŏ-far-in-jē'-al). Behind the pharynx.

Retroversion (rĕ-trŏ-ver'-shun). Turning backward. **R. of Uterus,** displacement of the whole of the uterus backward with the cervix pointing forward.

Reversion (rĕ-ver'-shun). A return to the original form.

Rhabdomyoma (rab-dŏ-mĭ-ō'-mă). A rare benign tumour composed of striped muscle fibres.

Rhagades (rag'-a-dēz). Linear fissures or cracks appearing in the skin, particularly at the corner of the mouth; if due to syphilis, they form a radiating scar on healing.

Rheostat (rē'-ŏ-stat). An instrument used for testing the resistance of an electrical current.

Rh. antigen. An antigen found in 85% of human bloods (identical with that found in the blood of the Rhesus monkey—hence the name of the antigen). The antibody produced by it in pregnant Rh. negative women bearing Rh. positive offspring is the main cause of erythroblastosis fœtalis in these children.

Rheum. (1) (rē'-um) Rhubarb. (2) (room) Catarrh.

Rheumatic (roo-mat'-ik). Relating to rheumatism.

Rheumatism (roo'-mat-izm). A disease of uncertain origin attacking the joints or muscles, causing acute pain, fever, and impairment of the part; may be acute or chronic. Heart disease is a dangerous complication, especially among children.

Rhinencephalon (rīn-en-kef'-a-lon). The olfactory lobe of the brain.

Rhinitis (rīn-ī'-tis). Inflammation of the nose.

Rhinolith (rīn'-ō-lith). A nasal calculus; a stone formed in the nose.

299

Rhinologist (rīn-ol'-o-jist). One who is an expert in the diagnosis and treatment of nasal disorders.

Rhinology (rīn-ol'-o-ji). The science which deals with the nose and its diseases.

Rhinophyma (rī-nō-fī'-mà). A tumour of the nose, usually a sebaceous adenoma, causing a " cauliflower nose."

Rhinoplasty (rīn-ō-plas'-ti). Plastic surgery of the nose.

Rhinorrhœa (rīn-ō-rē'-à). A nasal discharge.

Rhinosporidium (rīn-ō-spor-id-i-um). A sporing parasitic fungus causing tumours of the septum nasi.

Rhizome (rī'-zōm). A stem growing beneath the soil.

Rhodopsin (rō-dop'-sin). The visual purple contained in the rods of the retina.

Rhonchus (rong'-kus). A rattling sound in the bronchi heard during auscultation.

Rhubarb (roo'-bä(r)b). Rheum; the rhizome of *Rheum Palmatum* and other species of rheum cultivated in China and Tibet; is a favourite purgative.

Rhythm (rithm). A measured, periodic movement. **Gallop R.**, heart action in which the sounds recur in groups of three, like the hoof-beats of a galloping horse.

Ribs. The twelve pairs of bones which articulate with the twelve dorsal vertebræ.

The upper seven pairs are **True R.**, and, by means of the costal cartilage, are attached to the sternum. The remaining five pairs are the **False R.** The first three pairs of these do not attach to the sternum but to the costal cartilage above each. The lower two pairs are the **Floating R.**, which have no articulation in front, but are left free.

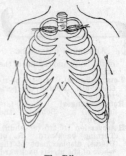

The Ribs.

Rice-water Stools. The stool which is characteristic of Asiatic cholera; it is pale in colour, and resembles the water in which rice has been boiled.

Richter's Hernia. Strangulated

hernia with only partial involvement of the lumen of the intestine.

Rickets (rik'-ets). A deficiency disease of childhood caused by lack of sunlight, insanitary environment, deficient or unsuitable food, and, above all, lack of vitamins in the diet, especially *Vitamin D*. The chief symptoms are deformity of the chest, pelvis, and long bones, with bossing of the frontal bones, delayed closure of the fontanelles, and enlargement of the epiphyseal ends of the long bones. Sweating, especially of the head, and abdominal enlargement are also common. Synonym, *Rachitis*.

Rickettsia (ri-ket'-si-á). A group of filter-passing viruses, members of which are the causative agents in typhus and trench fever.

Rickety (rik'-et-i). Affected with rickets.

Rider's Bone. An osteophyte or bony mass formed in the ligamentous attachments of the adductor muscles of the thigh, caused by repeated minor trauma in horse-riding.

Riedel's Lobe. A tongue-shaped process of the liver, frequently found protruding over the gall-bladder in cases of chronic cholecystitis.

Rigg's Disease. Pyorrhœa alveolaris; an inflammatory condition of the gums with the formation of pus in the teeth sockets.

Rigidity (rij-id'-it-i). Immovability; tenseness.

Rigor (rī'-gaw(r)). A sudden chill, especially one accompanied by severe shivering. A rapidly rising and high temperature and profuse perspiration, followed by a fall in temperature and a state of weakness. A rigor often ushers in a fever or accompanies severe toxæmias or septicæmias.

Rigor Mortis (rī'-gaw(r) maw(r)'-tis). The stiffening of the body after death.

Rima (rī'-má). A fissure or opening. R. Glottidis, the opening between the vocal cords.

Ringer's Solution. An isotonic solution containing sodium, potassium and calcium chloride.

Ringworm (ring'-wurm). *Tinea tonsurans*. A parasitic disease resulting in circular bald patches.

Risus Sardonicus (rī'-sus sá(r)-don'-i-kus). Contortion of the face into a grin, caused by acute spasm of the facial muscles in the disease of tetanus.

Rochelle Salt (ro-shel'). Tartrate of sodium and potassium; an aperient salt. Dose, 120-240 gr.

Rodent Ulcer (rō'-dent). A slow-growing form of cancer

which slowly but steadily eats into the tissues, causing great destruction. If treated early (usually by applications of " *snow*," *i.e.*, condensed CO_2, or with radium, or by excision) is curable. The most usual sites for the ulcer are on the outer angle of the eye ; also near the side of the nose and on the tip of the nose. Synonym, *Basal Cell Carcinoma*.

Roentgen Rays or Röntgen. X-rays ; discovered by *William Conrad Röntgen* in 1895. The first X-ray plate of the hand was published a year later.

Romberg's Sign (rom´-berg). Inability to maintain the body balance when the eyes are shut and the feet close together ; a characteristic sign of locomotor ataxy.

Rongeur (ron-zhur´). A gouge forceps.

Rosacea (rŏz-ā´-si-å or -shi-å). *See* Acne Rosacea.

Roseola (rŏz-i-ōl-å). A rose-coloured rash ; an erythema ; non-infectious.

Rostellum (ros-tel´-um). The small beak-like process on the head of a tapeworm, around which the hooklets are fixed.

Rotation (rŏ-tā´-shun). Turning or twisting.

Rotator (rŏ-tā´-tor). A muscle having the action of turning a part.

302

Rötheln (ro´-teln). Same as *German Measles*.

Rouleaux (roo´-lŏ). Clumps of red blood-corpuscles formed like a roll of coins.

Round Ligament. Two round cords passing from the front of the body of the uterus below the Fallopian tube, in the anterior wall of the broad ligament, outwards through the inguinal canals to the soft tissues of the labia majora. **R. L. of Liver,** the fibrous cord running from the umbilicus to the anterior border of the liver.

Round Worm. *See* Ascaris.

Rubber. Indiarubber. **R. Dam,** a thin sheet of rubber used for packing wounds.

Rubber Air Ring.

Rubefacients (roo-bi-fās´-i-ents). Substances which, when applied to the skin, cause redness.

Rubella (roo-bel´-å). German measles.

Rubeola (roo-bē´-o-lå). Measles : characterized by a red blotchy rash, coryza, and fever ; incubation period, ten to fourteen days ; rash appears on the fourth day.

Rudimentary (roo-di-ment'-a-ri). Undeveloped ; primitive.

Rugæ (roo'-gi). Wrinkles ; corrugations.

Rupia (roo'-pi-å). Syphilitic eruption of foul, encrusted ulcers.

Rupture (rup'-tūr). Literally means a burst or split ; the popular name for hernia. **Perineal R.**, a torn perineum. **R. of the Uterus**, tearing of the uterine muscle during parturition, due to faulty or careless midwifery ; very rare. **R. of the Membranes**, tearing of the membranes when the os is fully dilated. **R. of a Tubal Pregnancy**, when pregnancy occurs within the Fallopian tube, it usually ruptures if unrecognized and therefore left untreated ; the embryo is projected from the tube into the pelvis and severe bleeding may result, which necessitates prompt surgical measures.

S.

Sac. A small pouch or cyst-like cavity. **Hernial S.**, the pouch of peritoneum forming the covering of a hernia.

Saccharide Group ($C_6H_{10}O_5$). (sak'-a-rīd). The carbo-
hydrate grouping contained in each of the three main classes of sugars, e.g., polysaccharides, $C_6H_{10}O_5 \times$ many times ; disaccharides $C_6H_{10}O_5$ twice over $+H_2O = C_{21}H_{22}O_{11}$; monosaccharides, $C_6H_{10}O_5 + H_2O = C_6H_{12}O_6$. See **Carbohydrates**.

Sacchariferous (sak-a-rif'-e-rus). Containing sugar.

Saccharin (sak'-ar-in) ($C_6H_4CO.SO_2NH$). A sweet synthetic product derived from coaltar. A light white crystalline powder ; usually prepared in tablet form, each containing ½ gr. ; two of these is sufficient to sweeten 4 oz. of fluid.

Saccharolytic (sak-ar-ō-lit'-ik). Having the capacity of fermenting or disintegrating sugar.

Saccharomyces (sak-ar-ō-mī'-sēz). The yeast fungus.

Saccharose (sak'-ar-ōs). Cane sugar ; sucrose.

Saccharum (sak'-ar-um). Sugar. **S. Lactis**, milk sugar, i.e., lactose.

Sacculated (sak'-ū-lā-ted). The state of having sacs.

Saccule (sak'-ūl). (1) A minute sac. (2) The lower portion of the vestibule of the internal part of the ear.

Sacral (sā'-kral). Pertaining to the sacrum.

Sacrum (sā'-krum). The triangular-shaped bone lying between the fifth lumbar vertebra and the coccyx. It consists of five vertebræ fused together. It articulates on either side with the innominate bones of the pelvis, forming the sacro-iliac joints.

Saddle-nose. A nose with a deep or absent bridge ; often a sign of congenital syphilis.

Sadism (sā′-dizm). A sexual perversion in which the pervert obtains stimulation and gratification by inflicting pain, cruelty, or degradation on others.

Sagittal (saj′-it-al). Resembling an arrow. S. Suture, the suture joint formed by the articulation of the two parietal bones.

St Anthony's Fire. *See* Erysipelas.

St Vitus' Dance. Chorea.

Sal. Latin for salt. S. Alembroth, a salt of perchloride of mercury and chloride of ammonium ; gauze impregnated with this solution is coloured sky-blue to distinguish it. S. Volatile (sal vol-at′-i-li), aromatic spirit of ammonia ; smelling salts ; a stimulant. Dose, 15-60 minims in water.

Salicylate (sal-is′-il-āt). A salt of salicylic acid.

Saline (sā′-līn or sā′-lēn). Salty. A solution of salt and water. **Normal S.,** a 0·9% solution of salt ; *i.e.*, one consisting of 1 drachm of common salt to 1 pint of water. This is also known as *physiological saline solution*, since it exerts the same osmotic pressure as the blood.

Salisbury Diet. A diet used in the treatment of obesity.

Saliva (sal-ī′-vå). The secretion of the salivary glands ; spittle.

Salivary (sal′-iv-a-ri). Pertaining to saliva. S. Calculus, a stone formed in the salivary ducts. S. Glands, the glands which secrete saliva, viz., *parotids, submaxillary,* and *sublingual.*

Salivation (sal-i-vā′-shun). An increased secretion of saliva. Also called *Ptyalism.*

Salol (sāl′-ol). A drug compounded of salicylic acid and phenol ; is an intestinal antiseptic, and is also administered internally for rheumatism. Dose, 5-20 gr.

Salpingectomy (sal-pin-jek′-to-mi). Excision of a Fallopian tube.

Salpingitis (sal-pin-jī′-tis). Inflammation of a Fallopian tube.

Salpingo-oophorectomy (sal-ping-gō-oo-ō-for-ek′-to-mi). Excision of the Fallopian tubes and ovaries.

Salpingotomy (sal-ping-got′-o-mi). An opening into the Fallopian tube.

Salpinx (sal′-pinks). (1) The Fallopian tube. (2) Eustachian tube.

Salt (solt or sawlt). A compound formed by the chemical combination of an acid and a base. **Common S.**, sodium chloride (NaCl), **Epsom S.**, magnesium sulphate. **Glauber's S.**, sodium sulphate. **Rochelle S.**, sodium and potassium tartrate. **Rock S.**, native sodium chloride.

Saltpetre (solt-pē'-ter). Potassium nitrate ; chiefly used for the treatment of asthma. Blotting paper is soaked in a strong solution and dried ; when ignited the fumes are inhaled. It is a common ingredient of many asthma cures.

Salubrious (sal-ū'-bri-us). Healthful.

Salutary (sal'-ū-ta-ri). Conducing to health.

Salvarsan (sal-vår'-san). An arsenical preparation used in the treatment of syphilis ; popularly known as " 606 " ; it is administered intramuscularly and/or intravenously. *See also* **Galyl**.

Salve (såv). An ointment.

Sanatorium (san-a-taw'-ri-um). (1) A building set apart for the special care of convalescent patients. (2) Hospitals so constructed that open-air treatment can be carried out, *e.g.*, in tuberculosis.

Sand-flea. The jigger or chikoe flea which burrows into the skin, causing irritation and infection : found mainly in tropical countries.

Sane (sān). Of sound mentality.

Sanguine (sang'-gwin). (1) Pertaining to blood. (2) Hopeful.

Sanguineous (sang-gwin'-i-us). Bloody.

Sanious (sān'-i-us). Watery, foetid, greenish. (Refers to discharges.)

Sanitary (san'-it-a-ri). Pertaining to health.

Sanitation (san-i-tā'-shun). The methods by which health is promoted and disease prevented.

Sanity (san'-it-i). Mental soundness.

Santonin (san'-tō-nin). An anthelmintic drug used in the destruction of the *Ascaris lumbricoides*. Dose, 1-3 gr. Is apt to produce yellow vision.

Santorini's Duct (san-to-rē'-ni). The accessory pancreatic duct.

Saphenous (saf-ē'-nus). The name given to the two main veins of the leg.

Sapo (sap'-ō). Soap ; a compound of a fatty acid with a base like sodium, potassium or calcium.

Saponaceous (sap-on-ā'-shus). Pertaining to or resembling soap.

Saponification (sap-on'-i-fi-kā'-shun). Conversion into a soapy substance.

Saponin (sap-ō-nin). A glucoside with expectorant and emetic properties ; it also lakes blood.

Sapphism (saf'-izm). Un-

305

natural sexual intercourse between women.

Sapræmia (sap-rē'-mi-á). A toxic condition caused by the absorption into the blood of toxins or poisons produced by saprophytes which themselves remain localized, e.g., in the placental tissues. In a purturient woman the condition is known as **Puerperal S.**

Saprophyte (sap'-rō-fīt). A vegetable organism or bacterium which exists and thrives on dead organic matter.

Saprophytic (sap-rō-fit'-ik). Pertaining to saprophytes.

Sarcocele (sá(r)'-kō-sēl). A fleshy tumour of the testicle.

Sarcoid (sá(r)'-koid). Resembling flesh; a fleshy fibrous tumour resembling a sarcoma.

Sarcoidosis (sá(r)-koid-ō'-sis). A granulomatous condition, having some resemblance to hyperplastic tuberculosis, which affects the skin and some viscera; usually referred to as the **S. of Boeck.**

Sarcolemma (sá(r)-kō-lem'-á). The delicate outer membraneous covering of the muscle fibrils.

Sarcoma (sá(r)-kō'-má). A malignant growth derived from connective tissues; it is non-encapsuled, and spreads mainly by way of the blood-stream. There are several types, viz.: **Round-celled S.; Spindle-celled S.; Pleomorphic or Mixed-celled S.; Fibro-S.; Osteogenic S.,** etc.

Sarcomatous (sá(r)-kō'-ma-tus). Affected with or resembling sarcoma.

Sarcoplasm (sá(r)'-kō-plazm). The connective substance between the fibrillæ or sarcostyles of a muscle fibril.

Sarcoptes Scabiei. Another name for the itch-mite, the cause of scabies (q.v.).

Sarcostyle (sá(r)'-kō-stīl). One of the fine microscopic longitudinal elements seen on examination of a muscle fibril.

Sarsaparilla (sá(r)-sa-pa-ril'-á). A drug derived from the root of several species of *Smilax*; it is diuretic, tonic, and alterative. Dose: Decoction sarsæ co., ½-1 fl. oz.

Satiety (sat-ī'-et-i). Full to repletion.

Saturated (sat'-ū-rā-ted). Filled to excess. **S. Solution,** one in which as much of the drug is dissolved as will be held in solution by the fluid without depositing or floating.

Satyriasis (sat-ir-ī-a-sis). Excessive sexual desire.

Saw. An instrument with a

Amputation Saw.

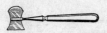

Hey's Skull Saw.

Gigli's Saw.

serrated edge designed for cutting through hard substances, *e.g.*, bone.

Sayre's Method (să'-erz). A method of strapping a fractured clavicle after it has been reduced. **S. Jacket,** a plaster of paris jacket used for tuberculosis of the spine.

Scab. A dried crust forming over an open wound.

Scabies (skā'-bēz). A parasitic skin disease caused by the itch mite or *Acurus* (or *sarcoptes*) *scabiei*; highly contagious.

Scald (skawld). A burn due to moist heat.

Scalp (skalp). The tissues covering the cranium.

Scalpel (skal'-pel). A small straight surgical knife.

Scaly (skā'-li). Covered with scales.

Scanning Speech. Slow and

hesitating speech; a symptom of *disseminated sclerosis*.

Scaphoid (skă'-foid). Shaped like a boat.

Scapula (skap'-ū-lă). The shoulder-blade.

Scar (skă(r). Cicatrix; the dense, avascular white fibrous tissue formed as the end result of healing of wounds or other injuries, especially in the skin.

Scarf-skin. A popular name for the epidermis.

Scarification (skar-i-fi-kā'-shun). The making of small cuts in a part, *e.g.*, the skin.

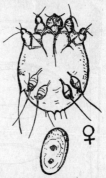

Acarus scabiei (itch mite), with Ovum.

307

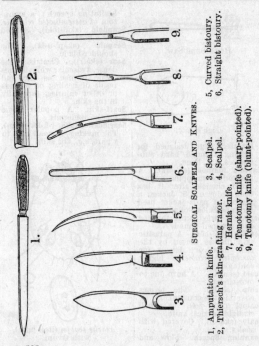

SURGICAL SCALPELS AND KNIVES.

1, Amputation knife.   3, Scalpel.   5, Curved bistoury.
2, Thiersch's skin-grafting razor.   4, Scalpel.   6, Straight bistoury.
                    7, Hernia knife.
                    8, Tenotomy knife (sharp-pointed).
                    9, Tenotomy knife (blunt-pointed).

Scarificator (skar-i-fi-kā'-tor). An instrument used for scarification.

Scarlatina (ská(r)-la-tē'-ná). Scarlet fever; an epidemic disease of childhood characterized by a rise of temperature, rapid pulse, fine red punctate rash, which gives rise to the name. Circumoral pallor is a distinguishing feature of the facial appearance.

Scarlet Fever. See **Scarlatina.**

Schafer's Method (shā'-fer's). A method of resuscitation from drowning. The patient is laid prone, with the head resting on the left arm and the face turned to the right. The rescuer (if a man) kneels astride the patient, or (if a woman) at the side. The hands are placed over the lower ribs, with the thumbs facing towards the vertebral column. By bending forward, so that the weight of the body is transmitted to the ribs, the chest of the patient is compressed and air driven out of the lungs. The rescuer now suddenly straightens up, releasing his hold, and this movement allows the lungs to expand and fill. The movements are repeated about 18 times per minute.

Schatz's Method. A method adopted in obstetrics of converting a face presentation into that of a vertex.

Schema (skē'-má). A plan or diagram.

Schick Test. A test used to determine a person's susceptibility or immunity to diphtheria. It consists in the injection of 2 or 3 minims of freshly prepared toxin beneath the skin of the left arm. A similar test is made into the right arm, but in this the serum is heated to 75° C. for 10 minutes, in order to destroy the toxin but not the protein. A *positive* reaction is recognized by the appearance of a round red area on the left arm within 24 to 48 hours, reaching its maximum intensity on the fourth day, then gradually fading with slight pigmentation and desquamation. This reaction indicates susceptibility or absence of immunity. *No reaction* indicates that the subject is immune to diphtheria. Occasionally a *pseudo-reaction* occurs, caused by the protein of the toxin; in this case the redness appears on both arms, hence the value of the control.

Schistocyte (shis'-tō-sīt). A small fragmentary red blood corpuscle.

Schistosomum (shis-tō-sō'-mum). A genus of trematode worms or flukes which infest and inflame the bladder or rectum. Synonym, *Bil-*

309

harzia. The disease caused is known as schistosomiasis or bilharziasis.

Schizomycetes (skī-zō-mī-sē'-tēz). A term which includes all genera of algæ, bacteria, and fission fungi.

Schizophrenia (skī-zō-frēn'-i-à). Dementia præcox. A cleavage of the mental functions.

Schlemm's Canal. A lymphatico-venous canal in the inner part of the sclera, close to its junction with the cornea, which it encircles.

Schneiderian Membrane (shnī-dier'-ri-an). The lining membrane of the nasal cavities.

Schonlein's Disease (shon'-līn). Purpura rheumatica ; peliosis rheumatica.

Schott's Treatment (shot's). A method of treating cardiac disease by means of warm baths and carefully graduated exercises.

Schultz - Charlton Reaction. When blood serum from a convalescent patient is injected into the skin of a scarlet fever patient, it causes local blanching of the rash ; a valuable diagnostic aid.

Schultze's Method. A method of resuscitating an asphyxiated infant at birth. The first and second fingers are placed in the child's axillæ, with the thumbs over the shoulders. In this way the child is held firmly, and

310

swung at arm's length above the head of the nurse. This brings the legs of the infant on to the abdomen, thereby compressing the chest. On swinging the child down again, the chest becomes expanded, and so inspiration takes place.

Schwann, Sheath of. The neurilemma of a nerve fibre. **S., White Substance of,** the myelin sheath of a nerve fibre.

Sciatica (sī-at'-ik-à). Inflammation of the sciatic nerve.

Scillæ (sil'-ē). The same as *Squills.*

Scirrhus (skir'-us). A hard, cancerous swelling. Adjective, *scirrhous*=hard, fibrosed.

Scissor-leg Deformity. Crossing of the legs while walking, due to disease of both hips.

Sclavo's Serum (sklā'-vō's). A serum used in the treatment of anthrax. It should be administered as early as possible after the onset of disease in doses up to 100 c.c. ; this can be repeated in smaller doses.

Sclera (sklier'-rà). The " white " of the eye ; the opaque bluish-white outer coat of the eyeball ; it merges into the cornea at the front.

Scleroderma (sklier-rō-der'-mà). A chronic skin disease characterized by hardening.

Scleroma (sklier-rō'-má). Hardening of the tissues.

Sclerosis (skle-rō'-sis). An abnormal condition of hardening of the tissues. **Disseminated S.**, a disease characterized by the presence of inflammatory patches, which later become sclerosed, scattered freely throughout the brain and spinal cord.

Sclerotic (sklier-rot'-ik). (1) Indurated; hardened. (2) Pertaining to the sclera.

Sclerotomy (sklier-rot'-o-mi). Incision of the edge of the sclera where it meets the cornea; an operation performed for the relief of glaucoma.

Scolex (skō'-leks). The knotlike head of the tape worm from which the segments or proglottides develop.

Scoliosis (skōl-i-ō'-sis). Lateral curvature of the spine.

Scopolamine (skō-pol'-a-mēn). Hyoscine; combined with morphine, it is used to diminish sensibility during labour, but does not interfere with the normal uterine contractions. This treatment is synonymous with *Twilight Sleep*. Dose, 1/200-1/100.

Scorbutic (skaw(r)-bū'-tik). Relating to scorbutus; affected with scurvy.

Scorbutus (skaw(r)-bū'-tus). The old name for scurvy.

Scotoma (skot-ō'-má). A blind spot in the field of vision.

Scott's Dressing. Scott's ointment spread on lint, which is cut into strips before applying. **S. Ointment**, *unguentum hydrargyri compositum*; it consists of camphor, olive oil, mercurial ointment, and beeswax.

Scrofula (skrof'-ū-là). A constitutional predisposition to tuberculosis.

Scrotum (skrō'-tum). The pouch in the male which contains the testicles.

Scruple (skroo-p'l). In the apothecaries' measure equals 20 gr.; 3 scruples equal 1 drachm. Symbol, ℈.

Scurvy (skur'-vi). A deficiency disease due to lack of sufficient fresh fruit and vegetables containing *Vitamin C*. The gums become soft and spongy, and bleed readily. Hæmorrhages occur in the subcutaneous tissue and muscle, causing ecchymosis and tenderness. There is also a tendency to subperiosteal hæmorrhage, epistaxis, and hæmaturia. **Infantile S.**, the characteristic symptoms differ slightly from the adult type, the most prominent being extreme tenderness of the limbs, which causes the infant to cry with apprehension if the cot is approached. The child is also very thin and pale. Synonym, *Barlow's Disease*.

Scybala (sib'-a-là). Rounded,

hard fæcal lumps which are passed in states of constipation.

Sebaceous (se-bā'-shus). Pertaining to fat or suet. **S. Glands**, the cutaneous glands which secrete an oily substance called *sebum*. The ducts of these glands are short and straight, and open into the hair-follicles. **S. Cysts**, rounded dilatations of the ducts of the sebaceous glands resulting from blockage ; the cysts are filled with fatty material and may grow to a large size and cause much inconvenience and unsightliness.

Seborrhœa (seb-o-rē'-á). An abnormal secretion of sebum. There are several different varieties, but the most commonly known are **S. Oleosa**, in which the skin and hair become excessively greasy ; **S. Sicca**, or dry seborrhœa, in which the epidermis is shed in dry flaky scales.

Seborrhœic (seb-o-rē'-ik). Affected with seborrhœa.

Sebum (sē'-bum). The normal secretion of the sebaceous glands ; it is not a true fat, but consists of fatty acids and cholesterol.

Secondary (sek'-on-da-ri). Following a primary condition. **S. Anæmia**, anæmia following some other disease ; not primary. **S. Areola**, a darker pigmentation of the area surrounding the nipple during pregnancy. **S. Hæmorrhage**, bleeding resulting as the cause of some primary injury, etc., but occurring after a lapse of 24 hours, commonly about the seventh day, and is always due to sepsis. **S. Tumour**, a metastasis.

Secretin (sē'-krē-tin). A hormone which is secreted in the cells of the mucous lining of the duodenum and carried by the blood to the pancreas, which it stimulates to produce pancreatic juice. For this reason it is sometimes called the *key* of the pancreas. In a similar way it excites the liver to produce bile.

Secretion (se-krē'-shun). A substance which is built up by certain glands from materials obtained from the blood. These are known as *true secretions*, and include gastric juice, milk, saliva, sweat, tears, and urine.

Secretory (se-krē'-to-ri). Pertaining to secretion.

Section (sek'-shun). Division by cutting ; a dissection ; a midline incision into the abdomen.

Sedative (sed'-a-tiv). An agent which allays or soothes pain.

Sedentary (sed'-en-ta-ri). Inactive ; resting, as in sitting.

Sediment (sed'-i-ment). The particles which settle at the

bottom of a fluid; a pre-
cipitate.

Segment (seg'-ment). A small
section; a part.

Segmental (seg-men'-tal). Having segments.

Segregation (seg-rē-gā'-shun).
A setting apart; a collection
of persons set apart by
themselves.

Seidlitz Powder (sed'-lits). An
aperient prepared in two
powders, each put up in a
separate packet. The *blue
paper* contains a mixture
of Rochelle salt, 120 gr. +
sodium bicarbonate, 40 grs.
The *white packet* contains
40 gr. of tartaric acid.
When the contents of the blue
packet followed by the white
are added to half a tumbler
of water, effervescence takes
place.

Sella Turcica (sel'-à tur'-sik-à).
The pituitary fossa; a
depression in the sphenoid
bone, which contains the
pituitary gland.

Semen (sē'-men). The secretion from the testicles, and
which contains the spermatozoa.

Semilunar (sem-i-loon'-à(r)).
Shaped like a crescent or
new moon. **S. Bone,** one of
the bones of the carpus. **S.
Cartilages,** the crescentic
interarticular cartilages of
the knee joint.

Seminal (sem'-in-al). Pertaining to semen.

Seminiferous (sem-in-if'-e-rus).
Carrying or producing semen.

Seminoma (sem-i-nō'-mà). A
malignant tumour of the
testis.

Senescence (sē-nes'-ens). The
state of growing old.

Senile (sēn'-īl). Old; aged.

Senility (sen-il'-it-i). Old age;
the bodily and mental weakness of old age.

Senna (sen-à). An aperient
drug, the chief preparations
of which are the *confection,*
60-120 gr.; *infusion, conc.,*
30-120 minims; *inf. recens,*
½-2 fl. ozs.; *syrup,* ½-2
drachms; and *tincture,* 30-60
minims.

Sensible (sen'-sib-'l). Endowed
with the sense of feeling.

Sensitive (sen'-sit-iv). Capable
of feeling; acutely sus-
ceptible to stimulation.

Sensitized (sen'-si-tīz'd. Having been made sensitive.

Sensory Nerves. Those nerves
which convey impressions to
the brain or spinal cord.

Sepsis (sep'-sis). The state of
being infected with pyogenic
organisms; putrefaction.

Septic (sep'-tik). Relating to
sepsis; infected; putrefying.

Septicæmia (sep-ti-sēm'-i-à).
A serious condition in which
the blood is infected with
living pathogenic bacteria.
Puerperal S., that which
occurs during the puerperium.

Septum (sep'-tum). A partition
between two cavities, *e.g.,*

313

between the nasal cavities, and also the two halves of the heart.

Sequela (sē-kwē'-là). A morbid state which may follow or persist after the original disease has disappeared.

Sequestrum (sē-kwes'-trum). A small piece of necrosed bone which separates and forms a foreign body.

Serofibrinous (sē-rō-fī'-brin-us). Containing both serum and fibrin.

Serology (sē-rol'-o-ji). The science of serum diagnosis and treatment.

Seropurulent (sē-rō-pūr'-ū-lent). Composed of serum and pus.

Serosa (sē-rōz'-à). A serous membrane, *e.g.,* the peritoneal lining of the abdominal viscera.

Serous (sē'-rus). Pertaining to serum. **S. Membrane,** a membrane lining a cavity which has no communication with the external air.

Serpiginous (ser-pij'-in-us). Creeping; resembling ringworm (= *serpigo*).

Serrated (se-rā'-ted). Notched like a saw.

Serum (sē'-rum). Defibrinated blood-plasma formed during the coagulation of blood. **S. Albumin,** the albumin found in serum. **S. Sickness,** the symptoms arising as a reaction after the administration of serum; includes headache, vomiting, rash,

painful inflammatory swelling of the tissues at the site of injection, and pyrexia. **S. Therapy,** the use of serum in the prevention and cure of disease. *See also* **Anaphylaxis.**

Sesamoid (ses'-a-moid). Resembling a grain. **S. Bones,** small bony masses formed in tendons.

Sessile (ses'-īl). Non-pedunculated, having a broad base.

Seton (sē'-ton). A silk thread passed through the skin in order to drain lymph from a certain area.

Sex. The state of being either male or female.

Sexual (seks'-ū-al). Pertaining to sex.

Shell-shock. *See* **Shock.**

Shin-bone. The tibia.

Shingles. The popular name for *herpes zoster.*

Shock. Complete bodily prostration accompanied by marked lowering of the blood-pressure, pallor, feeble pulse increasing in rate, shallow respiration, and restlessness; may result from accident or injury, loss of blood, burns, and psychic causes. **Delayed S.,** a form of shock which does not come on until some hours after the accident. **Shell-S.,** functional disturbance due to sudden loud noises, such as the firing of a gun, the bursting of bombs, etc.; this probably is a psychical phenomena brought about, not from injury but from repression of fear ; the symptoms are trembling of the limbs and head, stammering speech, disturbed sleep and appetite. **Spinal S.**, a condition following injury or transverse section of the spinal cord in which the reflex functions of the cord are abolished below the site of injury.

Shope's Papilloma. A warty growth, sometimes malignant, capable of transmission from animal to animal by cell-free filtrates ; *i.e.*, due to a virus.

Short-sightedness. Myopia (*q.v.*).

Show. A common term for the appearance of blood and mucus at the vulva during the commencement of labour.

Sialagogue (sī-al'-a-gog). An agent which increases salivation.

Sialorrhœa (sī-al-o-rē'-ä). Excessive flow of saliva.

Sibilus (sib'-il-us). Hissing or wheezing sounds heard in auscultation of the chest.

Siderosis (sīd-e-rō'-sis). The deposition of iron compounds in the tissues ; these compounds give the chemical and staining reactions of metallic iron.

Sigmoid (sig'-moid). Shaped like the letter S.

Sigmoidectomy (sig-moid-ek'-to-mi). Excision of the sigmoid flexure of the colon.

Sigmoidoscope (sig-moid'-os-

kōp). An instrument for examining the interior of the rectum and sigmoid flexure of the colon.

Sigmoidoscopy (sig-moid-os'-kop-i). The use of the sigmoidoscope.

Sign (sīn). Any objective evidence of disease.

Signature (sig'-na-tūr). That part of a prescription which gives the directions or instructions to the patient.

Silicon (sil'-i-kon), Si. Next to oxygen the most abundant element on the earth, and forms a constituent of many different minerals, especially quartz.

Silicosis (sil-i-kō'-sis). A fibrosis of the lungs due to inhalation of siliceous particles among stone workers, etc.

Silk. Threads made of spun silk prepared in strands suitable for surgical sutures, numbering in thickness from 0 to 5. Chinese silk is generally used ; it is sterilized by boiling for half an hour. **Oil-S.**, a fine waterproof substance used for covering fomentations, etc.

Silkworm Gut. A very strong material used for external sutures ; is sterilized by boiling in carbolic lotion 1-20, and immersed in sterile water before use.

Silver Nitrate. *See* Nitrate.

Simple (sim-p'l). Consisting of

315

one substance; uncomplicated; innocent or non-malignant.

Simples (sim-p'lz). Medicinal herbs.

Sim's Posture. *See* **Position.** **S. Speculum,** the speculum used for vaginal examination.

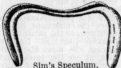

Sim's Speculum.

Sinapism (sin'-a-pizm). A mustard plaster.

Sinciput (sin'-si-put). The upper front part of the head.

Sinew (sin'-ū). A ligament or tendon.

Sinistral (sin'-is-tral). Pertaining to the left, or sinister, side.

Sinus (sī'-nus). (1) A channel for venous blood, *e.g.*, the sinuses of the brain. (2) A passage leading to a deep-seated abscess. (3) Any hollow or cavity. **Frontal S.,** two cavities in the frontal bone, one on either side of the medial line, and which open into the upper part of the nasal cavity. **Lateral S.,** one of the most important of the cranial venous sinuses.

Sinusitis (sīn-ū-sī'-tis). Inflammation of a sinus, especially the maxillary or frontal sinus.

Sinusoid (sīn'-ū-soid). A dilated channel into which arterioles open in some organs and which take the place of the usual capillaries.

Site (sīt). A situation, position or location.

Sitz-bath (sits'-bàth). A hip-bath, one in which the water covers the hips when in the sitting position; used in the treatment of vulvitis, vaginitis, etc.

Skatol (skă'-tol). A substance derived from tryptophane during digestion; a constituent of fæces.

Skeletal (skel-ē'-tal). Pertaining to the skeleton. **S. Muscle,** the muscular tissue covering the skeleton.

Skeleton (skel'-e-ton). The bony framework of the body; it is composed of over 200 bones.

Skene's Glands. Two small glands at the entrance to the female urethra; they are always infected in gonorrhœa, and exude pus if pressed.

Skiagram (skī'-a-gram). An X-ray photograph.

Skin. The tissue which forms the outer covering of the body; it consists of two main layers: (1) The *epidermis,* or cuticle, forming the outer coat; (2) the *dermis,* or cutis vera, the inner or true skin lying beneath the epidermis.

Skull. The bones forming the head. *See* **Cranium.**

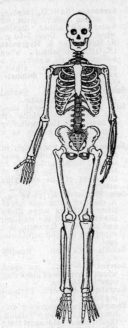

The Skeleton.

Sleeping Sickness. Trypanosomiasis (*q.v.*).

Sleepy Sickness. Encephalitis lethargica (*q.v.*).

Sling. A supporting bandage for a limb; generally made from a triangular bandage.

Slough (sluf). Septic tissue which becomes necrosed and separates from the healthy tissue.

Sloughing (sluf'-ing). The process of forming a slough.

Smallpox. A virulent infectious disease due to a virus; variola. The incubation period is twelve days. On the third day a rash appears which at first is papular, then vesicular, and finally pustular. These eventually dry up, forming scabs which, after falling off, tend to leave the skin pitted or scarred. Constitutional disturbance is marked, and there is a high temperature. **Confluent S.,** a type in which the pustules coalesce without healthy skin tissue between. **Malignant** or **Hæmorrhagic S.,** a black appearance of the pocks due to capillary hæmorrhage; usually fatal.

Smegma (smeg'-ma). The sebaceous secretion which accumulates beneath the prepuce.

Smelling Salts. Ammonium carbonate to which some scent has been added. The ammonia gas given off acts as a mild stimulant when sniffed.

Snare. A surgical instrument with a wire loop at the end ; used for the removal of polypi.

Snore. Noisy breathing during sleep.

Snow or **" CO₂-snow."** The powdery solidified CO_2 obtained by the sudden release of pressure of CO_2 escaping from compressed liquefied CO_2 in a steel cylinder. It can be formed into solid pencils, etc., and is used in the treatment of nævi and rodent ulcer. **S.-blindness,** partial blindness caused by the bright reflection of light from snow.

Snuffles (snuf'-'ls). Nasal catarrh in an infant, making breathing through the nose difficult ; commonly due to syphilis.

Soda (sō'-dà). Common washing-soda ; sodium carbonate.

Sodium (sō'-di-um) (Na). A metal. A soft, white, brilliant substance which, when placed in water, causes violent action to take place and the water is decomposed with the formation of caustic soda, or sodium hydroxide, and the liberation of hydrogen, e.g., $2Na + 2H_2O = 2NaOH + H_2$. For this reason, sodium is kept immersed in naphtha. **S. Carbonate** (Na_2CO_3), *common washing-soda.* **S. Bi-**

carbonate ($NaHCO_3$), *cooking or baking soda* ; gives off water and carbon dioxide when heated. Dose, 5-30 gr. **S. Hydrate** or **S. Hydroxide** (NaOH), obtained when sodium acts on water ; is a powerful caustic alkali ; *caustic soda.* **S. Sulphate,** *Glauber's salts.*

Sodomy (sod'-o-mi). Sexual connection by the anus.

Soft Sore. A venereal sore, but not due to syphilis ; it is caused by the *bacillus of Ducrey.* Also known as a *Chancroid.*

Softening. The conversion of tissue to a semi-fluid condition ; seen particularly in the brain as the result of thrombus of the supplying arteries.

Solar Plexus (sō'-là(r) pleks'-us). A mass of autonomic nerve tissue with its nerve fibres situated behind the stomach and in front of the aorta, and supplying the abdominal viscera.

Soluble (sol'-ū-bl). Readily dissolved.

Solvent (sol'-vent). An agent which is capable of dissolving other substances.

Somatic (sō-mat'-ik). Pertaining to the body.

Somnambulism (som-nam'-bū-lizm). (1) Sleep-walking. (2) An abnormal mental state indicating that the mind is in a condition of dissociation ;

generally occurs in emotional and hysterical persons; the condition is usually treated by psycho-analysis.

Somnifacient (som-ni-fā'-si-ent). A medicine producing sleep.

Somnolence (som'-nō-lens). Drowsiness.

Sonorous (son'-o-rus). Resonant; ringing.

Soporific (sop-or-if'-ik or sō-). An agent which induces profound sleep.

Sordes (saw(r)'-dēz). The formation of brown crusts on the lips and teeth of patients with a high temperature. Such concretions consist of particles of food, epithelial cells, and bacteria. This condition is preventable by careful and regular attention to mouth hygiene.

Souffle (soofl). A blowing, swishing sound heard during auscultation. **Funic S.,** heard on auscultation over the abdomen of a pregnant woman; the sound is probably produced by the course of the blood through the umbilical vessels, and is synchronous with the fœtal heart-beat. **Uterine** or **Placental S.,** a murmur heard during the latter end of pregnancy, and probably due to the passage of the blood through the dilated vessels of the placenta.

Sound. An instrument resembling a probe. **Uterine S.,** one which is used to indicate the size and position of the uterus.

Southey's Tubes (sow'-thēz). Small perforated metal tubes used for draining away the fluid from dropsical tissues; they are sterilized by boiling before insertion, and the fluid withdrawn should be measured.

Soxhlet Apparatus (soks'-let). An apparatus for sterilizing infant's milk; by this means several milk bottles can be prepared at one time.

Spanish Fly. A powder obtained by crushing the dried beetle, the *Cantharis vesicatoria*, used in the preparation of blistering fluid, and as an aphrodisiac.

Spasm. A violent muscular contraction, a sudden convulsive movement. **Clonic S.,** spasms alternating with short periods of relaxation. **Habit S.,** muscular spasms due to habit. **Tetanic S.,** the convulsions of tetanus. **Tonic S.,** spasms which occur without intervals of relaxation; persistent spasms.

Spasmodic (spaz-mod'-ik). Relating to spasm; convulsive.

Spasmophilia (spaz-mō-fil'-i-à). The condition in which there is a tendency to tetany and convulsions. Almost always associated with rickets.

Spastic (spas'-tik). In a condition of rigidity or spasm.

Spatula (spat'-ū-là). A flat,

flexible knife with blunt edges, used for making poultices and spreading ointment. **Throat S.,** a spatula made of glass, ivory, wood, or metal for holding down the tongue during examination of the throat.

Spay (spā). Castrate ; to remove the ovaries or testicles.

Specialist. One trained and skilled in the diagnosis and treatment of a special class of diseases.

Species (spē´-shēz). A group of individuals having common characteristics, but subordinate to a genus.

Specific (spe-sif´-ik). Special, characteristic, peculiar to ; e.g., a disease is said to be specific when it is always caused by the same special organism. **S. Disease,** syphilis. **S. Gravity,** the relative weight of a substance as compared with an equal volume of water. The weight of the water is regarded for convenience as represented by 1,000. Urine has a specific gravity ranging normally between 1,015 and 1,025.

Spectroscope (spek´-tros-kōp). An instrument for producing and examining the spectrum.

Spectrum (spek´-trum). The coloured band produced when light is dissociated into its constituent colour elements. The seven colours of which

white light is composed may be perceived when it is projected through a prism, and occur in the following order : Violet, indigo, blue, green, yellow, orange, red.

Speculum (spek´-ū-lum). An instrument used to hold the

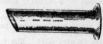

Ferguson's Speculum.

walls of a cavity apart, so that the interior of the cavity can be examined.

Sperm. Semen ; a seed.

Spermaceti (sperm-a-sē´-ti). A fatty substance obtained from the head of the sperm whale. After being separated from the oil with which it is combined, it is purified and used medicinally as an emollient.

Spermatic (sper-mat´-ik). Pertaining to the semen. **S. Cord,** a cord passing to the seminal vesicles from the testicles.

Spermatid (sper-mat´-id). A cell formed by the division of the spermatocyte.

Spermatocele (sper-mat´-ō-sēl). A cyst, attached to the testis or to the spermatic cord, which contains spermatozoa.

Spermatocyte (sper-mat´-ō-sīt). A cell formed by the division of the spermatogonia they ultimately develop into the spermatozoa vra spermatids.

Spermatorrhœa (sper-mat-o-rē'-à). An involuntary discharge of semen.

Spermatozoa (sper-mat-o-zō'-à). The male cells of reproduction which are developed from the spermatids about the age of puberty. They are minute organisms with a pointed head and a vibratile thread-like tail which enables the cell to become actively motile. The head of the spermatozoon pierces the envelope of the ovum and thereupon loses its tail. After fusion the two cells continue to develop as one cell.

Spes Phthisica (spez thī'-sik-à). An unnatural sense of well-being, happiness, and hopefulness in patients ill with phthisis who are making unsatisfactory progress. The cause of this state is an underlying fear from which the patient tries to escape, and accomplishes it by repression, which manifests itself by characteristic behaviour of the opposite extreme.

Sphenoid (sfē'-noid). A wedge-shaped bone at the base of the skull. It articulates with the *occipital* bone at the back, the *ethmoid* in the front, and the *parietals* and *temporal* bones at the sides.

Spherical (sfe'-rik-al). Round; like a sphere.

Sphincter (sfingk'-ter). A circular muscle guarding the entrance or exit of a cavity, *e.g.*, pylorus.

Sphygmocardiograph (sfig-mō-kà(r)'-di-ō-graf). An apparatus for taking a graphic tracing of the character of the heart-beat.

Sphygmogram (sfig'-mō-gram). The tracing of a pulse-beat.

Sphygmograph (sfig'-mō-graf). An apparatus attached to the wrist, over the radial artery, which records the movements of the pulse-beat.

Sphygmomanometer (sfig-mō-man-om'-e-ter). An instrument used for measuring the blood-pressure. *See* **Blood-pressure.**

Spica (spī'-kà). A term used for a method of applying a roller bandage; it is generally applied to the shoulder, groin or thumb. The bandage passes round the body and round the limb alternately, forming a figure of eight pattern.

Spicule (spik'-ūl). A small spike-like fragment of bone.

Spider-cells. The flattened, branched glial cells or astrocytes of the brain. **Spider nævus,** a small radiating capillary angioma; a telangiectasis resembling a small spider.

Spina Bifida (spī'-nà bif'-id-à).

L

321

An imperfect development of the spinal column in which there is a fissure in one or

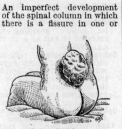

Spina Bifida.

more of the vertebræ, allowing the spinal membranes to bulge through ; generally has a fatal termination during childhood. **S.B. Occulta**, a minor form in which there is no obvious tumour on the back, though often marked by a growth of long hair over the site.

Spinal Anæsthesia. *See* **Anæsthesia. S. Cord**, the continuation of nervous tissue of the brain down the canal of the spinal column ; it commences at the medulla oblongata, passing through the foramen magnum, and terminates at the level of the first or second lumbar vertebra ; it weighs 1½ oz., and gives off 31 pairs of spinal nerves.

Spindle-celled. Composed of cells having a tapering or fusiform shape.

Spine. The vertebral column. **Railway S.**, a form of spinal neurosis resulting from a railway accident. **Typhoid S.**, a neurosis occurring during convalescence in typhoid fever ; there is pain and stiffness in the lumbar and sacral regions ; there is no temperature, but marked nervous disturbance.

Spirillum (spī-ril′-um). A genus of bacteria having a more or less spiral appearance, *e.g.*, the spirillum of Vincent's Angina.

Spirit (spir′-it). An alcoholic solution of a volatile substance.

Spirochæta Pallida (spī-rō-kē′-tà pal′-id-à). The microorganism causing syphilis ; it is a spirillum, actively motile, and found in great numbers in syphilitic lesions. Other spirochæta found in the blood are **S. Obermeieri**, the cause of relapsing fever ; **S. Duttoni**, causing tick fever ; **S. Icterohæmorrhagiæ**, the cause of infective jaundice, or Weil's disease.

Spirograph (spī′-rō-graf). An apparatus which records the movements of the lungs.

Spirometer (spī-rom′-et-er). An instrument for estimating the lung capacity.

Spittle (spit′-'l). Sputum ; that which is expectorated.

Splanchnic (splangk'-nik). Pertaining to the viscera.

Splanchnology (splangk-nol'-o-ji). The science which deals with the structure and function of the viscera.

Splay-foot. *See* **Flat Foot.**

Spleen (splēn). An oblong-shaped organ lying to the left of the stomach; anatomically, it lies behind the ninth, tenth, and eleventh ribs; popularly known as the *milt.* Enlargement of the spleen is an important symptom in many diseases.

Splenculus (splen'-kŭ-lus). An accessory spleen. Also **Spleniculus** and **Splenunculus.**

Splenectomy (splen-ek'-to-mi). Surgical removal of the spleen.

Splenitis (splen-ī'-tis). Inflammation of the spleen.

Splenomedullary Leukæmia (splēn-ō-me-dul'-a-ri lū-kēm'-i-å). A disease associated with a great increase in the number of leucocytes per cubic millimetre, hæmorrhage into the skin and from the mucous membranes, enlargement of the spleen, and changes in the bone marrow.

Splenomegaly (splēn-ō-meg'-a-li). Enlargement of the spleen.

Splinter (splin'-ter). A thin detached piece of bone; a sequestrum.

Splints. Apparatus used for immobilizing a fractured bone and for keeping the ends in

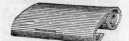

Thomas's Knee Splint.

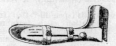

Gooch's Splinting.

Cline's Splint.

Internal Angular Splint.

Arm Splint.

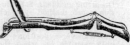

Macintyre (of Newcastle) Splint.

323

correct apposition to promote healing ; also used to prevent contracture or deformity in burns, etc. Splints are made from wood, aluminium, or other metals, poroplastic felt, plaster, and bandages. A limb is sometimes suspended upon strips of flannel adjusted to the shape of the limb and fastened securely to the sides of the splint.

Spondyle (spon'-dīl.) A vertebra.

Spondylitis (spon-dil-ī'-tis). Inflammation of a vertebra. **S. Deformans**, arthritis deformans of the spinal column.

Spondylolisthesis (spon-di-lō-lis'-thē-sis). Dislocation of the spine.

Sponge (spunzh). The porous skeleton of a marine species of animal ; readily absorbs water. *See* **Tepid Sponging**.

Spongioblastoma (spon-ji-ō-blas-tō-mà). A malignant tumour of the brain or cord composed of primitive neuroglial cells or spongioblasts.

Spongy (spun'-zhi). Soft and swollen, *e.g.*, spongy gums in scurvy and mercurial poisoning.

Spontaneous (spon-tā'-ni-us). Occurring unaided. **S. Evolution**, a rare method by which the fœtus is expelled from the uterus while it is lying in the transverse position ; is only possible (*a*) when the fœtus is very small and the

pelvis large, (*b*) when the fœtus is dead. **S. Fracture**, *see* **Fracture**. **S. Version**, the unaided conversion of a transverse presentation into either a vertex or breech presentation.

Sporadic (spo-rad'-ik). Scattered ; occurring in isolated cases ; not epidemic.

Spore (spaw(r). Any germ or reproductive element less organized than a true cell. Sporing is an asexual method of reproduction in many unicellular animals and plants. Certain bacteria also form spores, but this is more in the nature of a defensive mechanism than for reproduction. The spores of bacteria are difficult to destroy, as they are very resistant to heat and require prolonged exposure to high temperatures to destroy them.

Sport. A freak of nature ; an individual exhibiting some features abnormal to its species ; lusus naturæ.

Sporulation (spo-rū-lā'-shun). The act of forming spores.

Spotted Fever. Cerebro-spinal fever ; meningococcal meningitis.

Sprain (sprān). Tearing and stretching of tendinous insertions of muscles, the result of sudden violence applied to a joint either directly or indirectly.

Sprue (sproo). A tropical disease characterized by glossitis, a form of diarrhœa in which the stools are white and frothy, and a severe type of anæmia in which the blood picture closely resembles that of Addison's anæmia.

Spurious (spū'-ri-us). False. **S. Pains**, pains which sometimes precede the true pains of labour. These false pains generally commence in the abdomen, whereas true pains originate in the back and radiate round to the abdomen.

Sputum (spū'-tum). Matter which is expectorated from the lungs.

Squamous (skwā'-mus). Scaly. **S. Carcinoma**, carcinoma of the skin ; epithelioma.

Squills (skwilz). A drug obtained from the bulb of *Urginœa scilla* ; is diuretic and a cardiac tonic and expectorant. *Tincture*, 5-30 minims ; *syrup*, 30-60 minims.

Squint (skwint). Inco-ordinated action of the muscles of the eyeballs such that the visual axes of the two eyes fail to meet at the objective point ; strabismus. **Divergent S.**, when the eyes turn outwards. **Convergent S.**, when they turn towards the medial line.

Staccato Speech (stak-á'-tō). *See* **Scanning Speech**.

Stagnant (stag'-nant). Motionless.

Stagnation (stag-nä'-shun). A state of impurity due to lack of motion, *e.g.*, stagnation of air.

Stamina (stam'-in-à). **Innate** vigour.

Stammer (stam'-er). Difficult enunciation ; stutter.

Stanch. To stop or check the flow (as of blood).

Stapes (stā'-pēz). The stirrup-shaped bone of the middle ear.

Staphylococcus (staf-i-lō-kok'-us). A micrococcus capable of producing sepsis, *e.g.*, **S. Pyogenes Aureus**, commonly found on the skin and hair, a common cause of acute abscesses and boils. The staphylococci occur in group formation, resembling a bunch of grapes.

Staphyloma (staf-i-lō'-mà). A protrusion of the cornea or sclera of the eye.

Starch. A nutrient carbohydrate common to potatoes, cereals, etc. ; amylum ; $(C_6H_{10}O_5)n$. **Animal S.**, glycogen. **S. Enema**, an enema of starch-water.

Stasis (stā'-sis). Stagnation ; cessation of motion.

Static (stat'-ik). Stationary ; without movement.

Status (stāt'-us). A state. **S. Epilepticus**, an epileptic condition in which the fits are almost continuous. **S. Lymphaticus** or **S. Thymico-lymphaticus**. A condition in

325

which death occurs from apparently trivial causes. At one time believed to be due to or associated with an enlarged thymus or one persisting after puberty, at which age it normally becomes rudimentary. This view no longer generally accepted.

Steapsin (stē-ap'-sin). An enzyme of the pancreatic juice which during digestion splits fat into fatty acids and glycerine. Same as *Lipase*.

Stearic Acid (stē'-a-rik). A fatty acid formed by the action of steapsin on stearin. *See also* **Palmitic Acid.**

Stearin (stē'-a-rin). One of the commoner fats, a compound of glycerol and stearic acid.

Steatoma (stē-a-tō'-mà). *See* **Sebaceous Cysts.**

Steatorrhœa (stē-at-o-rē'-à). Increased secretion of sebaceous or fatty material ; the passing of large, loose, fatty stools.

Stegomyia (steg-ō-mī-i-à). A genus of mosquitoes which causes the dissemination of yellow fever from infected to healthy individuals.

Steinach Operation. A rejuvenating operation performed on senile persons by ligating the vas deferens.

Steinmann's Pin (stīn'-man). A narrow steel rod used for extension purposes in fractures of the femur. It is

passed right through the shaft of the bone just above the condyles. The strictest asepsis must be observed with the use of this pin.

Stellate (stel'-āt). Star-shaped.

Stellwag's Sign. Spasm or retraction of the upper eyelid ; a symptom of exophthalmic goitre.

Steno's Duct (stē-nō). *See* **Stenson.**

Stenosis (sten-ō'-sis). A narrowing.

Stensen's Duct (sten'-sen's). The duct leading from the parotid gland, and opening in the cheek opposite the upper second molar tooth.

Stercobilin (ster-kō-bī'-lin). The brown pigment of fæces ; it is derived from the bile pigments.

Stercoraceous (ster-ko-rā'-shi-us). Resembling or pertaining to fæces.

Stereoscopic (ste-ri-ō-skop'-ik). Pertaining to the perception of the depth of objects when viewed with binocular vision ; not flat.

Sterile (stē'-rīl). (1) Barren ; unable to reproduce ; nonfertile. (2) Free from contamination with living organisms, such as bacteria, protozoa, etc.

Sterility (ste-ril'-i-ti). The state of being sterile.

Sterilization (ste-ril-i-zā'-shun). The process or method of attaining sterility. After being thoroughly cleaned, instruments are sterilized by placing them into boiling water to which a little soda has been added. This prevents the formation of rust. Heavy instruments are placed at the bottom, lighter ones on top. Delicate or sharp instruments are first wrapped in lint to save them from injury. Boiling should continue for 20 minutes. Rubber tubing must not be boiled, as a chemical reaction occurs with the metal, and this tends to turn the instruments black. Soda has a deleterious effect upon rubber. Sharp instruments, such as scalpels and needles, are generally immersed in pure lysol, since boiling blunts them.

Sterilizer (ste'-ril-ĭ-zer). The apparatus used for rendering objects sterile, either by means of boiling or by steam pressure. *See* **Autoclave**.

Sternum (ster'-num). The breast-bone.

Sternutation (ster-nū-tā'-shun). The act of sneezing.

Stertor (ster'-taw(r)). Loud snoring ; sonorous breathing.

Stertorous (ster'-to-rus). Pertaining to stertor.

Stethometer (steth-om'-et-er). An instrument for estimating the maximum amount of chest expansion.

Stethoscope (steth'-o-skŏp). An

instrument used for listening to the various body sounds, especially those of the heart and chest.

Sthenic (sthen'-ik). Strong ; forceful.

Sticking-plaster. Resin plaster. Adhesive bandage or dressing.

Stiff. Hard and unbending.

Stigmata (stig'-ma-tă). (1) Blemishes on the skin. (2) Physical deformities, such as malposition of eyes, ears, etc., the so-called " *stigmata of mental deficiency.*"

Stilette (stil-et'). A sharp-pointed instrument ; medically, a thin piece of metal or wire for passing into a hypodermic or lumbar puncture needle to prevent blockage. In sterilizing the needle, the stilette is removed and boiled with the needle, so that it can be used if necessary.

Still-born. Born dead.

Stimulant (stim'-ū-lant). (1) Increasing some functional process. (2) The agent which excites or increases function.

Stimulus (stim'-ū-lus). Anything which excites or activates an organ.

Stokes-Adams Syndrome. A series of symptoms occurring in patients suffering from heart-block. The onset is sudden, resembling an attack of epilepsy, for which it is sometimes mistaken. It is due to stoppage or extreme slowness of ventricular contraction.

Stoma (stŏ'-mà). The mouth; any opening. Pl.: *stomata*.

Stomachic (stom-ak'-ik). An agent which increases the appetite.

Stomatitis (stŏ-ma-tī'-tis). Inflammation of the mouth. **Aphthous S.**, thrush (*q.v.*). **Mercurial S.**, produced by mercurial poisoning. **Gangrenous S.**, cancrum oris (*q.v.*).

Stomodeum (stom-ō-di'-um). The primitive mouth or oral cavity of the embryo.

Stone (stōn). Calculus.

Stool. The fæces. An evacuation of the bowels.

Stovain (stŏ'-vān). A local anæsthetic used for intrathecal anæsthesia.

Strabismus (stra-biz'-mus). *See* **Squint**.

Strabotomy (stra-bot'-o-mi). The operation for the cure of squint.

Strain (strān). (1) A sprain. (2) Tension. (3) To filter.

Stramonium (stra-mōn'-i-um). A drug obtained from the dried leaves of *Datura S.* It acts similarly to belladonna, and has a powerful action in relaxing the muscular spasm of the bronchi, and is therefore much prescribed for asthma. Dose: *Tincture*, 5-30 minims. The leaves are often smoked in the form of cigarettes or in the form of

powder; when ignited, the fumes are inhaled.

Strangulated (strang'-gū-lā-ted). Constricted so as to impede the circulation. *See* **S. Hernia**.

Strangury (strang'-gū-ri). Painful and difficult micturition, such as occurs with urethral calculus, enlarged prostate gland, etc., so that the urine is only passed out a drop at a time.

Strapping (strap'-ing). Various kinds of sticking-plaster used for covering or holding together the edges of wounds, for applying extension to a limb, or for keeping splints, etc., in position.

Stratified (strat'-i-fīd). Arranged in plate-like layers. *See* **Epithelium**.

Stratum (strā-tum). A layer or lamina, *e.g.*, the various layers of the epithelium of the skin, viz., **S. granulosum**, **S. lucidum**, etc.

Strawberry Tongue. The typical appearance of the tongue in scarlet fever; at first the tongue is covered with a whitish fur, through which projects the red papilli, resembling an unripe strawberry; later the fur disappears, leaving the tongue vividly red, like an overripe strawberry.

Streptococcus (strep-tō-kok'-us). A micrococcus measuring 0·5-1 μ in diameter, which forms shorter or longer chains. The commonest example is *S. Pyogenes* ; causes spreading inflammations such as erysipelas, cellulitis, suppuration, septicæmia, lymphangitis, etc.

Streptothrix (strep'-tō-thriks). A filamentous higher form of bacterium which is more or less intermediate between the lower bacteria and the higher fungi. An important member of this group is the *ray fungus* or *actinomyces*, the cause of actinomycosis. On culture, the organism grows in a radiating branched fashion and is Gram-positive.

Stretcher (strech'-er). A portable frame or cot for carrying the sick or injured.

Striæ (strī'-ē). Fine lineal marks which appear in skin which has been overstretched, with resultant rupture of the minute papillary muscles. Capillary bleeding occurs, giving the marks a purplish colour. Old scars are white. They are commonly seen on the thighs, abdomen, and breasts of pregnant women, but may result from any sudden enlargement due to dropsy, tumours, or excessive obesity.

Striated (strī-ā'-ted). Having lines or furrows.

Stricture (strik'-tūr). A narrowing of a tube or canal, such as the urethra or œsophagus.

Stridor (strī'-daw(r)). A harsh sound in breathing, caused by air passing through constricted air-passages.

Stridulous (strid'-ū-lus). Pertaining to stridor ; harsh.

Stroke (strōk). A sudden and severe seizure ; an apoplectic fit.

Stroma (strō'-mà). The interstitial or foundation substance of a structure.

Strophanthin (strō-fan'-thin). A glucoside of strophanthus. Dose, 1/240-1/50 gr. hypodermically.

Strophanthus (strō-fan'-thus). A drug derived from the seeds of *Strophanthus Kombé*. The action of this drug is closely allied to that of digitalis. Dosage : Tincture, 2-5 minims.

Struma (stroo-mà). A goiter ; a scrofulous or glandular tumour.

Strychnine (strik'-nēn). An alkaloid of nux vomica. It acts chiefly on the cells of the anterior horn of the spinal cord, so that their reflex excitability is enormously increased if toxic doses are administered. This accounts for the violent muscular spasms produced in strychnine poisoning. It has a tonic and a stimulating effect upon the respiratory and cardio-vascular systems. It has an accumulative effect in the body, and is eliminated slowly by the kidneys. Dos-

L *

age : Hydrochlor., 1/32-1/8 gr.; liq. strychnine hydrochloridi, 3-12 minims.

Stupe (stūp). A piece of flannel folded two or three times, soaked in boiling water and wrung out tightly. It is applied to the skin to relieve inflammation and pain. **Opium S.,** 30-60 minims of opium are sprinkled over the stupe after it has been wrung out. **Turpentine S.,** 1-2 drachms of turpentine are sprinkled evenly over the dry flannel before the water is poured on. For further details of application, *see* **Fomentations.**

Stupor (stū-paw(r)). A state of depression of the senses not amounting to coma.

Stutter (stut'-er). *See* **Stammer.**

Stye (stī). An abscess of the eyelid ; hordeolum.

Styptic (stip'-tik). *See* **Hæmostatics.**

Sub. A prefix meaning beneath, below, or under.

Subacute (sub-ak-ūt'). Of moderate severity ; relatively gradual.

Subarachnoid Space (sub-a-rak'-noid). The space beneath the arachnoid membrane, between it and the pia mater.

Subclavian (sub-klā'-vi-an). Beneath the clavicle.

Subculture (sub-kul'-tūr). A secondary bacterial culture.

Suboutaneous (sub-kū-tā'-ni-us). Beneath the skin.

Subdural (sub-dū'-ral). Beneath the dura mater ; between the dura and arachnoid membranes.

Subinvolution (sub-in-vō-loo'-shun). A failure of the gravid uterus to return to its normal size within a normal time after child-birth ; this usually takes about six weeks.

Subjective (sub-jek'-tiv). Internal ; personal ; arising from the senses, as opposed to objective.

Sublimate (sub'-lim-āt). A solid deposit resulting from the condensation of a vapour.

Sublimation (sub-lim-ā'-shun). (1) Volatilization of solid substances like camphor, iodine, etc. (2) A Freudian term designating the unconscious mental process whereby a repressed instinct is diverted from its natural expression into other activities which are satisfactory substitutes, and also conform to the ethics of society, *e.g.*, the sex instinct may find its expression in creative work, such as art, literature, etc.

Sublingual (sub-ling'-gwal). Beneath the tongue.

Subluxation (sub-luks-ā'-shun). Incomplete dislocation.

Submucous (sub-mū'-kus). Beneath a mucous membrane.

Subperiosteal (sub-pe-ri-os'-ti-al). Beneath the periosteum of bone.

Subperitoneal (sub-pe-ri-to-ni'-al). Beneath the peritoneum.

Subphrenic (sub-fren'-ik). Beneath the phren or diaphragm.

Subsidence (sub'-sid-ens). A falling to the bottom; the gradual disappearance of a disease.

Substage (sub'-stāj). That part of a microscope which is below the stage.

Subsultus (sub-sul'-tus). Muscular tremor as the result of weakness.

Subtotal (sub-tō'-tal). Incomplete. **S. Hysterectomy,** *see* **Hysterectomy.**

Succus (suk'-us). A juice. **S. Entericus,** the intestinal juice; has a specific gravity about 1,010, and is alkaline; has five main enzymes: (1) *lactase*; (2) *invertin*; (3) *maltase*; (4) *enterokinase*; (5) *erepsin.*

Succussion (suk-ush'-'n). Shaking the body of a patient to detect the presence of fluid in a cavity, such as the abdomen, by the splashing sound produced.

S u d a m i n a (sū-dam'-i-nă). Sweat rash.

Sudor (sū'-daw(r)). Sweat. *See* Miliaria.

Sudoriferous (sū-do-rif'-e-rus). Pertaining to sweat.

Sudorific (sū-do-rif'-ik). An agent which induces sweating.

Suffocation (suf-ō-kā'-shun). Cessation of breathing through obstruction to the air-passages, *e.g.*, hanging, drowning, choking, strangling, œdema of the glottis, etc.

Suffusion (su-fū'-zhun). An extravasation or spreading flow of blood or other fluid into the tissues.

Sugar. A sweet soluble compound belonging to the group of carbohydrates (*q.v.*). **S. Diabetes,** diabetes mellitus. **Fruit S.,** fructose. **Grape S.,** dextrose. **S. of Milk,** lactose. **Sugar Test for Urine:** take ½ in. each of Fehling's solution No. 1 and No. 2 in a test-tube, and boil the mixture. If fresh, it should retain its bright blue colour. Now add half as much of the suspect urine and boil. If sugar is present, a brick-red colour develops.

Suggestion (su-jes'-chun). In the psychological sense, a non-critical acceptance of some outward influence; also a form of treatment for nervous disorders.

Sulcus (sul-kus). A furrow or groove, particularly those separating the gyri or convolutions of the cortex of the brain.

Sulphadiazine (sulf-a-dī'-a-zēn). One of the sulphonamides.

Sulphæmoglobinæmia (sulf-hēm-ō-glō-bin-ēm'-i-ă). The presence in the blood of sulphæmoglobin, *i.e.*, a compound formed by the combination of hæmoglobin with hydrogen sulphide.

Sulphanilamide (sulf-a-nil'-a-mīd). A synthetic dye used as a drug for the control of streptococcal and some other infections. This drug is marketed under various trade names but always consists of p - amino - benzene - sulphonamide. *See* **Sulphonamide.**

Sulphapyridine (sulf-a-pir'-i-dēn). One of the sulphonamides; trade name, M and B 693; particularly used in pneumococcal infections.

Sulphate (sul'-fāt). A salt of sulphuric acid.

Sulphathiazole (sulf-a-thī'-a-zōl). One of the sulphonamides; M & B 760; particularly used in staphylococcal infections.

Sulphonal (sul'-fō-nal). A colourless hypnotic powder. Dose, 5-20 grs.

Sulphonamide. Certain analine derivatives contain what is known as the sulphonamide group. Various preparations for clinical use are sold under trade names. They are given by mouth or intra-muscular injection. Streptococcal infections yield well to these preparations. The newer compounds can also be used for staphylococcal, pneumococcal and gonococcal infections.

Sulphur (sul'-fur). Symbol, S.

A yellow crystalline non-metal found free in nature and also combined with metals in many minerals. S. Granules, small yellow particles in the pus of actino-mycotic infections ; these granules contain the ray fungus. **Flowers of S.,** sulphur sublimatum, used in ointments and also for room fumigation, giving off sulphur dioxide gas. **Potassa Sulphurata,** used as an ingredient for ointment and for medicinal baths in parasitic or other skin complaints. When sulphur is used, the nurse should watch for and report any signs of eczema.

Sulphuric Acid (sul-fū'-rik). Oil of vitriol (H_2SO_4).

Summer Diarrhœa. A form of acute diarrhœa occurring among infants ; sometimes called *cholera infantum* ; it causes a very high mortality during the hot summer months.

Sunstroke (sun'-strōk). Heat-stroke caused by undue exposure to the rays of the sun. The main symptoms are very severe headache, vomiting, mental confusion, and hyper-pyrexia, in which the temperature may rise as high as 107° F.

Superciliary (soo-per-sil'-i-a-ri). Relating to the eyebrow.

Superfœtation (su-per-fē-tā'-shun). A new conception

superimposed upon an already pregnant condition.

Supernatant (soo-per-nā'-tant). The liquid above a solid deposit ; floating on the surface.

Supernumerary (soo-per-nūm'-e-ra-ri). In excess of the normal number ; additional (as of digits or nipples).

Supination (soo-pī-nā'-shun). (1) The attitude of lying face upward. (2) The act of turning the palm upward.

Supine (soo'-pīn). Lying face upwards.

Supplemental Air. The extra air expelled from the lungs during forced expiration ; it varies from 1,000 to 1,500 c.c.

Suppository (su-poz'-it-a-ri). Small solid, conical bodies composed of oil of theobroma, glycerine, gelatine, or soap, which serve as a vehicle for certain drugs ; they are inserted into the rectum or vagina, where they melt. **Morphia S.**, contain morph.-sulph. ¼-½ gr. ; inserted into the rectum for the relief of pain. **Soap S.**, a small conical piece of soap which, after being lubricated with vaseline, is inserted well into the rectum ; it acts as a purgative.

Suppression of Urine. A critical condition in which the kidneys cease to secrete urine.

Suppuration (sup-ū-rā'-shun). The formation of pus.

Supraorbital (soop-rå-aw(r)'-bit-al). Above the orbits. **S. Ridge,** the ridge covered by the eyebrows.

Suprapubic (soop-rå-pū'-bik). Above the pubis. **S. Cysto-**

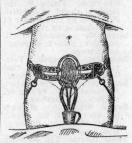

Hamilton Irving's Suprapubic Drainage Apparatus.

tomy, an operation for making an opening into the bladder above the pubis.

Suprarenal (soop-rå-rēn'-al). Above the kidney. **S. Gland,** a small gland, shaped like a cocked hat, situated just above each kidney ; it consists of an outer capsule or cortex and an inner soft medulla, which secretes a hormone known as adrenalin. *See also* **Addison's Disease.**

Surgery (sur'-je-ri). The branch of medicine dealing with

333

operative procedures. **Ortho-pædic S.,** originally that section of surgery which dealt with deformities of children ; now it includes all the surgery of the skeletal structures. **Plastic S.,** the repair of absent or defective structures by transference of tissue from other parts.

Susceptible (sus-sep'-tib-'l). Sensitive ; liable to infection ; not immune.

Suspended Animation. Temporary cessation of vital functions ; unconsciousness.

Suture (sū'-tūr). The junction of cranial bones ; in surgery, a stitch. *See* **Ligature.**

Swabs. Small pieces of gauze or wool used for wiping away blood or discharge from a wound.

Sweat (swet). The secretion from the sudoriferous glands.

Sycosis (sī-kō'-sis). Inflammation of the hair follicles, especially of the beard.

Symbiosis (sim-bi-ō'-sis). The association between different creatures which live together for their mutual benefit. They are in no sense parasitic upon each other, *e.g.*, a small fish, the bitterling, lays its eggs between the valves of a bivalve, such as the mussel. The fish hatch later, and are expelled into the sea, where they subsequently attach to the skin of the female fish.

Symblepharon (sim-blef'-a-ron).

Adhesion of the lid to the eyeball.

Syme's Amputation. Amputation of the foot through the ankle joint.

Sympathectomy (sim-path-ek'-to-mi). Excision of part of a sympathetic nerve.

Symphysiotomy (sim-fīz-i-ot'-o-mi). Cutting through the symphysis pubis.

Symphysis Pubis (sim'-fis-is pū'-bis). The junction of the pubic bones.

Symptom (simp'-tom). A subjective phenomenon or manifestation of disease ; sometimes also applied to the objective manifestations or signs.

Symptomatology (simp-tom-a-tol'-o-ji). The science which deals with the symptoms of disease.

Synæsthesalgia (sin-āz-thēz-al'-ji-à). Pain excited by stimulation of the opposite side of the body.

Synæsthesia (sin-āz-thēz'-i-à). Secondary sensations.

Synapse Synapsis (sin'-aps, sin-ap'-sis). The junction or structure at the junction between one neurone and another. There is no actual communication, but the synapse functions possibly by either modifying or intensifying the nerve impulse as it passes through.

Synarthrosis (sin-à(r)-thrō-sis). An immovable articulation of bones, *e.g.*, the suture joints.

Syncope (sing'-ko-pi). A faint; a suspension of animation due to ischæmia of the brain.

Syncytium (sin-sit'-i-um). A tissue or sheet of protoplasm containing nuclei but not divided into separate cells.

Syndactyly (sin-dak'-til-i). Webbed fingers.

Syndrome (sin-drŏm). A series of symptoms which in association with each other are typical of special diseases.

Synergism (sin'-er-jizm). Increased activity of a combination of drugs of different pharmacological action, or of different endocrine hormones, beyond addition of their individual actions.

Synonymous (sin-on'-i-mus). Having the same meaning.

Synostosis (sin-os-tŏ'-sis). Abnormal bony union of bones, *e.g.*, in a joint.

Synovial Fluid (sī-nŏv'-i-al). The clear fluid secreted by the synovial membrane of a joint. It serves to lubricate the ligaments, etc., and so prevents friction. **S. Membrane,** the membrane lining the capsule of a joint, but leaving the articular cartilage free.

Synovitis (sī-nō-vī'-tis). Inflammation of the synovial membrane.

Synthesis (sin'-the-sis). The chemical building up of complex substances from simpler constituents.

Synthetic (sin-thet'-ik). Formed by a process of synthesis.

Syphilis (sif'-il-is). A venereal disease caused by the *Spirochæta pallida* (*Treponema pallidum*), discovered by Schaudinn and Hoffman in 1905. The disease is either congenital or acquired. **Congenital S.** accounts for many cases of premature and still-births; symptoms usually appear shortly after birth. The infant has a wizened appearance, suffers from snuffles and rashes. Later, depression of the bridge of the nose occurs through gummatous erosion of the nasal bones, wasting, and bone changes in the head and tibia are common, and dentition shows the appearance of notched teeth (*Hutchinson's teeth*). **Acquired S.:** three stages are recognized—(1) The development of the primary sore, which appears after an interval of 3-4 weeks at the site of inoculation, usually the genitals, although accidental infection may occur on other sites. (2) The second stage commences six to eight weeks later, and is ushered in by pyrexia, malaise, headache, and sore throat, and the appearance of a rash and condylomata and other symptoms. (3) The third or tertiary stage may not appear for some time, varying from a few weeks to as much as 20 years. It is characterized by the development of gummata. See **Locomotor Ataxy** and **G.P.I.**

Syphilophobia (sif-il-ō-fō-bi-à). A morbid fear of syphilis.

Syringe (sir-inzh). An instrument used for injecting substances into the body. **Hypodermic S.**, a small syringe used for subcutaneous injections. **Serum S.**, a larger syringe used for injecting sera, etc., into the veins or the deep muscular structures of the body. Special syringes are used for special procedures, such as spinal anæsthesia, blood transfusion, etc.

Syringomyelia (sir-ing-gō-mī-ēl'-i-à). A disease characterized by the development of cavities within the spinal cord. It occurs in early adult life, and runs a very chronic course, during which pain, paralysis, and disturbed sensibility are prominent features. Treatment is unavailing, and death supervenes sooner or later.

Syringomyelocele (sir-ing-gō-mī'-el-ō-sēl). The presence of cysts in the spinal cord; one of the forms of spina bifida.

Syringotomy (sir-ing-got'-o-mi). Making an incision into a fistula.

Syrup, Syrupus (sir'-up, sir-ū'-pus). A concentrated solution of sugar in water.

System (sis'-tem). (1) A group of organs or structures which are interdependent upon each other for their actions. (2) Method or order.

Systemic (sis-tem'-ik). Pertaining to a system.

Systole (sis'-to-li). The term used for the period during which the heart is in a state of contraction.

Systolic (sis-tol'-ik). Pertaining to the systole.

T.

T-bandage. A bandage used for keeping perineal dressings in position. The transverse strip is pinned or tied round the waist, while the vertical strip is passed between the legs and fastened to the transverse strip in front of the abdomen.

T-fracture. One in which a bone splits both transversely and longitudinally.

T.A.B. Abbreviation for a mixed vaccine containing the organisms of typhoid and paratyphoid A and B.

Tabes (tā'-bēz). Progressive wasting. **T. Dorsalis**, see **Locomotor Ataxy**. **T. Mesenterica**, tuberculous infection of the glands of the mesentery in children.

Tabetic (ta-bĕt'-ik or ta-bet'-ik). Affected with tabes.

Table (tā'-bl). A plate of bone, *e.g.*, the inner and outer tables of the cranial bones.

Tablet (tab'-let). A substance reduced to a fine powder and compressed, after being rendered coherent by liquid, into a small disc or lozenge ; a troche or trochicus.

Tachycardia (tak-i-kà(r)'-di-à). A persistently abnormal rapidity of cardiac action. **Extrinsic T.**, that caused by factors which lie outside the heart itself, *e.g.*, instability of the nervous system or increased metabolism. **Intrinsic T.**, caused by infective states, such as the common infectious fevers, rheumatism, or pneumonia, etc. **Paroxysmal T.**, a very rapid action of the heart, persisting for a short period, and commencing and terminating suddenly.

Tachypnœa (tak-ip-nē'-à). Abnormal frequency of respiration.

Tactile (tak'-tīl). Pertaining to the sense of touch.

Tænia (tēn'-i-à). (1) A flat band. (2) A genus of flat parasitic worms the Cestodes or tapeworms. **T. Coli,** three flat bands running the length of the large intestine and consisting of the longi-tudinal muscle fibres of the colon. **T. Solium,** the common tapeworm.

T.A.F. Abbreviation for *toxoid antitoxin floccules.*

Talc, Talcum (talk, tal'-kum). A soft, greasy dusting powder composed of magnesium silicate.

Talipes (tal'-i-pēz). Club-foot. **T. Calcaneus,** the foot rests entirely on the heel, D. **T. Cavus,** increased curvature of the arch of the foot ; the same as *Pes Cavus.* **T. Equinus,** the foot rests on the toes with the heel raised, A. **T. Planus,** flat-foot, E. **T. Valgus,** deformity with the foot turned outward, B. **T. Varus,** the foot turns inward, C. These two latter forms may be associated either with *T. Calcaneus* or *T. Equinus.*

Talus (tāl'-us). The astragalus ; the second largest bone of the ankle.

Tampon (tam'-pon). A plug made of wool and surrounded by gauze. A piece of tape is tied round the middle, and the ends left hanging for 4-6 in. to facilitate removal. They are inserted into the vagina to absorb discharge or as a means of bringing medicaments into contact with the vaginal walls. In this case they may be dipped into ichthyol and glycerine, picric acid, etc. They are renewed daily.

337

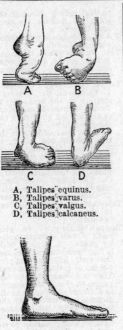

A, Talipes equinus.
B, Talipes varus.
C, Talipes valgus.
D, Talipes calcaneus.

E, Flat Foot.

Tamponade (tam'-pon-ād). Treatment by the use of tampons; compression of the heart by the escaped blood in a hæmopericardium.

Tannin (tan'-in). Tannic acid; derived from oak-galls; is astringent and styptic, and is given as an antidote to strychnine poisoning.

Tansy (tan'-zi). The plant *tanacetum vulgare*, the leaves and tops of which are used as an emmenagogue.

Tap. To withdraw fluid. *See* **Paracentesis.**

Tapeworms. Flat worms; parasites belonging to the class *Cestoda*. The front end is thin and small, possessing suckers. The worm is segmented and of great length. The segments or proglottides break off when ripe, and the worm increases in length by a budding process from the front. Each segment or proglottis is hermaphrodite. The larval and cystic stages of the life-cycle are developed in secondary hosts.

Tapotement (ta-pōt'-mon(g)). A beating or tapping movement used in massage.

Tardieu's Spots (tȧ(r)'-dū). Small ecchymoses on the pericardium and the pleural surfaces of the lungs, especially in the interlobar fissures, indicative of asphyxia.

Tarsal (tȧ(r)'-sal). Pertaining to the tarsus.

Tarsalgia (tà(r)-sal'-ji-à). Pain in the tarsus, particularly in the heel.

Tarsectomy (tà(r)-sek'-to-mi). Removal of the bones of the tarsus.

Tarsus (tà(r)'-sus). The seven small bones of the foot: Os

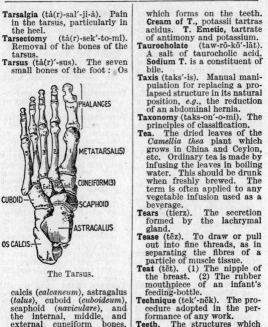

The Tarsus.

calcis (*calcaneum*), astragalus (*talus*), cuboid (*cuboideum*), scaphoid (*naviculare*), and the internal, middle, and external cuneiform bones. *See diagram.*

Tartar (tà(r)'-ter). The deposit which forms on the teeth. **Cream of T.,** potassii tartras acidus. **T. Emetic,** tartrate of antimony and potassium.

Taurocholate (taw-rō-kō'-lāt). A salt of taurocholic acid. **Sodium T.** is a constituent of bile.

Taxis (taks'-is). Manual manipulation for replacing a prolapsed structure in its natural position, *e.g.*, the reduction of an abdominal hernia.

Taxonomy (taks-on'-o-mi). The principles of classification.

Tea. The dried leaves of the *Camellia thea* plant which grows in China and Ceylon, etc. Ordinary tea is made by infusing the leaves in boiling water. This should be drunk when freshly brewed. The term is often applied to any vegetable infusion used as a beverage.

Tears (tierz). The secretion formed by the lachrymal gland.

Tease (tēz). To draw or pull out into fine threads, as in separating the fibres of a particle of muscle tissue.

Teat (tēt). (1) The nipple of the breast. (2) The rubber mouthpiece of an infant's feeding-bottle.

Technique (tek'-nēk). The procedure adopted in the performance of any work.

Teeth. The structures which are used for mastication. There are two sets in the human being : (1) **Temporary or Milk T.**, these first begin to erupt about the sixth month, and are shed about the age of seven years ; usually the two lower incisors appear first ; the total number of teeth is ten in each jaw ; rarely, one or more teeth are present at birth. (2) **Permanent T.**, these are already formed in the gum, and by growing push the temporary teeth out ; altogether there are thirty-two, sixteen in each jaw, thus :—

4 incisors = biting teeth.
2 canines = fangs or " eye " teeth.
4 bicuspids = premolars.
6 molars = grinding or double teeth.

The teeth of man are the same as for anthropoid apes, and are represented by the following *dental formula* :—

$$\frac{2.1.2.3}{2.1.2.3}$$

Teething (tēth'-ing). Eruption of the teeth ; dentition.

Tegmen (teg'-men). A roof or cover.

Tegument (teg'-ū-ment). Same as *Integument*.

Telangiectasis (tēl-an-ji-ek'-ta-sis). A mass of small dilated arterioles and capillaries ; a superficial angioma.

Teleology (tēl-i-ol'-o-ji). The doctrine of final causes.

Telepathist (tel-ep'-a-thist). One who believes in or practises telepathy.

Telepathy (tel - ep' - a - thi). Thought transference between two persons, said to occur even when the individuals are many miles apart, the *modus operandi* being unknown.

Temperament (tem'-per-ra-ment). Individual nature or characteristic.

Temperature (tem'-per-ra-tūr). The state a body is with regard to its hotness or coldness. It is recorded by a clinical thermometer. The exact **Normal T.** = 98·4° F., but in a healthy subject any temperature between 97° and 99° is considered normal. **Subnormal T.** = 97° F. and below. **Ward T.** should range between 60°-65° F. ; slightly higher than this is allowable for old people and infants because of their lowered vitality.

Temple (tem'-pl). That part of the head lying between the outer angle of the eye and the top of the ear-flap.

Temporal Bone (tem'-por-al). The bone at the side of the head in which the middle ear is situated.

Tenacious (ten-ā'-shus). Adhesive ; tough ; sticky.

Tenderness (ten'-der-nes). (1) Gentleness. (2) Pain on

pressure; sensitiveness to touch.

Tendinous (ten'-din-us). Pertaining to a tendon.

Tendon (ten'-don). A firm, white, fibrous inelastic cord which attaches muscle to bone. **T. of Achilles**, the large tendon at the lower end of the gastrocnemius muscle; it inserts into the os calcis bone of the foot.

Tenesmus (ten-ez'-mus). Pain and straining on defæcation.

Tenosynovitis (tēn-ō-sīn-ō-vī'-tis). Inflammation of a tendon and its sheath.

Tenotomy (ten-ot'-o-mi). Division of a tendon.

Tension (ten'-shun). A condition of being stretched. **Mental T.**, anxiety and apprehension; a state of being on the *qui vive*.

Tensor (ten'-saw(r)). A muscle which causes tension of adjacent structures.

Tentorium (ten-taw'-ri-um). That part of the dura mater which lies between the cerebrum and the cerebellum.

Tents. Small cylindrical rods made of compressed absorbent material which swell to double their thickness in the presence of moisture; used to dilate the mouth of a hollow organ, such as the cervix uteri. The natural secretion of cervix provides the moisture, so that when one or two tents are inserted

into the canal they swell steadily and strongly. A piece of thread is passed through a hole at the lower end of the tent, and this facilitates removal. Tents are sterilized by keeping them immersed in an alcoholic solution of biniodide. **Sea-tangle T.**, same as *Laminaria Tents*. **Laminaria T.**, made from a form of compressed seaweed. *See p.* 204.

Tepid (tep'-id). Lukewarm. **T. Bath**, a bath prepared at 85°-95° F.

Ter in Die. Three times in a day.

Teratoid (te'-ra-toid). (1) Resembling a monster. (2) Resembling teratoma.

Teratoma (te-ra-tō'-mȧ). A complex embryonic tumour containing a variety of different tissues, such as hair, teeth, brain, etc. Such tumours may be found in any part of the body but are commonest in the ovary and testis. As a rule they are easily removed and seldom recur.

Terebene (tĕ'-re-bēn). A colourless antiseptic fluid obtained from oil of turpentine by distillation; it stimulates expectoration, and if inhaled, assists respiration in bronchial diseases.

Terebinthina (te-re-binth'-i-nȧ). Turpentine.

Teres (tĕ'-rēz). Round and smooth.

Term. A definite period. Usually refers to the period of gestation.

Terminal (ter'-min-al). Ending.

Terminal Ileitis. *See* **Regional Ileitis.**

Terpene (ter-pēn). Any hydrocarbon of the formula $C_{10}H_{16}$, many of which occur in the volatile oils of plants, especially the conifers.

Tertian (ter'-shun). Occurring every third day.

Tertiary (ter'-shi-a-ri). Of the third order. **T. Syphilis,** the third and most advanced stage of syphilis. **T. Order of St Francis,** a religious order founded by St Francis of Assisi; the members, who were known as "*Tertiaries*," were chiefly concerned with nursing, and although taking vows they were not under strict discipline and were not enclosed.

Test. To try out; to examine. **Mental T.,** a series of tests for measuring intelligence; were first devised for mental defectives, but are also of value for the normal and supernormal type of individual. The **Binet-Simon T.** are most commonly used, or some modification of them. There are also special tests for tracing repressed mental complexes, and for measuring such things as memory, observation, etc. **T. Meal,** special meals given to determine the quality and quantity of the gastric juice. **T. Tube,** a thin glass tube for testing small quantities of fluid. **T. Types,** letters of graduated sizes for testing the sight, *e.g.*, *Snellen's types.*

Testicle (tes'-tik-'l). *See* **Testis.**

Testis (tes'-tis). One of the two glandular bodies contained in

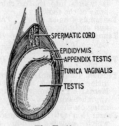

SPERMATIC CORD

EPIDIDYMIS

APPENDIX TESTIS

TUNICA VAGINALIS

TESTIS

The Testis.

the scrotum of the male; they secrete semen.

Tetanospasmin (tet-an-ō-spaz'-min). The constituent of tetanus toxin which is responsible for the convulsions in tetanus.

Tetanus (tet'-a-nus). A virulent disease caused by the tetanus bacillus, discovered by *Nicolaier*; characterized by violent muscular convulsions.

Tetany (tet'-an-i). A condition

associated with spasms of the hands and feet, and general muscular irritability. It is associated with a low calcium content of the blood.

Tetra (tet'-rá). A prefix signifying four.

Thalamus (thal'-a-mus). The large posterior ganglion of the brain lying mesial to the internal capsule.

Thebain (thē'-bān). An alkaloid of opium.

Thebesius's Valve. The valve guarding the opening of the Thebesian vein as it empties into the right auricle.

Theca (thē'-ká). An enveloping sheath, e.g., the meninges of the spinal cord.

Thecal (thē'-kal). Pertaining to the theca.

Theine (thē'-in). An alkaloid of the tea plant, *Camellia*.

Thenar (thē'-ná(r)). The palm of the hand and the sole of the foot. **T. Eminence,** the palmar eminence below the thumb.

Theobroma (thē-ō-brō'-má). Cacao butter; used as a foundation for suppositories.

Therapeutic (the-ra-pū'-tik). Relating to therapeutics.

Therapeutics (the-ra-pū'-tiks). The science which deals with the treatment of disease and the application of remedies.

Therapy (the'-ra-pi). Treatment. *See* **Therapeutics.**

Therm. A small calorie (*q.v.*).

Thermocautery (ther-mō-kaw'-te-ri). A method of cauterizing by means of heat, e.g., Pacquelin's cautery.

Thermogene (ther'-mō-jēn). Medicated wool for use next to the skin in bronchitis, rheumatism, etc.

Thermogenic (ther-mō-jen'-ik). Producing heat.

Thermolabile (ther-mō-lā'-bĭl). Capable of being altered by heat.

Thermometer (ther-mom'-et-er). An instrument for recording the degree of temperature. *See diagram. See also* **Réaumur T.,** and **Kata-T.**

Thermostat (ther'-mō-stat). An automatic device for regulating the temperature.

Thesis (thē'-sis). The essay of a candidate for a degree; it usually embodies the result of original research.

Thiersch's Razor (tiersh). A razor specially designed for skin-grafting (*q.v.*).

Thigh (thī). That part of the lower limb between the hip and the knee.

Thoracentesis (thaw-rō-sen-tē'-sis). Puncture of the chest wall to withdraw fluid.

Thoracic (thaw-ras'-ik). Pertaining to the thorax. **T. Duct,** the main channel for conveying lymph; it commences as a pear-shaped enlargement, the *receptaculum chyli*, at the level of the

THERMOMETERS

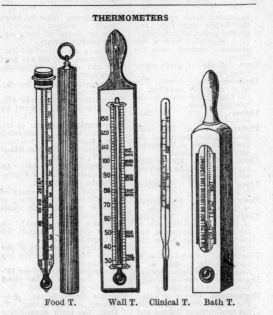

Food T.   Wall T.   Clinical T.   Bath T.

second lumbar vertebra, and passes up the abdomen, through the diaphragm, to the chest, where it empties into the innominate vein at the junction of the left jugular and subclavian veins. **Thoracoplasty** (thaw-ra-kō-plas'-ti). Any plastic operation on the chest.

Thorax (thaw'-raks). The chest cavity.

Thread-worm. The *Oxyuris vermicularis*.

Thrill. Vibration as perceived by the sense of touch.

Thrombin (throm'-bin). A substance derived from the interaction of prothrombin with thrombokinase and calcium salts in the blood. It is concerned with the conversion of fibrinogen into fibrin during the coagulation of blood.

Thrombocyte (throm'-bō-sīt). The same as blood platelet.

Thrombocytopenia (throm-bō-sīt-ō-pĕn'-i-ä). A reduction in the platelet count in the blood.

Thrombocytosis (throm-bō-sīt-ō'-sis). An increase in the number of platelets in the blood.

Thrombogen (throm'-bō-jen). Same as *Prothrombin. See* **Coagulation.**

Thrombokinase (throm-bō-kī'-nāz). A substance formed on the disintegration of the blood platelets and tissue cells. It activates prothrombin in the presence of calcium ions with the formation of thrombin.

Thrombophlebitis (throm-bō-fle-bī'-tis). Inflammation of a vein associated with the formation of a thrombus.

Thrombosis (throm-bō'-sis). The intravascular formation of a blood clot.

Thrombus (throm'-bus). A blood clot formed intravascularly during life.

Thrush. A disease associated with the presence of small white ulcers on the mucous membrane of the mouth. The cause is a *fungus*, the *Oidium albicans*.

Thymol (thī'-mol). Obtained from oil of thyme ; it is antiseptic, antiparasitic, and anthelmintic.

Thymoma (thī-mō'-mä). A tumour of the thymus.

Thymus (thī'-mus). A gland lying behind the manubrium of the sternum ; is large and well developed in infancy, but gradually decreases in size as puberty approaches, and has become rudimentary by the time adult age is reached.

Thyroglossal (thī-rō-glos'-al). Pertaining to the thyroid gland and the tongue. **T. Cyst,** a congenital cystic dilatation in the course of the thyroglossal duct. **T. Duct,** the fœtal passage from the thyroid gland to the back of the tongue where its vestigial end remains as the foramen cæcum.

Thyroid Cartilage (thī'-roid). The large anterior cartilage of the larynx. **T. Gland,** one of the endocrine glands situated in front and below the thyroid cartilage; it secretes a hormone called thyroxin. **T. Extract,** extract of sheep's thyroid gland; given for myxœdema, some types of goitre, obesity, etc. Dosage, ½-5 gr.

Thyroidectomy (thī-roid-ek'-to-mi). Excision of part of the thyroid gland.

Thyroidism (thī-roid'-izm). A group of symptoms caused by an excessive outpouring of thyroid secretion into the blood, *e.g.*, tachycardia, sweating, wasting, tremor, exophthalmos, etc.

Thyroiditis (thī-roid-ī'-tis). Inflammation of the thyroid gland. **Riedel's T.**, a chronic fibrosis of the thyroid gland of woody hardness; ligneous goitre.

Thyroidotomy (thī-roid-ot'-o-mi). Incision of the thyroid cartilage or gland.

Thyroxin (thī-roks'-in). The internal secretion or hormone of the thyroid gland.

Tibia (tib'-i-à). The shin-bone.

Tibial (tib'-i-al). Pertaining to the tibia.

Tic. Purposeless and involuntary muscular movements and twitchings due partly to habit, but often associated with a psychological factor.

Tic Douloureux (tik doo-loo-rur'). Trigeminal neuralgia of unknown origin. Par-

oxysms of intense pain affecting the fifth cranial nerve. The attacks occur at shorter intervals and with greater severity as the years advance.

Tidal Air. The air which is inhaled and exhaled during ordinary quiet breathing.

Tincture (tingk-tūer or tingk-cher). A solution of a medicinal substance in alcohol.

Tinea (tin'-i-à). A cutaneous eruption of fungoid origin. **T. Furfuracea,** dry seborrhœa. **T. Sycosis,** barber's rash. **T. Tonsurans,** ringworm of the head.

Tinnitus (tin'-i-tus). A buzzing, thumping, or ringing sound in the head.

Tissue (tish'-oo or tis'-ū). The conglomeration of cells which unite to form a definite structure.

Titration (tī-trā'-shun). Volumetric analysis by aid of standard solutions.

Titre (tē'-ter or tī'-ter). A standard of fineness or strength.

T.N.T. Abbreviation for trinitrotoluene, a highly explosive substance.

Toluene, Toluol (tol'-u-ēn, tol'-ū - ol). A hydrocarbon, $C_6H_5CH_3$, from coal-tar.

Tone, Tonus (tōn, tōn'-us). Normal activity or vigour; the natural healthy state of tension.

Tongue (tung). The flexible organ contained in the

mouth; it is concerned with speech and taste. *See* **Strawberry Tongue.**

Tonic (ton'-ik). An agent which increases the tonicity of a muscular structure.

Tonsillectomy (ton-sil-ek'-to-mi). Excision of the tonsils.

Tonsillitis (ton-sil-ī'-tis). Inflammation of the tonsils. **Follicular T.**, having the appearance of numerous small septic foci filling the crypts of the tonsil. **Peri-T.**, quinsy.

Tonsilloliths (ton-sil'-ō-liths). Calculi in the tonsil.

Tonsillotome (ton-sil'-ō-tōm). An instrument for abscission of tonsils.

Tonsils (ton'-sils). (1) The small glandular bodies embedded in the fauces between the palatine arches. (2) Two small lobes of the cerebellum.

Tophus (tō'-fus). A small, hard concretion forming on the helix of the ear, and on the joints of the phalanges, toes, etc., in gout. Pl.: *tophi.*

Topography (tō-pog'-raf-i). A description of the regions of the body.

Torpid (taw(r)'-pid). Relating to torpor; inactive.

Torpor (taw(r)'-paw(r)). A state of abnormal inactivity.

Torsion (taw(r)'-shun). Twisting.

Torticollis (taw(r)-ti-kol'-is). Wry-neck (*q.v.*).

Tourniquet (turn'-i-kā or -ket).

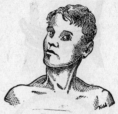

Torticollis.

An apparatus which arrests bleeding by causing compression of the injured vessel. In arterial bleeding it should be placed *above* the bleeding point, and in venous bleeding *below* the bleeding point.

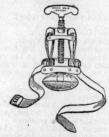

Petit's Tourniquet.

347

Tourniquet.

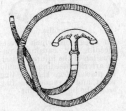

Samway's Tourniquet.

Tow (tō). Coarse flax.

Toxæmia (toks-ēm′-i-å). A poisoned state of the blood, usually the result of absorption into the blood of toxins from bacteria or necrotic tissues.

Toxic (toks′-ik). Poisonous.

Toxicology (toks-i-kol′-o-ji). The science which treats of the symptoms, action, and therapeutics of poisons.

Toxicosis (toks-i-kō′-sis). Any disease state due to poisoning.

Toxin (toks′-in). A poison of bacterial origin.

Toxoid (toks′-oid). A toxin which has been rendered non-poisonous, *e.g.*, by treatment with formalin. It still retains its power to stimulate the production of anti-toxin.

Trabeculæ (tra-bek′-ū-lē). The fibrous bands projecting into the interior of an organ, *e.g.*, the spleen ; they are extensions from the capsule surrounding the organ.

Trachea (trak-ē′-å). The wind-pipe.

Tracheal (trak-ē′-al). Pertaining to the trachea.

Tracheitis (trak-ē-ī′-tis). Inflammation of the trachea.

Tracheloplasty (trak-el-ō-plas′-ti). Operative repair of a lacerated cervix uteri.

Trachelorrhaphy (trak-el-o′-raf-i). Repair of a lacerated cervix by stitching.

Tracheotomy (trak-ē-ot′-o-mi). Making an opening into the trachea for the introduction of a tube which will assist in breathing ; performed chiefly in diphtheria. The tube must be kept free from mucus or diphtheritic membrane, or asphyxiation may result. **High T.,** one performed above the isthmus of the thyroid gland. **Low T.,** performed below the thyroid isthmus.

Trachoma (trak-ō′-må). A contagious type of conjunctivitis

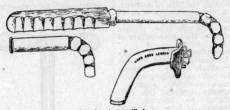

Tracheotomy Tube.

in which the inner surface of the eyelid becomes red and granulated.

Traction (trak'-shun). A drawing or pulling. **Axis T.,** traction in the direction of the axis of the channel through which a body is being drawn.

Tragacanth (trag'-a-kanth). A gum largely used as a demulcent.

Trait (trā). Any peculiarity or individual characteristic.

Trance. A prolonged state of insensibility due to psychic causes ; catalepsy.

Transformation (trans-faw(r)-mā'-shun). A complete change in appearance or attitude, etc.

Transfusion (trans-fū'-zhun). The transfer of fluid into a vein. **Saline T.,** the introduction of normal salt solution ; given by means of a cannula and tubing at temp.

100° F. **Blood T.,** the passing of blood into a vein. *See* **Blood T.**

Transillumination (trans-i-loo-min-ā'-shun). A method of detecting the presence of pus in the frontal sinus or antrum of Highmore. When a small bright electric bulb is placed in the mouth in a darkened room, the sinuses are shown up as illuminated spaces in the face. When pus is present, the transmission of light is diminished or even absent.

Translucent (trans-loo'-sent). Intermediate between opaque and transparent ; partly transparent.

Transmigration (trans-mī-grā'-shun). The transit of a cell through a membrane.

Transmission (trans-mish'-'n). The transfer of disease.

Transpiration (trans-pi-rā'-shun). The passage of fluid

349

through the cells of a tissue, *e.g.*, the elimination of sweat through the skin, or water lost through the minute pores on the under-surface of a leaf.

Transudation(trans-ū-dā'-shun). The oozing of fluid through membrane, *e.g.*, plasma through the capillary walls.

Trauma (traw'-mă). Injury.

Traumatic (traw-mat'-ik). Pertaining to trauma. **T. Neurosis**, a form of mental disturbance which occurs as the result of an accident or injury.

Traumatotherapy (traw-mat-ō-the'-ra-pi). The special branch of medical science which deals with the treatment of accidents and injuries.

Trematode (tre'-ma-tōd). One of the parasitic, unsegmented worms.

Tremor (trem-aw(r)). Involuntary trembling. **Coarse T.,** violent trembling. **Fine T.,** slight trembling; often seen in the hands in exophthalmic goitre. **Intentional T.,** tremor which only occurs on voluntary movement, *e.g.*, in disseminated sclerosis.

Trendelenburg's Position. The patient lies on the back, inclined at an angle of about 45° with the pelvis higher than the head.

Trephine (tre-fīn'). A surgical

instrument for removing a circular piece of bone from the skull.

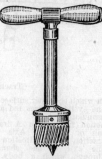

Trephine.

Treponema Pallidum (trep-o-nē'-mă pal'-id-um). The causative organism of syphilis; also known as the *Spirochæta pallida.*

Trichinosis (trik-in-ō'-sis). A disease caused by eating pork which is infested with the *Trichina spiralis*. Also known as *Trichiniasis.*

Trichiuris (trīk-i-ūr'-is). The thread-worm. Also known as *Trichocephalus.*

Trichology (trīk-ol'-o-ji). The science dealing with hair.

Trichomonas Vaginalis (trī-kō-mōn'-as vaj-in-āl'-is). A

flagellated unicellular parasite which causes vaginal inflammation.

Trichophytosis (trĭ-kō-fī-tō′-sĭs). Infection of the hair with the *Trichophyton*, the parasitic fungus causing ringworm.

Trichosis (trĭ-kō-sĭs). Any disease of the hair.

Tricuspid (trī-kus′-pĭd). Having three cusps. **T. Disease,** inflammation of the tricuspid valve. **T. Valve,** the valve situated between the right auricle and ventricle.

Trigeminal (trī-jem′-in-al). Triple. Also relates to the **T. Nerve,** *i.e.,* the fifth cranial nerve, which has three branches, supplying the skin of the face, the tongue and teeth. **T. Neuralgia,** *see* Tic Douloureux.

Trigone (trī′-gōn). A triangular-shaped area.

Trinitrin (trī-nī′-trĕn). Nitroglycerine.

Trinitrotoluene (trī-nī-trō-tol′-ū-ēn). One of the high explosives largely used in modern warfare; it is a yellow powder and those who handle it are liable to some harmful effects, *e.g.,* anilism (cyanosis), dyspepsia, and dermatitis. Occasionally it produces acute liver necrosis and aplastic anæmia.

Trional (trī′-ō-nal). Methyl sulphonal; a hypnotic which acts quickly. Dosage, 5-20 gr.

Triplets (trip′-lets). Three children delivered at one birth.

Trismus (triz′-mus). Spasmodic contractions of the muscles of mastication; a prominent symptom of tetanus.

Triturate (trit′-ū-rāt). To pulverize by a process of rubbing.

Trocar (trō′-kă(r)). The sharp instrument which fits inside a cannula for piercing the tissues.

Trochanter (trō-kan′-ter). Two processes, one larger than the other, between the shaft and neck of the femur; they serve for the attachment of muscles.

Troche (trō′-kē) or **Trochiseus** (trō-kis′-kus). A medicinal lozenge.

Trophic (trō-fĭk). Pertaining to nutrition.

Trophoneurosis (trō-fō-nū-rō′-sĭs). Impairment of nutrition due to defective nervous action.

Tropistic Action (trō-pis′-tik) or **Tropism** (trō′-pizm). The directional response of an organism to certain external influences, *e.g.,* **Chemio-T.,** the influence exerted by chemicals on the organism. **Geo-T.,** the tendency of an organism to turn towards the earth. **Helio-T.,** a tendency to turn towards the sun. **Photo-T.,** a turning towards light.

Truncated (trung'-kā-ted). Deprived of limbs ; amputated.

Truss. An appliance designed for keeping a hernia in place.

Trypanosome (trip'-an-ō-sōm). A genus of infusoria, some of which are parasites of the blood and cause such diseases as sleeping sickness.

Trypanosomiasis (trip-an-ō-sō-mī'-a-sis). Infection with trypanosomes.

Trypsin (trip'-sin). An enzyme of the pancreatic juice ; it exerts a proteolytic action, converting peptones into amino-acids.

Trypsinogen (trip - sin' - o - jen). An inert precursor of trypsin ; it is activated by contact with enterokinase, an enzyme of the succus entericus.

Tryptophane (trip'-tō-fān). One of the essential amino-acids.

Tsetse Fly (tse'-tsi or set'-si). A species of fly which carries the infective protozoon of trypanosomiasis.

Tubal (tū'-bal). Pertaining to a tube.

Tube (tūb). A long, hollow cylindrical structure. **Drainage T.,** a glass or rubber tube which, when inserted into a cavity, drains away its fluid contents. **Eustachian T.,** the tube passing from the throat to the middle ear. **Fallopian T.,** see **Fallopian.** **Intubation T.,** a tube for passing into the larynx to facilitate breathing. **Œsophageal T.,** same as *Stomach T.* **Stomach T.,** a rubber tube, 16 in. in length, for introducing food or other fluid into the stomach. **Tracheotomy T.,** a tube for inserting into the trachea. *See* **Tracheotomy.**

Tuber (tū-ber). A nodule, prominence, or tuberosity.

Tubercle (tū'-ber-kl). A small prominence or a tuberculous nodule, such as occurs in miliary tuberculosis.

Tubercular (tū-ber'-kū-lá(r)). Nodular; pertaining to or containing tubercles or nodules.

Tuberculin (tū-ber'-kū-lin). An extract from cultures of the tubercle bacillus.

Tuberculoma (tū-ber-kū-lō'-mà). A granulomatous tumour caused by tuberculosis ; most typically and commonly found in the brain.

Tuberculosis (tū-ber-kū-lō'-sis). A disease caused by infection with *Koch's tubercle bacillus.* There are four main types : (1) **Bovine T.,** occurring in cattle and communicable to man, causing disease of the lungs, joints, and glands ; (2) **Avian T.,** non-communicable to man, the type seen in birds ; (3) **Piscine T.,** not transferable to man ; the form affecting fish ; (4) **Human T.,** the form most common to man resulting from infection with the

Bacillus tuberculosis hominis. See **Phthisis.**

Tuberculous (tū-ber'-kŭ-lus). Pertaining to tuberculosis.

Tuberosity (tū-ber-ros'-it-i). A large bony prominence.

Tubular (tūb-ū-là(r)). Having the form or properties of a tube. **T. Breathing,** bronchial respiration. **T. Gestation,** pregnancy implanted in the Fallopian tube: the commonest form of extra-uterine or ectopic pregnancy.

Tularaemia (tūl-a-rēm'-i-à). A fever associated with swelling of lymph glands due to infection with *Pasteurella tularensis;* usually contracted by handling infected animals, *e.g.,* rabbits and hares, or from bites by mites or other parasites from such animals.

Tumefaction (tū-mi-fak'-shun). Formation of a swelling.

Tumescence (tū-mes'-ens). A state of swelling; turgidity.

Tumour (tūm'-er). A swelling or enlargement; a pathological localized overgrowth of tissue, not being the result of inflammation and fulfilling no function. **Benign T.,** not malignant, nor having a tendency to recur. **Cystic T.,** one which is made up of cysts. **Fibroid T.,** one containing fibrous tissue. **Innocent T.,** *see* **Benign Tumour. Malignant T.,** one which will recur and which will destroy life; a cancer. **Phantom T.,** a swelling of the abdomen due to hysteria. **Sebaceous T.,** one caused by a sebaceous gland.

Tunica (tūn'-ik-à). A lining membrane; a coat. **T. Adventitia,** the outer coat of an artery. **T. Media,** the middle muscular coat of an artery. **T. Intima,** the internal or lining coat of an artery.

Turbinated Bones (turb-in-ā-ted). The L-shaped bones forming the floor of the nose.

Turbinectomy (turb-in-ek'-to-mi). Removal of a turbinated bone.

Turgescence (tur-jes'-ens). Swelling caused by congestion of a part.

Turgid (tur'-jid). Swollen; firmly distended, as with blood by congestion.

Turpentine (tur'-pen-tīn). An oleoresin much used medicinally. *See* **Enema** and **Stupe. T. Liniment,** a liniment containing turpentine as one of its ingredients.

Tussis (tus'-is). A cough.

Twilight Sleep. *See* **Scopolamine.**

Twin. One of two children born at the same birth.

Twinge (twinzh). A momentarily sharp, stabbing pain.

Twitch, Twitching. A sudden, sharp pull or jerk; an irregular minor spasm.

Tympanic (tim-pan'-ik). Pertaining to the tympanum. **T. Membrane,** the eardrum.

M

Tympanites (tim-pan-ī'-tēz). Abdominal distension due to accumulation of gas in the intestine. Also *Tympanism*.

Tympanitis (tim-pan-ī'-tis). Inflammation of the membrana tympani or of the tympanum itself.

Tympanum (tim'-pan-um). The cavity of the middle ear. **Membrana Tympani,** the eardrum.

Typhlitis (tif-lī'-tis). Inflammation of the mucous lining of the cæcum ; cæcitis ; often used to include appendicitis.

Typhlotomy (tif-lot'-o-mi). A temporary opening into the cæcum.

Typhoid (tī'-foid). Resembling typhus. **T. Fever,** an acute infectious fever commonly running a three-weeks' course, and caused by the *B. typhosus*, which is found in practically all the tissues and especially the Peyer's patches of the intestine, which become inflamed and thinned out. A rose-coloured rash appears on the abdomen, chest, or back about the seventh day.

Typhus (tī'-fus). An acute epidemic disease caused by a filter-passing virus, one of the rickettsias, carried by the body-louse. It is accompanied by fever, great prostration, and the appearance of a mulberry-coloured rash. Also known as *Gaol Fever.*

Tyrosin (tī'-rō-sin). An amino-acid formed by the breaking down of protein matter during digestion.

Tyson's Glands (tī'-son's). Glands of the prepuce of the penis which secrete a sebaceous matter called smegma.

U.

Ulcer (ul'-ser). A superficial open sore with a discharging surface. **Duodenal U.,** one formed in the mucous lining of the duodenum. **Gastric U.,** formed in the gastric mucous lining. **Indolent U.,** chronic ulcer of slow development ; occurs generally in old people. **Perforating U.,** one that penetrates deeply through underlying tissues. **Rodent U.,** a malignant type of ulcer which forms on the head at the outer angle of the eye, etc., and involves in time all soft and hard tissues alike. **Tuberculous U.,** one caused by tuberculosis. **Varicose U.,** ulceration of the skin over a varicose vein.

Ulceration (ul-ser-rā-shun). The formation of an ulcer.

Ulna (ul'-nà). The bone of the internal side of the forearm.

Ulnar (ul-nà(r)). Pertaining to or on the side of the ulna.

Ultramicroscope. A microscope for the examination by reflected light of objects too small to be seen by ordinary microscopes.

Umbilical (um-bil-ĭ-kal). Pertaining to the umbilicus. **U. Cord**, the cord passing from the abdomen of the child to the placenta. **U. Hernia**, the development of a hernia in the region of the umbilicus.

Umbilicated (um-bil′-i-kā-ted). Having a depression like an umbilicus.

Umbilicus (um-bil-ī′-cus). The abdominal scar left by the separation of the umbilical cord after birth; popularly known as the *Navel*.

Unavoidable Hæmorrhage. That which results from placenta prævia.

Unciform, Uncinate (un′-si-fawm, un′-si-nāt). Hooked; hook-shaped.

Uncinaria (un-sin-ē′-ri-à). The hook-worms.

Uncinariasis (un-sin-a-rī′-a-sis). Infestation with the hook-worm.

Unconsciousness (un-kon′-shus-ness). A state of deep insensibility.

Unction (ungk′-shun). Ointment.

Undine (un′-dēn). A small, thin, glass flask with a long and a short spout. The flask is filled through the latter with warm boracic lotion; used for irrigating the eyes.

Undulant Fever (un′-dū-lant). A fever alternating with

quiescent periods, giving the recorded temperature a wave-like appearance on the chart.

Ungual (ung′-gwil). Pertaining to a nail. Also **Unguinal**.

Unguentum (ung-gwen′-tum). An ointment.

Unicellular (ŭ-ni-sel′-ŭ-là(r)). Consisting of only one cell.

Unilateral (ŭ-ni-lat′-e-ral). Pertaining to one side only.

Union (u′-ni-un). A uniting or joining. *See* Healing.

Unipara (ŭ-nip′-à′-rà). A woman who has borne only one child.

Uniparous (ŭ-nip′-a-rus). Producing one at a birth.

Unipolar (ŭ-ni-pō-là(r)). Having one process, *e.g.*, unipolar cells.

Unit (ū′-nit). A single quantity used as a standard by which other quantities are measured or expressed.

Unna's Paste (un′-à). A paste used in the treatment of varicose ulcers, etc.; it includes the following constituents : Gelatine, 15 parts ; zinc oxide, 15 parts ; glycerine, 35 parts ; distilled water, 35 parts.

Unorganized (un-aw(r)′-gan-īzd). Without organs but not necessarily lifeless ; without definite scheme or pattern.

Unstriated Muscle (un-strī′-ā-ted). Involuntary muscle fibres without cross striations.

Unwell. Ill ; a popular term

for the occurrence of the menses.

Urachus (ū′-rak-us). A fibrous cord from the bladder to the umbilicus.

Uræmia (ū-rēm′-i-à). The symptoms due to the accumulation in the blood of poisonous substances normally excreted by the kidneys.

Urate (ū-rāt). A salt of uric acid with a base.

Urea (ū-rē′-à). The end waste product of protein metabolism; it is excreted in the urine at the rate of 300-600 gr. in 24 hours. **U. Clearance Test,** a test for renal efficiency depending on an estimation of the number of c.c. of blood cleared of urea in a given time by the kidneys. **U. Concentration Test,** a simpler test for estimating the renal efficiency; it depends upon the fact that when healthy kidneys are presented with an extra amount of urea in the blood, they will excrete an equal amount of urea into the urine. *Method—*The patient is asked to urinate, and is then given a solution of 15 grm. of urea in 2 or 3 oz. of water to drink. After one hour the patient urinates again, and also after the second hour. The two specimens are then tested for the amount of urea,

which should rise above 2 %, provided the urea has not provoked an undue diuresis.

Uresis (ū-rē-sis). The passing of urine; urination; micturition.

Ureter (ū′-re-ter). The tube passing from the kidneys to the bladder for the conveyance of urine into the bladder.

Ureteral (ū-rē′-te-ral). Pertaining to the ureter.

Ureteritis (ū-re-te-rī′-tis). Inflammation of the ureters.

Ureterolith (ū-rē′-te-rō-lith). A calculus within a ureter.

Urethane (ū′-re-thăn). Ethyl carbamate, a white crystalline compound used as a hypnotic.

Urethra (ū-rē′-thrà). The passage from the bladder through which urine is voided; in the female it measures 1-1½ in., and in the male 10 in.

Urethral (ū-rē′-thral). Pertaining to the urethra.

Urethritis (ū-re-thrī′-tis). Inflammation of the urethra.

Urethroscope (ū-rē′-thrō-skop). An instrument used for examining the urethra.

Urethrotome (ū-rē′-thrō-tōm). An instrument for performing urethrotomy.

Urethrotomy (ū-re-throt′-o-mi). The operation of making an incision into the urethra for the relief of stricture.

Uric Acid. The end product of the action of various

enzymes on nucleic acid; that which appears in the urine is of both endogenous and exogenous origin. The uric acid of the blood becomes increased in persons suffering from gout.

Uridrosis (ū-ri-drō′-sis). The presence of urea in the sweat.

Urinal (ū-rin-al). A vessel into which urine can be passed.

Urinalysis (ū-ri-nal′-i-sis). The examination and analysis of urine.

Urinary (ū′-rin-a-ri). Pertaining to urine.

Urination (ū-rin-ā′-shun). *See* **Micturition.**

Urine (ū′-rin). The amber-coloured fluid which is excreted from the kidneys at the rate of about 50 oz. every 24 hours in the adult; it is slightly acid, and has a normal specific gravity of 1,015-1,025.

Uriniferous Tubules (ū-rin-if′-e-rus). The minute tubules which conduct the urine from the glomeruli to the pelves of the kidney, and in which the urine is concentrated. *See* Diagram.

Urinometer (ū-rin-om′-e-ter). An instrument for estimating the specific gravity of urine.

Urobilin (ū-rō-bīl′-in). A pigment contained in urine, derived from bilirubin.

Urobilinogen (ū-rō-bī-lin′-o-jen). A precursor of urobilin.

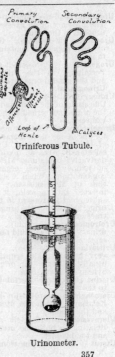

Uriniferous Tubule.

Urinometer.

357

Urobilinuria (ū-rō-bĭl-in-ū-ri-à). The presence of an excess of urobilin in the urine.

Urochrome (ū'-rō-krōm). One of the pigments contained in urine.

Urogenital (ū-rō-jen'-it-al). Pertaining to the urinary and the genital organs ; also **Urinogenital**.

Urology (ū-rol'-o-ji). The scientific study of the urine and of the organs concerned with its excretion.

Uroselectan. A contrast agent for the X-ray demonstration of the urinary tract. Uroselectan-B. is a pyridin derivative containing 51·5% of iodine in close organic combination. When a solution of the substance is injected into a vein, it is subsequently excreted in the urine, and renders the urinary tract opaque to X-rays.

Urotropine (ū-rot'-ro-pin). A urinary and spinal fluid antiseptic. See **Hexamine**.

Urticaria (ur-ti-kĕ'-ri-à). A very irritable skin eruption usually allergic in origin. Synonym, *Nettle-rash.*

Uterine (ū'-te-rīn). Pertaining to the uterus.

Uterovaginal (ū-te-rō-va-jīn'-al). Relating to both the uterus and the vagina.

Uterovesical (ū-te-rō-ve-sīk'-al). Relating to both the uterus and the bladder.

Uterus (ū'-te-rus). The womb.

Bicornuate U., a double uterus ; one possessing two horns. **Gravid U.,** a pregnant uterus.

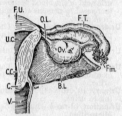

Right half of Uterus in section, with Appendages (posterior view).

F.U., Fundus of uterus.
O.L., Ovarian ligament.
F.T., Fallopian tube.
Fim., Fimbria.
B.L., Broad ligament.
V., Vagina.
C., Cervix.
C.C., Cervical canal.
U.C., Uterine cavity.

Utricle (ū'-trik-l). 1. A little sac or pocket. 2. One of the aural cavities.

Uvea (ū'-vi-à). The pigmented part of the iris.

Uveitis (ū-vi-ī'-tis). Inflammation of the uvea.

Uvula (ū'-vū-là). The tag-like

structure hanging down from the free edge of the soft palate.

Uvulitis (ū-vū-lī´-tis). Inflammation of the uvula.

Uvulotomy (ū-vū-lot´-o-mi). Excision of a piece of the uvula.

V.

Vaccination (vak-sin-ā´-shun). Inoculation with vaccinia or cowpox for the purpose of protecting the individual from a severe attack of smallpox. The lymph is usually introduced by scarification into the upper part of the left arm, or into the calf of the leg.

Vaccine (vak´-sēn). A preparation containing attenuated or dead bacteria which, after introduction into the patient, induces the body to produce its own antibodies, and thus raises the resistance of the body to disease. **Autogenous V.**, one made from bacteria from the patient's own body.

Vaccinia (vak-sin´-i-à). Cowpox ; is a disease of the cow and horse. It is a modification of smallpox.

Vacuole (vak´-ū-ōl). A clear space filled with fluid, such as is found in the amœba, *e.g.*, **Food V.**, for feeding. The pseudopodia flow all round the particle of food, finally fuse, and the particle is enclosed in a bubble of fluid. **Contractile V.**, this fills up with fluid, bursts, and fills up again ; the fluid excreted contains nitrogen and is closely allied to urea, and this is therefore an excretory organ.

Vacuum (vak´-ū-um). A space without atmosphere.

Vagal (vā´-gal). Pertaining to the vagus nerve.

Vagina (va-jīn´-à). A tubular structure into the top of which projects the cervix uteri. The vaginal entrance is guarded by the hymen. The anterior wall measures 3 in., while the posterior is 3½ in.

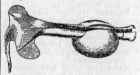

Auvard's Vaginal Speculum.

Vaginal (va-jīn´-al). Relating to the vagina.

Vaginismus (vaj-in-iz´-mus). Painful muscular spasm of the vaginal walls.

Vaginitis (vaj-in-ī´-tis). Inflammation of the vagina.

Vagitus (vaj-ī-tus). The cry of an infant.

Vagotonia (vā-gō-tōn´-i-à).

359

Increased tonus or activity of the parasympathetic nervous system.

Vagus (vā'-gus). The pneumogastric nerve; the tenth cranial nerve, composed of both motor and sensory fibres, with a very wide distribution in the neck, thorax, and abdomen; sends important branches to the heart, lungs, and stomach, etc.

Valency (vāl'-en-si). The combining power of an element. Hydrogen (H) and chlorine (Cl) each have one valency, hence their combination produces HCl; iron (Fe), on the other hand, has three valencies, hence FeCl₃.

Valerian (val-ier'-ri-an). A sedative drug prepared from the dried root of *Valeriana officinalis*. Dose: ammoniated tincture, ½-1 drachm.

Valgus (val'-gus). *See* **Genu V.** and **Talipes V.**

Valve (valv). A fold across a canal obstructing movement of contents in one direction.

Valvulæ Conniventes (val'-vū-li con-i-ven'-tēz). Circular membraneous folds projecting into the lumen of the small intestine; they do not disappear on distension of the bowel, and act by retarding the passage of the food along the bowel; they also provide a greater absorbing area.

Vaporization (vā-por-i-zā'-shun).

The conversion of a liquid to vapour.

Varicella (var-i-sel'-å). Chicken-pox. A mild infectious fever characterized by a crop of vesicles which scab and heal without leaving scars.

Varicocele (var'-i-kō-sēl). A dilated condition of the veins of the spermatic cord.

Varicose (var-i-kōs). Dilated, congested. **V. Veins**, tortuous, dilated veins, commonest in the lower rectum (hæmorrhoids) and the legs; treatment by injections into the vein has largely superseded the operative method. **V. Ulcer**, an ulcer caused by a varicose condition of the veins.

Variola (var-ī'-ō-lå). Smallpox (*q.v.*).

Varix (vē'-riks). A vein showing a varicose state.

Varus (vē'-rus). *See* **Genu V.**

Vas. A vessel or tube.

Vasa Vasorum. The minute vessels supplying the walls of arteries and veins with blood.

Vascular (vas'-kū-là(r)). Highly supplied with blood-vessels. **V. System**, the blood-vessels of the body, *i.e.*, arteries, capillaries, and veins.

Vasectomy (vas-ek'-to-mi). Resection of part of the vas deferens.

Vaseline (vas'-el-ēn). *Paraffinum molle*; a soft grease prepared from petroleum and used medically mainly as a lubricant and base for ointments.

Vasoconstriction (vă - zō - kon-strik'-shun). A state of contraction of the blood-vessels.

Vasodilation (vă-zō-dī-lā'-shun). Dilation of the lumen of the blood-vessels.

Vasomotor Nerves (vă-zo-mō'-ter). Nerves which cause either contraction or dilation of the blood-vessels.

Vector (vek-taw(r)). The carrier of a parasite or infection, e.g., the body-louse is the vector of typhus.

Vegetarian (vej-e-tē'-ri-an). A person who lives entirely on vegetable foods.

Vegetations (vej-e-tā'-shuns). Growths or accretions composed of fibrin and platelets occurring on the edge of the cardiac valves in acute endocarditis.

Vegetative (vej-e-tā'-tiv). Having the power of growth.

Vein (văn). A vessel conveying blood from the tissues to the heart; the bluish colour of venous blood is due to displacement of oxygen by CO_2.

Velum (vē'-lum). A veil or veil-like structure.

Venæ Cavæ. Two large veins which empty their contents into the right auricle of the heart. **Superior Vena Cava,** the large vein which collects blood from the head, chest, and upper extremities; it is formed by the junction of the two innominate veins. **Inferior Vena Cava,** the vein which receives blood from the trunk of the body and lower extremities; is formed by union of the two common iliac veins.

Venereal (ven-ier'-ri-al). Pertaining to sexual intercourse. **V. Diseases,** gonorrhœa, syphilis, and soft sore.

Venepuncture (vē-ni-pungk'-tūr). The introduction of a needle into a vein for injection of fluids or for withdrawing of blood.

Venesection (vē-ni-sek'-shun). Blood-letting.

Venom (ven'-um). The poison secreted by certain insects and reptiles. **Russell's Viper Venom,** used as a hæmostatic, especially in hæmophilia.

Venous (vē'-nus). Pertaining to the veins.

Ventilation (ven-ti-lā'-shun). The supplying of fresh air, e.g., by movement of air in a room. **Pulmonary V.,** the exchange of stale air for fresh by the movement of the lungs.

Ventral (ven'-tral). (1) The anterior surface of the body. (2) Pertaining to the belly.

Ventricle (ven'-trik-l). A small belly-like cavity. **V.'s of the Brain,** five cavities filled with cerebro-spinal fluid within the brain: the 3rd, 4th, 5th, and two lateral ventricles. **V.'s of the Heart,** the two lower, strongly muscled cavities of the heart. **V. of the Larynx,** the pouch-like cavity between the true and false vocal cords.

Ventriculography (ven-trik-ū-log'-raf-i). X-ray examination of the ventricles of the brain after the fluid in them has been wholly or partly displaced by air injected through the brain.

Ventrofixation (ven-trō-fiks-ā'-shun). An operation for the relief of uterine prolapse. The abdomen is opened and the fundus of the uterus securely sutured to the anterior abdominal wall.

Venule (vēn-ūl or ven-). A small vein.

Veratrum (ve'-ra-trum). A drug obtained from the dried roots of *Veratrum viride*; sedative. Dosage: Tincture, 5-15 minims.

Vermicide (ver'-mi-sīd). An agent which destroys worms.

Vermiform (ver-mi-faw(r)m). Resembling a worm. **V. Appendix,** the small vestigial hollow organ attached to the lower end of the cæcum. It measures 1 to 6 in. in length by ¼ in. in diameter and is closed at its free end. **V. Process,** the elongated middle lobe of the cerebellum.

Vermifuge (ver'-mi-fūj). An agent which expels worms.

Verminous (ver'-min-us). In-

fested with worms or with any obnoxious parasitic insects, especially lice.

Vernix Caseosa (ver'-niks kā-zi-ō'-zà). The fatty substance which covers the skin of the fœtus at birth.

Veronal (ve'-ro-nal). A hypnotic drug. Dose, 5-10 gr.

Verruca (ve-roo'-kà). A wart.

Verrucose (ve'-rū-kōs). Warty.

Version (ver'-shun). The method of changing the position of the fœtus so that some other part presents. **Cephalic V.,** causing the head to present. **Podalic V.,** converting the position into a foot presentation.

Vertebra (ver'-te-brà). One of the small bones forming the vertebral column. In children these are 33, but the bones of the coccyx and sacrum later unite to form 2 instead of 9, so that there are only 26 in the adult.

Vertex (ver'-teks). The top of the head.

Vertigo (ver'-tig-ō or ver-ti'-gō). Giddiness; dizziness.

Vesica (vēs-i-kà). The bladder.

Vesical (ves-ī'-kal). Pertaining to the vesica.

Vesicant (vēs'-i-kant). A blistering substance.

Vesicle (vēs'-ik-l). A small blister or sac.

Vesicular Mole (ves-ik'-ū-là(r) mōl). *See* **Hydatidiform Mole.**

Vesiculitis (ves-ik-ū-lī'-tis). Inflammation of a vesicle, particularly the seminal vesicles.

Vestibule (ves′-ti-būl). (1) The middle part of the internal ear, lying between the semicircular canals and the cochlea. (2) The triangular area between the labia minora.

Vestigia! (ves-tij′-i-al). Forming a trace; indicating a remnant of something formerly present.

Viable (vī′-a-b′l). Capable of living a separate existence.

Vial (vī′-al). A small bottle.

Vibratile, Vibratory (vī-brā-tĭl, -to-ri). Swaying to and fro.

Vibrio (vib′-ri-ō). A genus of curved motile micro-organisms.

Vicarious (vik-é′-ri-us). Substituting the function of one organ for another. **V. Menstruation,** menstrual bleeding from the nose, stomach, or any place other than the uterus during the menses.

Villous (vil′-us). Possessing or resembling villi.

Villus (vil′-us). Pl. *villi* (vil′-ī). A microscopical finger-like projection as seen in the mucous membrane of the small intestine or on the outside of the chorion of the embryonic sac.

Vincent's Angina. *See* Angina.

Vinegar (vin′-i-gá(r)). A dilute solution of acetic acid formed by the fermentation of wines and spirits.

Vinum (vīn′-um). Wine.

Virgin (ver′-jin). A woman who has never had sexual intercourse; unpolluted.

Virilism (vir′-il-izm). The appearance of secondary male characteristics in a female.

Virility (vir-il′-i-ti). The condition of mature manhood; masculinity.

Virulent (vir′-ū-lent). Malignant; noxious; poisonous.

Virus (vī′-rus). A disease-producing or poisonous substance; any protozoa or bacteria c.pable of causing disease. The term is chiefly applied to ultra-microscopic, filter-passing living agencies which cause a number of diseases, *e.g.*, Poliomyelitis, Chicken-pox, Smallpox, Influenza, etc.

Visceroptosis (vis-e-rop-tō′-sis). Downward displacement or dropping of the abdominal organs.

Viscid (vis′-id). Thick and sticky: viscid body fluids are blood and bile and mucus.

Viscopaste (vis′-kō-pāst). An adhesive gelatine bandage of the "Unna" type. It is used in varicose ulcers and allied conditions, varicose veins, lymphangitis, and fractures of the leg. It is quickly applied, and gives sufficient support to last two months if desired.

Viscose (vis′-kōz). A gummy

substance used for sealing bottles, etc.

Viscosity (vis-kos'-i-ti). The power of adhering; gumminess; viscidity.

Viscus (vis'-kus). An internal organ of the body. Pl. *viscera* (vis'-e-rá).

Visual (vizh'-ū-al or viz'-ū-al). Pertaining to vision. **V. Field,** the area within which objects can be seen. **V. Purple,** a purple pigment in the retina of the eye.

Vital (vī'-tal). (1) Pertaining to life. (2) Essential. **V. Capacity,** the volume of air that can be expelled after a full inspiration.

Vitamins (vit-a-mins or vīt-a-mēns). Essential food factors of a chemical nature present in small amounts in certain foodstuffs, the absence of which cause deficiency diseases. The first studies were made by Eykman in 1897 and by Hopkins in Cambridge in 1912. Some can now be synthesized on the commercial scale. They are indicated by letters, numerals, and names. The following vitamins are known: Vitamins A, B_1, B_2, C, D, E, and K.

Vitamin A. Diet deficient in this vitamin causes (1) xerophthalmia; this is characterized by absence of tears and dryness of the cornea, with consequent soreness and

ulceration, which may eventually terminate in blindness; (2) impairment of growth; (3) impairment of the power to resist infection. Vitamin A is found in animal fat, such as butter, meat fat, cream, and cod-liver oil, but not in vegetable fat; also in fresh watercress, cabbage, lettuce, and tomato. See also association of vitamin A with carotene.

Vitamin B. This is divided into B_1 and B_2. B_1 is called the antineuritic vitamin because it prevents certain nervous diseases, *e.g.,* beriberi, which develops among Eastern people who live on polished rice. The vitamin is found in the germ of cereals, yeast extracts, egg yolk, peas, nuts, and liver. It is slowly destroyed by heating. B_2 is the antipellagric vitamin because it prevents the disease of pellagra. This is characterized by the appearance of a raised purply red eruption on the skin of the hands and face when exposed to the sun; it is associated with serious gastric and mental disturbance. This vitamin is found in most fresh foods, especially peas, beans, lentils, eggs, and yeast. B_2 contains Riboflavin. It is not destroyed by heat. Minor deficiency in diet causes anorexia and dermatitis, first seen at the angles of the mouth (cheilosis).

Vitamin C (ascorbic acid) is known as the antiscorbutic vitamin because it prevents scurvy; this is recognized by bleeding from the gums and nose, bruising of the skin, pain and tenderness of the bones, while in severe cases even fractures may occur. The vitamin is found in all fresh fruits, particularly oranges, lemons, limes, black currants and rose-hips, fresh vegetables, especially cabbage and the juice of turnips; it also exists in milk and meat. Heat, as required in cooking and preserving foods, destroys the vitamin.

Vitamin D prevents rickets, and is therefore designated the antirachitic vitamin. It aids in the absorption of calcium and phosphorus through the usual channels. It is abundant in fish oils, especially cod-liver oil and halibut-liver oil, animal fats, and all foods containing vitamin A. It has been demonstrated that if ergosterol is exposed to sunlight or ultra-violet radiation, it becomes rich in vitamin D.

Vitamin E. Thought to be essential for reproduction, since experiments on rats suggest that lack of it results in sterility. Very little is known so far, but it probably exists in most fresh foods.

Vitamin K plays a part in the coagulation of blood. It is fat-soluble and the effects of its deprivation is seen in the increased tendency to bleeding evinced by patients with obstructive jaundice.

Vitelline (vi-tel′-īn). Relating to the yolk of an egg.

Vitiligo (vit-il-ī′-gō). *See* **Leucoderma.**

Vitreous (vit′-ri-us). Resembling jelly. **V. Chamber,** the cavity inside the eyeball. **V. Humor,** the jelly-like substance contained in the vitreous chamber.

Vitriol (vit′-ri-ol). Sulphuric acid. **Blue V.,** copper sulphate. **Green V.,** ferrous sulphate.

Viviparous (vī-vip′-a-rus). Bearing young which are formed and alive when born.

Vivisection (viv-i-sek′-shun). Scientific experimental work carried out on a living animal.

Vocal Cords. Membraneous folds stretched antero-posteriorly across the larynx. Sound is produced by the vibration of the cords as air from the lungs passes between them.

Void. To evacuate, to empty.

Volar (vō′-là(r)). Palmar; pertaining to the palm of the hand.

Volatile (vol-a-tīl). Having rapid evaporation, easily passing from the liquid to the gaseous state.

Volition (vŏ-lish'-'n). The will to act.

Volkmann, Richard von (1830-1899). German surgeon. **V. Deformity**, a muscular paralysis resulting from applying a splint too tightly. **V. Spoon**, a sharp-edged spoon used for scooping out a cavity, and for scraping a granulating surface.

Volkmann's Spoon.

Volsellum (vol-sel'-um). *See* Vulsellum.

Volt (vŏlt). The unit of electromotive force.

Voltaic (vol-tā-ik). Pertaining to galvanic electricity.

Voltmeter (vŏlt'-mē-ter). An apparatus for measuring voltage.

Voluntary (vol'-un-ta-ri). Under the control of the will ; free and unrestricted.

Volvulus (vol'-vŭ-lus). Rotation of a section of intestine upon its mesenteric axis, such as may result from the intercoiling of one loop of intestine with another. Circulation of the parts is seriously interfered with, causing strangulation.

Vomer (vŏ'-mer). The bone forming the septum of the nose.

Vomit (vom'-it). Ejection of the stomach contents through the mouth ; sickness.

Vomiting of Pregnancy. *See* Hyperemesis Gravidarum.

Vomitus (vom'-i-tus). The material vomited.

Von Pirquet's Test. A diagnostic test for tuberculosis, in which a little old tuberculin is applied to a scarified area of the skin of the arm. A positive reaction is seen if a red papular eruption appears at the site of inoculation.

Von Recklinghausen's Disease. (1) Multiple neurofibromata occurring on the skin along the course of the nerves ; is associated with marked cutaneous pigmentation. Synonym, *Molluscum Fibrosum*. (2) Generalized fibrocystic disease of the bones.

Vulcanite (vul'-kan-īt). A hard, black solid, made by heating 2 parts of indiarubber with 1 part of sulphur to a temperature of about 150° C.

Vulnerable (vul'-ner-ra-b'l). Liable or subject to damage or wounding.

Vulsellum (vul-sel-um). A long-pronged forceps with a catch at the handles to keep them in position ; used in gynæcological operations for holding the cervix uteri.

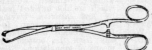

Vulsellum.

Vulva (vul'-vă). The external organs of generation in the female.

Vulvitis (vul-vī'-tis). Inflammation of the vulva.

W.

Walcher's Position. *See* Position.

Wane (wān). To decrease; to decline; to fade.

Wart (waw(r)t). A papilloma of the skin; verruca. Some warts are the result of a virus infection.

Washing-soda. Sodium carbonate, Na_2CO_3.

Wassermann Reaction (vas'-er-man). A blood-serum test performed for the diagnosis of syphilis.

Water-beds. Rubber mattresses which can be filled three parts full with warm water (temp. 100° F.); they must not be too full or they will be hard. Fracture boards are placed across the wire mattress to produce a firm foundation and prevent sagging; they are refilled every fortnight.

Water-brash. *See* Heartburn.

Watt. A unit of electrical energy.

Wean (wēn). The process of discontinuing breast-feeding; this should normally occur at the ninth month, but on the advice of a doctor may take place earlier.

Weil-Felix Reaction. *See* Felix-Weil Reaction.

Weil's Disease (vīl's). Acute infective jaundice, due to infection with a spirochæte; spirochætosis icterohæmorrhagica.

Weir-Mitchell Treatment. A method of treating neurasthenia. The patient is nursed in a room alone, and no visitors, books, etc., are allowed. A very generous diet is insisted upon; massage is usually given to tone up the muscles.

Wen. A sebaceous cyst.

Wertheim's Hysterectomy (vert'-hīm). *See* Hysterectomy.

Wet-nurse. A woman who breast-feeds another woman's child; she should be absolutely healthy, and particularly free from such diseases as syphilis and tuberculosis.

Wharton's Jelly. A jelly-like substance contained in the umbilical cord.

Wheal (wēl). A raised stripe or ridge on the skin.

Wheelhouse's Operation. External urethrotomy for impassable urethral stricture.

White Leg. Same as *Phlegmasia Alba Dolens.* **W. Mixture,** a purgative mixture, white in colour, and containing sulphate of magnesia in suspension. Synonym, *Mist. Alba.*

Whites. See Leucorrhœa.

Whitlow. See Onychia.

Whooping-cough. See Pertussis.

Widal Reaction (vē'-dal). A diagnostic blood-serum test of persons suffering from typhoid fever.

Wind-pipe. The trachea.

Winslow's Foramen. The aperture which connects the lesser with the greater peritoneal sac ; situated between the stomach and the liver.

Womb (woom). The uterus.

Woolsorters' Disease. Pulmonary anthrax.

Wound (woond). A breach in the continuity of the soft tissues of the body, which also involves either skin or mucous membrane. **Incised W.,** one which is caused by a sharp-cutting instrument, such as a knife or bayonet. **Lacerated W.,** one with jagged edges. **Punctured W.,** usually deep and narrow, as caused by a stab. **Poisoned W.,** those due to insect bites, snake-bite, wounds due to rabid animals, and bacterial infection of wounds, *e.g.*, whitlow. Incised wounds which are not infected heal by *first intention*, leaving only a thin lineal scar. Infected wounds heal gradually from the bottom by means of granulations. See **Granulations** and **Proud Flesh.**

Wrist (rist). The carpus (*q.v.*).

Writers' Cramp. Spasm of the muscles of the hand in writers ; may be due to faulty manipulation of the pen or to a psychoneurosis.

Wry-neck (rī'-nek). A condition in which the head is drawn down towards the shoulder, and is caused by contraction of the sternocleidomastoid and other muscles of the neck ; it may be either *congenital* or *acquired.* See **Torticollis.**

X.

Xanthelasma (zan-thel-az'-má). The appearance of new growths on the skin, which have a yellow pigmentation, and especially develop on the eyelids.

Xanthine (zan'-thēn). A nitrogenous extractive contained in the body, formed during the metabolism of nucleoproteins. Through the action of certain enzymes it becomes further converted into uric acid, and as such is passed into the urine.

Xanthochromia (zan-thō-krōm'-

i-à). A yellowish tinge of the cerebro-spinal fluid.

Xanthoderma (zan-thō-der′-mà). A yellow discoloration of the skin.

Xanthoma (zan-thō′-mà). *See* **Xanthelasma**.

Xanthopsia (zan-thop′-si-à). Yellow vision (*q.v.*).

Xanthosis (zan-thō′-sis). The yellow colour of the skin in cancerous conditions.

Xerophthalmia (zē-rof-thal′-mi-à). A disease of the eyes in which there is dryness and ulceration of the cornea, which in severe cases may terminate in blindness; the condition is associated with lack of Vitamin A.

Xerosis (ze-rō′-sis). Dryness.

Xerostomia (ze-ros-tō′-mi-à). A dry state of the mouth.

Xiphisternum (zif-i-ster′-num). The ensiform cartilage.

Xiphoid (zif′-oid). *See* **Xiphisternum**. Shaped like a sword.

X-rays. *See* **Rontgen Rays.**

Xylol, Xylene (zī-lol, zī-lēn). Dimethyl benzene. A hydrocarbon from coal-tar used medicinally and also as a fat solvent in laboratory work.

Y.

Yaws. The same as *Frambœsia.* A contagious tropical disease resembling syphilis and also due to a spirochætal infection.

Yeast (yēst). A species of fungus which will cause fermentation; on microscopic examination seen to consist of spores and branching filaments; said to be rich in vitamin B.

Yellow Fever (yel′-ō fē′-ver). An epidemic disease characterized by a marked degree of jaundice, hyperpyrexia, and black vomit. It is due to a virus and is mainly found in the tropics. **Y. Spot,** the macula lutea of the retina. **Y. Vision,** a disturbance in vision in which objects appear to be coloured yellow; a common symptom after an overdose of santonin, or in obstructive jaundice. **Y. Ointment,** ointment containing yellow oxide of mercury.

Yolk (yōk). The yellow part of an egg which serves as a store of food for the growing embryo.

Young's Rule. A rule by which the suitable dose can be estimated for children from the adult dose. *See* **Appendix.**

Z.

Zein (zē′-in). A protein found in maize; it is lacking in the amino-acids of *lysine* and *tryptophane,* and therefore will not support life.

Zenker's Degeneration of Muscle. A hyaline degenera-

369

tive change in the muscles, especially of the abdominal wall, which occurs in some acute infections, particularly typhoid fever.

Zero (zē'-rō). Nought. The point on a thermometer from which it is graduated. On the centigrade and Réaumur scales the zero or 0° is the temperature of melting ice. On the Fahrenheit it is a much lower temperature. To obtain this fixed point the thermometer is immersed in melting ice, and when the mercury column ceases to fall, the level at which it remains is fixed as 0° on the C. and R. scales and as 32° on the F. scale.

Zinc (zingk). A bluish-white metallic element. Symbol, Zn.

Zingiber (zin'-jib-er). Ginger; is carminative and stimulative.

Zona (zō'-nà). A zone; a term sometimes used for the girdle formation of herpes zoster. **Z. Pellucida**, the striated vitelline membrane which surrounds the ovum.

Zooglea (zō-og'-lē-à). The encystment stage in the life-cycle of certain minute organisms.

Zoology (zō-ol'-o-ji). That section of biology which specially studies the structure, life-cycles, habits, and functions of animal organisms.

Zoophyte (zō'-o-fīt). An organism which has the characteristics of both plant and animal.

Zoosperm (zō'-o-sperm). Same as *Spermatozoon*.

Zoster (zos'-ter). Herpes zoster (*q.v.*). Shingles.

Zygoma (zī-gō'-mà). The cheek-bone.

Zygomatic (zī-gō-mat'-ik). Pertaining to the zygoma. **Z. Arch,** the arch formed by the zygomatic processes of the *malar* and *temporal* bones.

Zygote (zī'-gōt). The union of two germ cells. The spermatozoon pierces the ovum, and the two nuclei completely fuse.

Zymogen (zī'-mō-jen). An enzyme of the pancreas and a precursor of trypsin, *i.e.*, *trypsinogen*.

Zymose (zī'-mōs). Same as *Invertin*; one of the sugars.

Zymosis (zi-mō'-sis). Fermentative action.

Zymotic Diseases (zī-mot'-ik). Any bacterial disease of an infectious or contagious nature, whether occurring sporadically or in epidemic form.

APPENDIX.

Diseases Designated by the Names of those who Discovered or First Described them.

ACOSTA'S DISEASE. *Mountain sickness.*

ADDISON'S ANÆMIA. *Pernicious anæmia; idiopathic anæmia; primary anæmia; Biermer's disease.*

ADDISON'S DISEASE. *Destruction of the suprarenal glands; usually due to T.B.*

ALBERS-SCHÖNBERG DISEASE. *Marble bone disease.*

ARAN - DUCHENNE or DU-CHENNE - ARAN DISEASE. *Progressive muscular atrophy; chronic anterior poliomyelitis.*

AYERZA'S DISEASE. *Cyanosis and erythrocytosis with chronic pulmonary disease.*

BANTI'S DISEASE. *Splenic anæmia with cirrhosis.*

BARLOW'S DISEASE. *Infantile scurvy.*

BASEDOW'S DISEASE. *Graves' disease, q.v.*

BELL'S PALSY. *Paralysis of the facial (seventh) nerve.*

BENNETT'S FRACTURE, or *Bennett's stave of thumb. Fracture of the first metacarpal.*

BOECK'S SARCOIDOSIS. *A nonbacterial granulomatous condition affecting skin, lymphglands and (less often) the viscera.*

BRIGHT'S DISEASE. *Nephritis, acute and chronic.*

BRILL'S DISEASE. *Typhus fever.*

BRODIE'S ABSCESS. *Formation of a chronic abscess inside a bone.*

BRUCELLOSIS. *Malta fever; undulant fever.*

BUHL'S DISEASE. *Icterus neonatorum.*

CALVE'S DISEASE. *Perthes' disease, q.v.*

CHARCOT'S DISEASE. *Neuropathic arthritis.*

CLUTTON'S JOINTS. *Congenital syphilitic symmetrical effusions into joints.*

COCK'S PECULIAR TUMOUR. *Ulcerated sebaceous cyst.*

COLLES' FRACTURE. *Fracture of the lower end of the radius.*

COOLEY'S ANÆMIA. *A leucoerythroblastic anæmia of children of Mediterranean stock.*

CORRIGAN'S DISEASE. *Aortic incompetency.*

CROHN'S DISEASE. *Regional or terminal ileitis.*

DERCUM'S DISEASE. *Adiposis dolorosa.*

DIETL'S CRISES. *Attacks of pain due to kinking of the ureter.*

DUCHENNE'S DISEASE. (1) *Locomotor ataxy; (2) pseudohypertrophy of muscles.*

DUKES' DISEASE. *Fourth disease, an infectious disease resembling rubella, scarlet fever, and measles.*

ERB'S or ERB-DUCHENNE'S PARALYSIS. *Upper arm brachial paralysis.*

ERB-GOLDFLAM'S DISEASE. *Myasthenia gravis.*

EWING'S SARCOMA. *A reticulo-sarcoma arising inside the shaft of bones of children.*

FLEXNER'S DYSENTERY. *One of the commoner types of bacillary dysentery.*

FRIEDREICH'S ATAXIA. *Hereditary ataxia.*

FRÖHLICH'S SYNDROME. *Dystrophia adiposo-genitalis; hypopituitarism.*

GAUCHER'S SPLENOMEGALY. *Primary infantile splenomegaly.*

GEE'S CŒLIAC AFFECTION. *Cœliac disease; cœliac infantilism.*

GLENARD'S DISEASE. *Visceroptosis.*

GRAVES' DISEASE. *Exophthalmic goitre; hyperthyroidism; also Basedow's or Parry's disease.*

GRAWITZ'S TUMOUR. *Hypernephroma.*

GULL'S DISEASE. *Myxœdema.*

HAND - SCHÜLLER - CHRISTIAN DISEASE. *Lipo-granuloma affecting the bones, especially of the skull.*

HANOT'S CIRRHOSIS. *Hypertrophic biliary cirrhosis.*

HEINE-MEDIN DISEASE. *Acute poliomyelitis.*

HENOCH'S PURPURA. *Purpura with colic.*

HIRSCHSPRUNG'S DISEASE. *Megacolon.*

HODGKIN'S DISEASE. *Lymphadenoma.*

HUNTERIAN CHANCRE. *Primary syphilitic chancre; hard chancre.*

HUNTINGTON'S CHOREA. *Chronic hereditary chorea.*

JACKSONIAN EPILEPSY. *Epilepsy of traumatic or tumour origin.*

JENNER'S EMPHYSEMA. *Hypertrophic emphysema.*

KIENBOCK'S DISEASE. *Rarefying osteitis of the semilunar of the wrist.*

KLUMPKE'S PARALYSIS. *Lower arm brachial palsy.*

KÖHLER'S DISEASE. *Chronic sclerosis of the scaphoid bone.*

LÆNNEC'S CIRRHOSIS. *Alcoholic or portal or multilobular cirrhosis of liver; gin-drinker's liver; hobnail liver.*

LANDRY'S DISEASE. *Acute ascending paralysis.*

LANE'S DISEASE. *Intestinal stasis.*

LEGG'S DISEASE. *Perthes' disease, q.v.*

LEISHMANIASIS. *Kala-azar; tropical sore; Delhi boil.*

LITTLE'S DISEASE. *Cerebral diplegia; spastic paralysis of infants.*

LITTRE'S HERNIA. *Strangulation of a herniated diverticulum.*

LOBSTEIN'S DISEASE. *Fragilitis ossium.*

LUDWIG'S ANGINA. *Cellulitis of neck.*

MADELUNG'S DEFORMITY. *Stunting of growth of radius following old separated lower epiphysis.*

MARIE'S DISEASE. (1) *Hereditary cerebellar ataxia;* (2) *acromegaly;* (3) *hypertrophic pulmonary osteoarthropathy;* (4) *spondylose rhizomelique.*

MARIE'S HEREDITARY CEREBELLAR ATAXIA. *Spinocerebellar ataxia.*

MARIE STRUMPELL'S ARTHRITIS. *Spondylitis deformans; spondylose rhizomelique.*

MÉNIÈRE'S DISEASE. *Auditory vertigo.*

MIKULICZ'S DISEASE. *Chronic hypertrophic enlargement of the lachrymal and salivary glands.*

MILROY'S DISEASE. *Hereditary œdema of the legs; chronic trophœdema.*

MONCKEBERG'S SCLEROSIS. *Calcific hardening of the middle coats of the arteries.*

MORTON'S DISEASE. *Metatarsalgia.*

MORVAN'S DISEASE. *Syringomyelia with painless whitlows.*

NIEMANN-PICK'S SPLENOMEGALY. *One of the lipoid-storage reticuloses causing enlargement of the spleen.*

OLLIER'S DISEASE. *Achondroplasia.*

OPPENHEIM'S DISEASE. *Amyotonia congenita.*

OSGOOD-SCHLATTER'S DISEASE.

Rarefying osteitis of the tubercle of the tibia.

OSLER'S DISEASE. *Polycythæmia rubra or vera; erythræmia; Vaquez's disease.*

PAGET'S DISEASE. (1) *Osteitis deformans;* (2) *cancerous eczema of the nipple.*

PARKINSON'S DISEASE. *Paralysis agitans; shaking palsy.*

PARRY'S DISEASE. *Graves' disease, q.v.*

PERTHES' DISEASE. *Pseudo-coxalgia; Legg's disease; osteochondritis deformans; Calve's disease.*

PICK'S DISEASE. *Enlargement of the liver with recurring ascites, but without jaundice.*

POTT'S DISEASE. *T.B. spine; spinal caries.*

POTT'S FRACTURE. *Fracture of the lower end of the fibula.*

POTT'S PUFFY TUMOUR. *Swelling of the scalp over the site of an extra-dural abscess.*

RAYNAUD'S DISEASE. *Idiopathic trophoneurosis.*

RICHTER'S HERNIA. *Strangulation of part of the gut with only partial obstruction of the lumen.*

RIEDEL'S THYROIDITIS. *Fibrosis of the thyroid gland; ligneous goitre.*

RIGG'S DISEASE. *Pyorrhœa alveolaris.*

SCHIMMELBUSCH'S DISEASE. *Chronic cystic mastitis.*

SCHLATTER'S DISEASE. *Avulsion of the projection of the tubercle of the tibia with inflammation of the insertion of the ligamentum patellæ.*

SCHONLEIN'S DISEASE. *Purpura rheumatica.*

SHIGA DYSENTERY. *A severe form of bacillary dysentery, chiefly tropical.*

SIMMONDS' DISEASE. *Emaciation following destruction of the pituitary gland.*

SONNE'S DYSENTERY. *A mild type of bacillary dysentery.*

STILL'S DISEASE. *Arthritis deformans in children.*

STOKES - ADAMS' DISEASE. *Heart-block.*

STRUMPELL-MARIE'S DISEASE. *See MARIE STRUMPELL.*

SYDENHAM'S CHOREA. *Rheumatic chorea ; St Vitus' dance.*

TAY-SACH'S DISEASE. *Amaurotic familial idiocy.*

THOMSEN'S DISEASE. *Myotonia congenita.*

VAQUEZ'S DISEASE. *Osler's disease,* q.v.

VINCENT'S ANGINA. *Membraneous tonsillitis.*

VOLKMANN'S CONTRACTURE. *Contracture of the muscles of* *the hand and forearm due to ischæmia, usually following splinting or bandaging.*

VON BECHTEREW'S ARTHRITIS. *Spondylitis deformans.*

VON ECONOMO'S DISEASE. *Encephalitis lethargica.*

VON JAKSCH'S ANÆMIA. *Splenic anæmia of infants.*

VON RECKLINGHAUSEN'S DISEASE. *(1) Generalised neuro-fibromatosis ; molluscum fibrosum ; (2) generalised osteitis fibro-cystica.*

WEIL'S DISEASE. *Epidemic jaundice, spirochætosis ictero-hæmorrhagica.*

WERDNIG - HOFFMANN'S MUSCULAR ATROPHY. *Progressive muscular atrophy of childhood.*

WERLHOF'S MORBUS MACULOSIS. *Purpura hæmorrhagica.*

WILMS' TUMOUR. *Renal tumour of childhood ; renal adenosarcoma ; embryonal adeno-myo-sarcoma of the kidney.*

WILSON'S DISEASE. *Progressive hepato-lenticular degeneration.*

WITTS' ANÆMIA. *Hypochromic, microcytic anæmia.*

TRAYS PREPARED FOR NURSING TECHNIQUES

*T*HE following pages show trays prepared for nursing techniques. It should be realized that these purport to be only the foundation, therefore any special appliance used in a particular hospital can be added or substituted. The apparatus for the more complicated techniques can be placed on a dressing trolley if desired. All instruments, gloves, etc., must lie flat in the dish, but for the sake of clarity this rule has not been rigidly adhered to in the drawings.

In each case articles not required can be omitted.

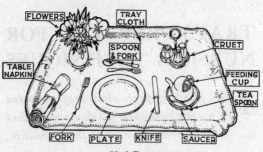

Meal Tray.

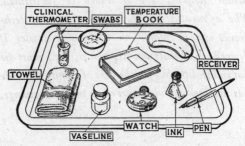

Temperature, etc.

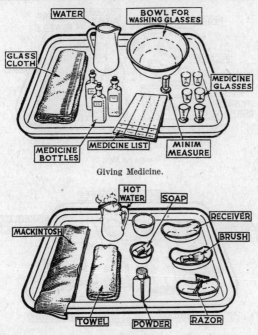

WATER

BOWL FOR
WASHING GLASSES

GLASS
CLOTH

MEDICINE
GLASSES

MEDICINE
BOTTLES

MEDICINE LIST

MINIM
MEASURE

Giving Medicine.

HOT
WATER

SOAP

RECEIVER

MACKINTOSH

BRUSH

TOWEL

POWDER

RAZOR

Shaving.

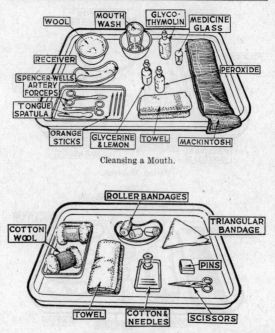

Cleansing a Mouth.

Applying a Bandage.

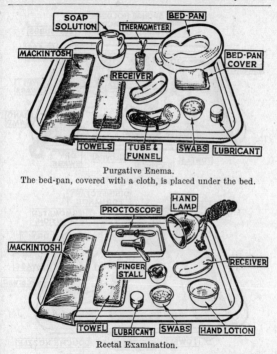

Purgative Enema.
The bed-pan, covered with a cloth, is placed under the bed.

Rectal Examination.

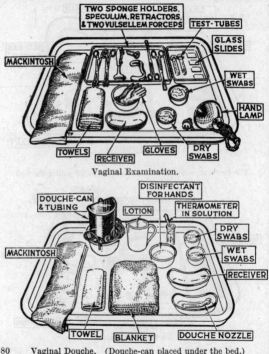

TWO SPONGE HOLDERS, SPECULUM, RETRACTORS, & TWO VULSELLEM FORCEPS

TEST-TUBES

GLASS SLIDES

MACKINTOSH

WET SWABS

HAND LAMP

TOWELS

RECEIVER

GLOVES

DRY SWABS

Vaginal Examination.

DISINFECTANT FOR HANDS

DOUCHE-CAN & TUBING

LOTION

THERMOMETER IN SOLUTION

DRY SWABS

MACKINTOSH

WET SWABS

RECEIVER

TOWEL

BLANKET

DOUCHE NOZZLE

380   Vaginal Douche.   (Douche-can placed under the bed.)

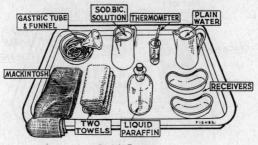

Gastric Lavage.

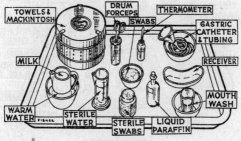

Gastric Feed.

381

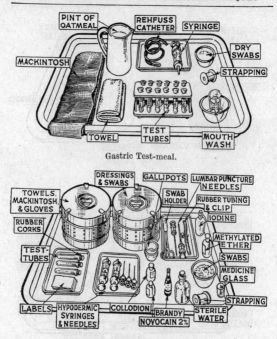

Gastric Test-meal.

Lumbar Puncture.

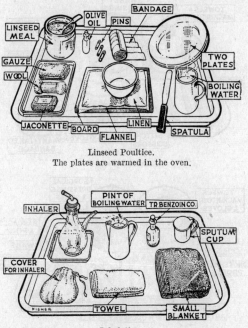

Linseed Poultice.
The plates are warmed in the oven.

Inhalation.

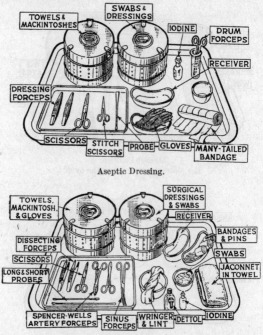

Aseptic Dressing.

Septic Dressing.

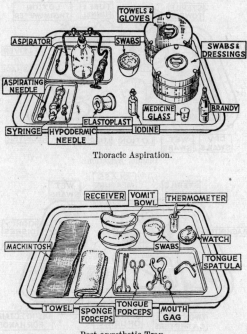

Thoracic Aspiration.

Post-anæsthetic Tray.

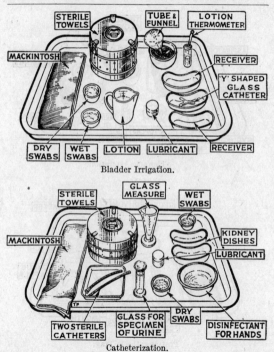

Bladder Irrigation.

Catheterization.

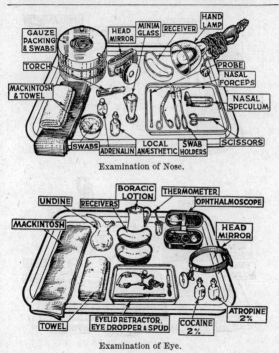

Examination of Nose.

Examination of Eye.

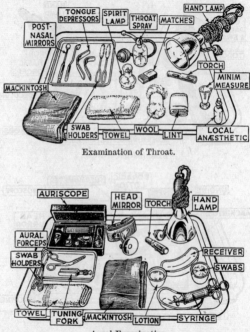

Examination of Throat.

Aural Examination.

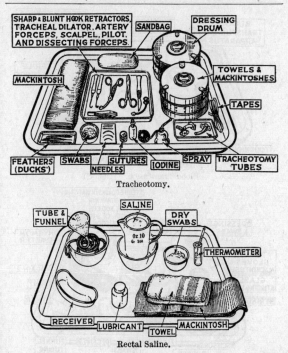

SHARP & BLUNT HOOK RETRACTORS, TRACHEAL DILATOR, ARTERY FORCEPS, SCALPEL, PILOT, AND DISSECTING FORCEPS.

SANDBAG

DRESSING DRUM

MACKINTOSH

TOWELS & MACKINTOSHES

TAPES

FEATHERS (DUCKS')

SWABS

NEEDLES

SUTURES

IODINE

SPRAY

TRACHEOTOMY TUBES

Tracheotomy.

TUBE & FUNNEL

SALINE

DRY SWABS

Oz 10 Gr 300

THERMOMETER

RECEIVER

LUBRICANT

TOWEL

MACKINTOSH

Rectal Saline.

389

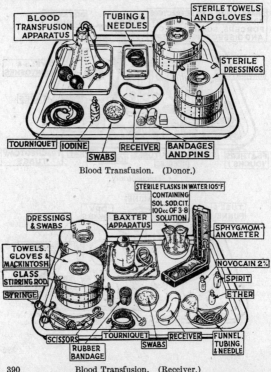

BLOOD TRANSFUSION APPARATUS

TUBING & NEEDLES

STERILE TOWELS AND GLOVES

STERILE DRESSINGS

TOURNIQUET

IODINE

SWABS

RECEIVER

BANDAGES AND PINS

Blood Transfusion. (Donor.)

DRESSINGS & SWABS

BAXTER APPARATUS

STERILE FLASKS IN WATER 105°F CONTAINING SOL. SOD CIT. 100cc OF 3·8 SOLUTION

SPHYGMOM-ANOMETER

TOWELS. GLOVES & MACKINTOSH

GLASS STIRRING ROD

SYRINGE

NOVOCAIN 2%

SPIRIT

ETHER

SCISSORS

RUBBER BANDAGE

TOURNIQUET

SWABS

RECEIVER

FUNNEL, TUBING, & NEEDLE

Blood Transfusion. (Receiver.)

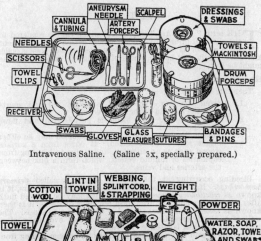

Intravenous Saline. (Saline 3x, specially prepared.)

Fracture of Extension Tray.

FIRST AID.

THE term "First Aid" implies aid which can be rendered to the sick and injured by a non-medical person until treatment by a doctor is available. Every one should possess such knowledge, as it may be the means of saving life, which otherwise might be lost.

Hæmorrhage.

There are three types :—

1. *Arterial Bleeding.*—The blood is bright red and spurts from the cut end of the blood-vessel.
2. *Venous Bleeding.*—The blood is purplish-red and flows from the wound.
3. *Capillary Bleeding.*—The colour of the blood may be either bright red, dark, or mixed. It oozes from a surface wound such as an abrasion, and is due to bleeding from capillaries or minute vessels, which form a link between the arteries and veins.

Bleeding occurring at the time of injury is called *primary hæmorrhage.* If it begins later, but within twenty-four hours, it is known as *reactionary hæmorrhage.* Bleeding may be delayed until after twenty-four hours or even for a few days or weeks, it is then known as *secondary hæmorrhage* and is always due to sepsis. The wall of a blood-vessel is gradually eroded, and eventually gives way ; such bleeding is often very severe.

Bleeding is said to be *external* when it can be seen issuing from the body. It may, however, be unseen as when it escapes into a body cavity such as the chest, and can then only be recognized by signs and symptoms ; this is *internal hæmorrhage.*

Signs and Symptoms of Hæmorrhage.

Signs—

1. An increasingly rapid and feeble pulse.
2. Pallor.
3. Sweating.
4. Extreme restlessness.
5. Dilated pupils.
6. Cold clammy skin.

Symptoms—
  1. Gasping, sighing respiration (air-hunger).
  2. Extreme thirst.
  3. Faintness.
  4. Failing sight.
  5. Nausea.
  6. Fear of death.

Treatment of Hœmorrhage.—Bleeding can be arrested by natural or artificial means. The former is only possible in the case of small vessels, where a clot forms in the opening of the cut end, while at the same time the muscle fibres contract and lessen the size of the opening. In a large vessel the flow is generally too forceful to allow a clot to form, and recourse must be had to artificial arrest, of which there are several methods :—

  1. Digital pressure.
  2. The use of a tourniquet.
  3. The use of pads.
  4. The use of styptics (hæmostatics).
  5. Posture.
  6. The application of heat or cold.
  7. Forcipressure.
  8. Torsion.
  9. Ligation.

Digital Pressure.—The fingers are placed over the artery which is compressed against an adjacent bone, but never against elastic tissues such as muscle. In the case of arterial bleeding pressure is applied above the bleeding spot ; in venous bleeding below, and in capillary bleeding immediately over the wound. The common arterial pressure points are as follows :—

Temporal Artery—
  (a) Place the thumb on the temporal region and press hard where the pulsation can be felt.
  (b) Place the thumb over the zygoma, immediately in front of the ear. This will prevent blood passing upwards to the temple.

Facial Artery.—Place the thumb over the vessel where it passes over the edge of the lower jaw, $\frac{1}{2}$ in. from the angle. This arrests bleeding from the cheek and lips. If the latter are badly cut, pressure must be applied to both facial arteries. Alternatively,

N *

grasp the wound between fingers and thumbs. For bleeding after extraction of a tooth, plug the socket with cotton-wool, then place a larger pad between the jaws and ask the patient to bite hard upon it. If bleeding still persists, consult the dentist again.

Common Carotid Artery.—Place the thumb on the side of the neck and press backwards against the cervical vertebræ. (The fingers are placed behind the neck to give support.)

Subclavian Artery.—Standing opposite the point of the patient's shoulder, place the fingers of one hand on the chest, the fingers of the other hand on the back. Then put one thumb above the other and press firmly downwards behind the clavicle, on the vessel where it passes over the first rib. (The pressure is made slightly to the sternal side of the centre of the clavicle.) This will cut off the blood supply to the whole of the arm on the same side. Pain may be caused owing to the position of important nerves ; it is also difficult to exert sufficient pressure with the thumbs because of the powerful muscles in this region. An alternative method, therefore, is to use a hard object such as a key, the head of which is protected with a handkerchief wrapped around it to prevent injury to the tissues.

Auxiliary Artery.—It is difficult and indeed almost impossible to compress this artery with the fingers. The best procedure is to compress the subclavian artery and so cut off the blood supply ; or place a large firm pad in the axilla and bind the arm tightly to the chest.

Brachial Artery.—Standing behind the patient place our fingers along the course of the vessel and compress it against the upper end of the humerus. If this is done correctly, no pulse should be felt at the wrist.

Ulnar and Radial Arteries.—Owing to their position between the bones it is impossible to apply pressure directly to these vessels at any point above the wrist. Two methods are available to stop bleeding in the forearm : (1) Application of a tourniquet above the elbow. (2) Placing a large pad in the bend of the elbow, flexing the arm and tying the wrist to the humerus.

Palmar Arch.—Apply pressure with the thumbs placed over the site of the ulnar and radial arteries at the wrist. Each vessel crosses the end of the bone of the same name. The radial artery is quickly recognized by its pulsation. Another method of arresting bleeding from the palm is to give the patient a firm pad to grasp and bind the fingers tightly over it.

External Iliac Artery.—This can be found slightly internal to a point midway between the anterior, superior, iliac spine and the pubic spine. The vessel passes over the pectineal eminence against which it can be compressed. This point is useful for arresting hæmorrhage in the groin.

Femoral Artery.—With the patient in the recumbent position, grasp the upper part of the thigh between the hands and place the thumbs one on top of the other, over the vessel, on the upper, inner side of the upper part of the thigh, and press backwards against the femur. As this causes great fatigue, the nurse may need a relief. In changing over, the thumbs of the assistant are slipped gently under the thumbs of the first person before she releases her grasp. In this way a constant pressure is maintained and the exact position is not lost.

Dorsalis Pedis.—Place the thumb over the lower end of the tibia.

Plantar Artery.—This is found midway between the external malleolus (fibula) and the os calcis (heel bone), against which it is pressed. Compression of these last two vessels simultaneously arrests bleeding in the foot. Alternatively, a large pad can be applied to the sole of the foot and firmly bandaged.

Tourniquet.—This is made of rubber with an attachment for preventing it slipping when in position. A simple tourniquet is made by knotting a handkerchief round the limb, passing a pencil or small stick through, twisting it to tighten the handkerchief, then tying it in position. Points to remember about a tourniquet :—

1. It should not be placed next the skin because of the danger of bruising ; also it would cause unnecessary pain.
2. It should not be left on tightly for longer than twenty minutes at a time.
3. It should be applied gently but firmly.
4. It must be sufficiently tight to arrest bleeding.
5. It is applied above the wound in arterial hæmorrhage, but below in venous bleeding.
6. If made of rubber it should be stretched fully whilst being applied.
7. Owing to the position of the vessels in the forearm and lower leg, a tourniquet is useless in these parts, and must always be applied above the elbow or knee.

Pads.—In addition to their use already mentioned, capillary bleeding is stopped by applying pads in graduated sizes, commencing with the largest and binding them firmly over the bleeding part. Scalp wounds generally show capillary bleeding.

Styptics.—These are chemical substances, such as tincture of iron. which have the property of arresting capillary hæmorrhage when applied to a bleeding surface. They are not used as much as formerly, as they tend to cause sloughing of the tissues.

Posture.—A bleeding limb should be supported in an elevated position. For burst varicose veins, lay the patient flat and raise the leg on a chair. This generally stops the bleeding, but if not, apply a firm pad directly over the bleeding spot.

Internal Hæmorrhage.—Put the patient to bed, the foot of which should be raised. Bandage the limbs firmly from below upwards in order to keep the blood as much as possible in the trunk of the body. Keep the patient warm with extra blankets. If hot water bottles are used, be cautious of burns. Open the window wide to give as much air as possible. Oxygen inhalation is given if available. Water *ad lib* is allowed if the alimentary canal is not affected, but if this is unknown, do not give anything by mouth. Stimulants are strictly forbidden, as by raising the blood-pressure, bleeding is increased. Should fainting occur, do not attempt to revive the patient as this is nature's attempt at lessening the bleeding by reducing the force of the heart beat. While awaiting the arrival of the physician, the apparatus for intravenous saline should be prepared ; also morphia ($\frac{1}{4}$ gr.). Alarm should not be shown in front of the patient, but every effort made to calm his fear.

Epistaxis (see p 136.).—Seat the patient on a chair. Keep the head slightly back. Apply pressure and ice-cold water to the bridge of the nose and nape of the neck. Hold the arms above the head. If the bleeding persists, prepare apparatus for plugging the nose with adrenalin (1-1000) while awaiting the physician.

Hæmatemesis (see p. 169).—Bleeding from the stomach. The blood is dark and " coffee-ground " in appearance and is vomited. It is acid in reaction. Keep the patient flat and warm. Give nothing through the mouth. Apply an ice-bag to the stomach.

Hæmoptysis (see p. 170).—Bleeding from the lungs. The blood is bright red and is coughed up, or flows. It is frothy, being mixed with air, and is alkaline in reaction. Keep the patient flat with the head and shoulders raised. Turn the face to the affected side to avoid suffocation with blood. Keep warm. Do not permit talking. Give cold mouth washes and ice to suck. Cold drinks are allowed as desired.

Unconsciousness.

This is a state of deep insensibility and may be due to different causes :—

1. Fainting.
2. Concussion.
3. Fits.
4. Poisoning.
5. Coma (diabetic or uræmic).

The first thing to do is to determine the cause if possible.

1. *Fainting.*—Lay the patient flat with the head low. Loosen tight clothing. Give plenty of fresh air. Smelling salts must be used with caution. Recovery usually occurs in a few minutes, but if delayed unduly send for the doctor.

2. *Concussion.*—Keep the patient flat in a semi-darkened room. Apply ice to the head.

3. *Fits.*—

  (a) *Apoplexy.*—Raise the head and loosen tight clothing, especially round the neck. Keep the patient warm, but remember the danger of burning a paralysed patient with hot bottles. Keep the head turned to one side to allow saliva to run out freely.

  (b) *Epilepsy.*—Place the patient on the floor and loosen tight clothing. Remove furniture, etc., against which the patient might injure himself. Insert a spoon handle (covered with rubber or linen) between the teeth to prevent the tongue being bitten. Make no attempt to control the limb movements. The fit passes off in a short time and the patient then sleeps for some hours. He should not be left alone during this period.

4. *Poisoning.*—Endeavour to waken up patient. If able to swallow, give emetic or stimulant (see pp. 417-418).

5. *Coma.*—Very little in the way of first aid can be done for these patients unless it be due to diabetes or poisoning. The latter is dealt with on p. 417. In diabetes, if the condition is one of sus-

pected hyperglycæmia, as evidenced by sugar in the urine, prepare insulin for the immediate use of the doctor. In hypoglycæmia give the patient sugar and orange juice if he can swallow at all ; if not a solution of glucose is given per rectum.

Fractures.

A fracture is a broken bone. It may be caused by violence, direct or indirect, or by disease of the bone.

Fractures are recognized by :—

1. Unnatural mobility of the part.
2. Swelling.
3. Pain.
4. Bruising.
5. Deformity.
6. Shortening of a limb.
7. Crepitus.
8. Shock.

There are many types of fractures (see p. 155), but the most important are the simple, compound, and complicated.

When handling the patient it is extremely important to avoid converting a simple fracture into a compound one, as in this case an open wound has to be dealt with in addition to the fracture. If the wound should become septic it greatly delays union.

Complicated fractures are most serious as the fractured ends of the bone injure adjacent organs or tissues. Common examples are a broken rib penetrating the lung ; a depressed fracture of the skull causes injury to the brain substance.

First Aid.—The first thing is to arrest hæmorrhage, if any ; secondly, apply an antiseptic dressing if required ; thirdly, render the fractured part immovable by means of improvised splints before moving the patient, if the leg or body is injured ; finally, treat the patient for shock by keeping him warm and giving hot drinks and stimulants.

Fractured Femur.—As a person with this type of fracture always suffers severely from shock he must be handled very carefully. While one person steadies the limb at the hip, another should exert a steady pull on the limb to correct any gross deformity. A long splint is then adjusted to the outer side of the limb. This should reach from the armpit to below the foot. It is secured in

398

position by bandages tied above and below the fracture. Another is tied at hip level and another round the chest. The lower part of the leg is fixed by a bandage below the knee; while another holds the feet and splint together. A short splint placed on the inner side of the thigh is helpful in giving extra support. The two limbs are held securely together by a bandage passed around both knees and ankles.

N.B.—The word bandage refers to triangular ones, but if these are not available, handkerchiefs, scarves, etc., may be used.

Fracture of the Tibia and Fibula.—Apply splints to the outer and inner sides of the leg. Secure by bandages, placing one above and one below the site of fracture. Secure the knees and feet as already described.

Fracture of the Patella.—Place the limb on a straight splint. Apply bandages above and below the knee and at the centre of the thigh, while another secures the ankle and foot.

Fracture of the Ankle or Foot.—Treat as for fracture of the lower leg, but do not attempt to correct deformity.

Fracture of the Clavicle.—One method is to place a large pad in the axilla, pull the shoulders well back, place the arm across the chest, and bandage in position. A piece of lint or linen should always be placed between the skin surfaces to prevent soreness.

Fracture of the Humerus.—Apply a short splint to the inner side and a longer one to the outer side of the upper arm. Bandage them in position and secure the arm to the body by a broad bandage. Then support the lower arm in a narrow sling. Gooch splinting, if available, makes a good first-aid splint.

Fracture of Ulna and Radius.—Bandage the arm on a straight splint, palm upwards, and support it in a broad sling.

Colles' Fracture.—Do not try to reduce this, but treat as for fractured forearm.

Fractured Hand.—Wrap the hand in plenty of wool and bandage lightly to a splint.

Fractured Ribs.—Instruct the patient to expel the breath as much as possible. Then apply a broad bandage tightly round the chest. This gives some support and limits respiratory movements.

Fracture of the Sternum.—Lay the patient flat with a small sandbag or hard pillow placed between the shoulders. As this fracture may be associated with a fractured spine, it needs very careful handling.

Fracture of the Spine.—This is possibly the most serious of all forms of fracture and is accompanied by severe shock. It is especially dangerous on account of the possibility of injury to the spinal cord. There may be paralysis below the site of injury. The thighs, knees, legs, and feet are bandaged together and the patient kept absolutely flat. A rigid stretcher is obtained, and four assistants are necessary for lifting. This should be done at a given signal to avoid jolting or further damage. Assistant No. 1 places his hands gently above and below the suspected site of the fracture, No. 2 places his hands beneath the hips, No. 3 lifts the head and shoulders, while No. 4 lifts the legs. Keep the patient warm with blankets and hot bottles, and remove him to hospital as quickly as possible. If the accident occurs in the middle of a busy street, the traffic must be held up until the patient can be moved with safety. This remark applies to all fractures, which must be rendered immobile with splints before removal is allowed.

Fracture of the Pelvis.—This generally results from being crushed or run over. Pass a broad binder, such as a roller towel, tightly round the pelvis. Bandage the thighs and legs together and lift on to the stretcher as in the case of a fractured spine. It is important to prevent the patient from passing urine until he has been examined by a doctor. Treat for shock.

Fractured Skull.—Remember there may be no external sign of fracture. It is recognized by a gradual onset of insensibility with stertorous breathing caused by pressure of a piece of bone or by blood-clot. Protect the wound, if any, by a clean dressing. If bleeding is severe, apply a ring pad between the dressing and the bandage. The patient is kept in the lying position with the head slightly raised.

Fractured Lower Jaw.—Gently close the mouth and firmly apply a four-tailed bandage.

400

Dislocation of the Lower Jaw.

Place the thumb, protected by a handkerchief, inside the mouth, while the fingers grasp the angle of the jaw. Press quickly downwards and backwards, when the condyle of the jaw will slip into place and the mouth will shut with a snap.

Other Dislocations.

Should be treated on the same lines as a fracture.

Sprains and Strains.

If there is much pain and swelling apply cold water bandages or an evaporating lotion such as lead lotion. Severe sprains must be treated by a doctor.

Bruises.

Apply cold pads as quickly as possible and a firm bandage.

Impacted Fish Hook.

If possible push the hook onwards through the skin, break off the barb, then withdraw the stem. Apply iodine and a clean dressing and bandage.

Wounds.

Arrest any bleeding first. Next bathe the part with a warm antiseptic lotion such as dettol to cleanse it, then apply a clean dressing. If the wound is extensive or likely to become septic a doctor should be consulted without delay.

Drowning and Suffocation.

In a case of drowning, as soon as the patient is rescued place him prone, with the face turned to the right and the head resting on the left arm. Clear the mouth and nose of mud and weeds, then compress the chest to empty the air passages of water. This can also be accomplished by raising the body at the hips, while an assistant compresses the chest. Artificial respiration is then commenced. This should be carried out rhythmically at the normal rate of respiration. Schafer's method is most generally adopted (see p. 309). An assistant in the meantime secures a doctor, hot

401

bottles, and stimulants. Artificial respiration must be kept up if there is the slightest sign of a pulse beat. When the breathing is well established, wet clothing is removed, and the patient wrapped in blankets. The limbs are rubbed to restore circulation and stimulants are administered. On no account should the patient be allowed to walk home, however well he may feel, as secondary failure of the respiration sometimes occurs later. A doctor should always be consulted.

Hanging and Strangulation.

Having cut the body down, remove the cord and any tight clothing. Then start artificial respiration. Send an assistant for a doctor.

Foreign Bodies in the Throat.

Open the mouth widely and try to hook up the obstruction with the finger. Failing this, place the patient downward and slap him smartly between the shoulders. This often dislodges the particle. If not, send for the doctor immediately

Burns and Scalds.

Burns may be caused by dry or moist heat and may vary from a slight reddening of the skin to complete destruction of the tissues. First aid obviously aims at preventing primary shock and suffocation. The flames are best extinguished by excluding air. To do this wrap a rug, blanket, or coat around the victim. If the front is burning, lay him on his back on the floor. By doing so the flames will be confined to the front and so further injury avoided. Prevent him from rushing out of doors or to an open window. Having extinguished the flames, the patient must be treated for shock. Do not attempt to remove the burnt clothing, but keep him warm with blankets and hot bottles, and raise the foot of the bed. Send for the doctor, and in the meantime give oxygen if available. Prepare for giving a saline and also have morphia ($\frac{1}{4}$ gr.) ready. Do not use oil for the burns. Linen dipped in strong cold tea is best because of the tannin it contains. If the eyes are burnt, instil one or two drops of castor oil. Burnt children can be immediately immersed in a warm bath to which bicarbonate of soda has been added. This relieves pain and minimizes shock. If the burn is caused by acids or alkalis, remove clothing which is soaked in the solution. Then wash the part with running water to remove the corrosive. Afterwards for an acid burn apply an alkaline substance such as a solution of soda bicarbonate ; for an alkali burn, apply a solution of lemon juice or vinegar.

Electrical Burns.

When a severe electrical shock is experienced the patient becomes unconscious, with shallow breathing and feeble pulse. The skin at the point of contact will be burned. First turn off the electric current, but if this is impossible, insulate the hands with rubber gloves or a mackintosh, stand on a dry coat or piece of wood, which acts as an insulator between yourself and the earth, then with a rapid pull try and free the patient. He will then be treated for shock and burns. If the breathing has ceased, artificial respiration must be started.

GAS WARFARE PRECAUTIONS

THE lessons learnt from the Great War show that it is very difficult to prevent enemy aircraft from reaching their objective. At the present time these difficulties are greatly increased owing to (a) the fact that planes can travel at much higher speeds ; (b) that they can fly at much greater altitudes ; (c) they have greater weight-carrying possibilities.

In a war of the future, three types of bombs are to be feared :—

Gas bombs (gas or spray).
Incendiary bombs (thermite).
High explosive bombs.

With proper precautions the first of these will be the least dangerous, but without such precautions it may well be the most dangerous of the three. Panic will be the greatest problem, and to avoid this the population must be persuaded to stay in their homes or in shelters provided, and to keep the streets clear.

Measures of Protection include :—

1. A *Gas-proof room* in every private house, equipped with necessaries for a twenty-four hours' stay.
2. *Public shelters*, quickly and easily reached.
3. *Rapid evacuation of slum dwellers* by a well-organized transport system.
4. *Control of city lighting*, so that there could be a rapid "black-out."
5. *Plans for the maintenance of the essential services* upon which the life and health of the people depend.
6. *Provision of adequate protection* to the main industries to enable them to carry on, etc.

In addition to these :—

a) *Fire brigades* must be trained, equipped, and maintained for dealing with thermite and other outbreaks of fire.
(b) *Squads of highly trained chemists* will be necessary to detect the type of gas used, and advise as to the best methods of dealing with it.

404

    (c) *Decontamination centres* must be provided complete with shower-baths, clothing stores, decontamination plant, and highly trained personnel. These centres must be so situated that they can be reached within ten minutes.

    (d) *The organization of casualty and base hospitals.*

    (e) *The organization and control of first-aid squads.*

    (f) *The organization of road-repair and road-decontamination squads.*

    (g) *The maintenance of the sanitary services.*

Gas may be used as a liquid, spray, solid, or vapour. The solid is just as deadly as the liquid. Mustard gas will freeze into a white crystalline solid at 14·4° C. or 55° F., and in this solid state will not give off vapour, but will do so as soon as the atmospheric temperature rises. This insidious behaviour makes it dangerous to deal with. It will burn the hand if touched while frozen.

Gases are divided into two main groups :—

    1. Persistent gas (P.G.). Remains for long periods.

    2. Non-persistent gas (N.P.G.). Is soon dispersed by wind and air-currents.

Persistent Gas includes :—

    Ethyl-idoacetate (K.S.K.) } Tear gases
    Bromobenzyl cyanide (B.B.C.) } (lachrymators).
    Dichlor-ethyl (mustard gas) } Blister gases
    Lewisite (the dew of death) } (vesicants).

Non-persistent Gases include :—

    Phosgene (C.G.) } Choking gas
    Chlorine (Cl.) } (lung irritants).
    Diphenylchlorarsine (D.A.) } Nose irritant gas
    Dichlor-methyl-ether (D.M.) } (sternutators).
    Diphenyl-cyanarsine (D.C.) }
    Chloracetophenone (C.A.P.). Tear gas.
    Arsine (arseniuretted hydrogen).

Tear Gases are easily detected owing to their immediate irritant effect upon the eyes, giving rise to severe pain, profuse lachrymation, and, in some persons, nausea or even vomiting. The symptoms soon disappear after removal from the contaminated area.

C.A.P. is a white solid which vaporizes when heated, the gas being invisible. It causes slight skin irritation and is non-lethal.

K.S.K. A dark brown oily liquid when impure and smells of pear-drops. May be a respiratory irritant.

B.B.C. A brown liquid with a pungent odour. Is an invisible gas and very persistent.

No treatment is usually needed for tear gases, but if so, wash out the eyes with normal saline solution. A drop of castor oil may be inserted in the eye.

Choking Gases.

Phosgene.—In the natural state is a whitish cloud, the size of which is no indication of the amount of gas present, as it may be concentrated. It has a pungent smell resembling musty hay. All lung irritants cause the same kind of symptoms. The chief effect of the gas is in the deep substance of the lungs, involving the smaller bronchioles and the alveoli, which become inflamed, full of blood and inflammatory exudate, and air. This causes the lung substance to swell and become greatly congested. The bronchi and trachea are filled with coughed-up yellowish or blood-stained fluid which may be seen as bubbles of froth at the nose and mouth. There is immediate irritation of the respiratory passages, a feeling of tightness and constriction in the chest. These symptoms may quickly pass off until about twenty-four hours later, when they return with increased severity. Vomiting may occur at this stage. The subsequent course varies with the severity of the case :—

    (a) The milder type, with flushed face and rapid, panting respiration. He is very drowsy, but improved by sleep.

    (b) The severe or "blue" type with much mental distress, quick full pulse, rapid shallow breathing, cyanosis. This type may relapse into

    (c) The very severe or "grey" type. Collapse is extreme ; pulse rapid and thready ; the skin is cold and clammy, and the face is grey. The prognosis is very bad.

Treatment.—The three things of most importance are :—

    1. Rest, *i.e.*, absence of all exertion. The patient should be made to lie down. All cases must be removed on stretchers.

2. Warmth. Treat for shock—with blankets, hot-water bottles, etc.

3. Oxygen. Get patient quickly to hospital, where O_2 can be administered with the Haldane apparatus. (*N.B.—* The hospitals will probably provide O_2 units, the gas being given by specially trained nurses under medical supervision, who will concentrate on this to the exclusion of all other work.) The O_2 will be given twenty-five minutes on and five minutes off.

Venesection is often helpful, but there are difficulties to be remembered. Stimulants are useful. Also pituitrin 1/2 c.c. at intervals.

Morphia is contraindicated, while digitalis and strychnine are probably of very little value. Expectorants are forbidden. Emesis, if induced, is harmful, therefore apomorphine and ipecacuanha are both forbidden. Artificial respiration is distinctly dangerous, as it may force a large amount of fluid from the congested lungs into the bronchi and trachea, and so drown the patient. Posture to assist lung drainage is helpful. Turn the face to the side and raise the foot of the bed 3 ft. for a few minutes at a time. Mouth hygiene is also very important. To allay thirst, which may be extreme, give repeated sips of fluid. Food must be sparingly given.

Chlorine.—Symptoms and treatment the same as for phosgene, except that there is no " delay period."

The Nose Irritant Gases.

These are released as particulate clouds. *D.M.* is a yellow crystalline solid, the others are white, and they all contain arsenic in their composition. They have no smell. *Symptoms* include a burning pain in nose, mouth, and throat; sneezing; pain in the eyes and lachrymation; frontal headache and pain in the gums and jaws. Mental depression is severe and suicide must be guarded against. Temporary paralysis may ensue, but quickly passes off. On being removed from the infected area the symptoms may increase at first, but soon subside. Recovery is rapid. No treatment usually needed.

The Vesicants.

Mustard gas is the most dreaded and poisonous of all gases and produces casualties far in excess of its killing power. It is a dark, heavy, oily fluid which slowly vaporizes, and must be distinguished from *K.S.K.* and *B.B.C.*, which are similar in appearance. It is very persistent. Bursting bombs may scatter liquid or spray over a considerable area. It has an odour of garlic, mustard, or onions, and is easily recognizable at first. but after a few sniffs the nose appears to become insensible to it and this is an added danger, as it may give a sense of false security. The boiling-point of mustard gas is 417° F., 217° C. The freezing-point is 14·4° C., 55° F. Although only slightly soluble in water, it is highly soluble in animal fats, and animal fat in any form should be carefully avoided in treatment. The best solvents are alcohol, ether, and petrol. Mustard gas has great powers of penetration, except for glass, metals, and certain woods. It acts as a cell poison in the body, being five times as toxic as phosgene.

Intense irritation of the entire respiratory tract is caused and the necrosis of the mucous membrane may block the air-passages and encourage the breeding of bacteria, thus giving rise to pneumonia and other secondary infections.

The symptoms do not appear for from four to twenty-four hours, depending on the concentration and length of exposure. An early onset is of serious import. Affection of the eyes sets up conjunctivitis and photophobia. Ulceration is rare and only occurs if the eye is splashed with liquid. Blindness is uncommon. Recovery takes from two to four months. Cocaine is especially contraindicated in the treatment of these cases, since it tends to loosen the corneal epithelium. Atropine should be used instead.

The Skin.—The sweat glands are readily damaged and there is burning and itching of the skin, and blisters form. The burnt areas show a brown discoloration which may turn black, but which eventually disappears. The vesicles occur in crops, are reddish in colour, and filled with a yellow serum. The damaged epithelium may be shed, exposing a raw, red, painful surface, but this should be avoided if possible, as it serves as a natural protection. It is a characteristic feature of mustard-gas burns, that the deeper tissues become involved and the resulting ulcer shows an overhanging edge. If vesicles have not formed, dust the skin with dry dusting powder. If the skin had been exposed to mustard gas, two lines of action are possible :—

1. To destroy the poison by antidotes.
2. Washing it away before it penetrates too deeply.

To be effective, first-aid must be applied within the first five minutes. Apply the antidote first, *i.e.*, chloride of lime paste or bleach vaseline. These are prepared as follows :—

Bleach paste.—One part bleach to one part water.
Bleach vaseline.—Two parts bleach to one part vaseline.

Rub well in for one minute, then remove with a dry rag if ointment has been used, but well wash off the paste with hot soap and water. In either case the skin should be thoroughly cleaned by scrubbing with soap and water, under a shower if possible. If liquid is actually seen on the skin, it may be removed with petrol. If the clothing is contaminated, remove it carefully and send it to be decontaminated ; then treat the skin. If blisters have formed, puncture them, but do not remove the epithelium. Swab with 20 per cent. dettol or tannic acid.

For the respiratory system, inhalations of menthol, Friar's balsam, or creosote are useful. These cases are best kept in isolation owing to their susceptibility to secondary infection.

For gastro-intestinal symptoms the diet should consist of fluid only.

Lewisite.—Resembles mustard gas in its symptoms and treatment, but the following differences should be noted :—

1. There is no delayed action, the symptoms being felt immediately.
2. The vesicles only involve the epithelium and are pearly-white in appearance.
3. The serum contains arsenic and therefore must be evacuated quickly, or arsenical poisoning may ensue.
4. It has a strong smell of geraniums.

N.B.—The gas mask gives complete protection for the lachrymator, sternutator, and lung irritant gases ; also for the respiratory system and eyes in the vesicant gases. The skin must, however, be protected by clothing made of oilskin or other gas-proof material.

Arsine.—Invisible gas. Liberated by action of moisture on calcium arsenide. It is odourless in low concentration. The gas produces weakness, headache, nausea, gastric pain, and backache.

There is breathlessness on exertion. Severe symptoms may be delayed for an hour or two.

Treatment.—Patients must be treated as stretcher cases and medical aid procured quickly. Hot sweet tea is given, and rest and warmth are essential.

The Gas Mask.

This is designed to protect the eyes, nose, and throat, and there are at present two main types :—

1. The civilian duty respirator.
2. The service respirator.

Both give adequate protection and the same principles of construction underlie each, although the details vary somewhat.

The service respirator consists of :—

A *face-piece or mask.* This is made of rubber covered with stockinet, with elastic bands to pass over the head to keep it in position. There are two large eye-pieces made of triplex glass, and these are kept polished by " anti-dim." Expired air passes out through a valve, where it is discharged. From the valve holder *a flexible corrugated tube* connects with a *canister,* or metal box, containing activated nut-charcoal and a filter of cotton-wool pads. At the bottom of the container a rubber disc is fixed so that air can be drawn through the container during inspiration. The whole outfit is carried in a waterproof haversack.

Care of the Respirator.

1. After use the inside of the face-piece is carefully wiped out with a rag kept in the haversack for the purpose.

2. Disinfection.

    (*a*) The same procedure as before, but the rag used is first wrung out in a solution of Izal.

    (*b*) Turn the face-piece inside out and fill the hollow thus formed with about $\bar{3}$ii of Izal solution. Do not allow any of the fluid to run into the Tissot channel or it will escape into the canister and ruin it. To prevent this, place the thumb in it to block it.

    (*c*) After exposure to infection, or when passing the respirator on to another person, complete immersion of the face-piece will be necessary. Detach the tube from the container, then prepare the solution by adding 3 parts of Izal to 100 parts of water (roughly, 1 eggcupful to 1 bucket of water). This quantity should only be used for fifty face-pieces. The whole tube and face-piece is immersed for five minutes, after which it is rinsed in clear water and then thoroughly wiped. Place it in a draught to dry, and never use heat.

General Points in Care of Respirator.

1. Keep it clean.
2. Avoid moisture.
3. Avoid prolonged storage.
4. Avoid heat.
5. Avoid incorrect folding.
6. Avoid stretching of the head harness as this spoils the fit.
7. Avoid dents in the container, as these cause resistance in inhalation.
8. Avoid stretching or twisting of the tube.
9. Do not scrub the haversack, it destroys the proofing. If soiled with mud, etc., allow it to dry, then remove with a stiff brush.

Some Special Points to Remember.

1. The earlier decontamination is begun the more complete it will be. This applies to persons, clothing, apparatus, etc.
2. If in doubt whether the gas is in liquid or vapour form, treat it as vapour.
3. Do not touch any gas-contaminated surface with unprotected hands.
4. Pay great attention to the efficiency of the respirator and protective suit.
5. Do all that lies in your power to keep the people calm and avoid panic.

BLANKET FOLD

As designed by

ALDERSBROOK HOSPITAL FIRST-AID POST, WANSTEAD AND WOODFORD

Adaptations by S. F. Witchalls

The shoulder brace by E. C. Bailey

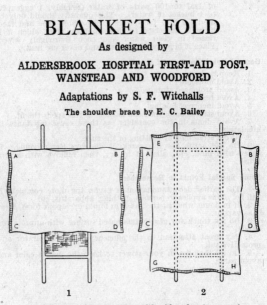

1

2

1, Lay first blanket crosswise with side edge to cross-bar at head.

2, Lay second blanket lengthwise with end edge half-way over handles at head.

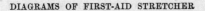

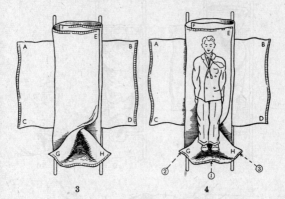

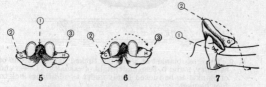

3, Fold back the corners of second blanket at foot.
4, Place casualty on stretcher.
5, 6, 7, Method of folding blanket over feet.

413

8, 9, The cross-blanket at A and C is tucked under left side of casualty, B and D, then under right of casualty. Lower end of blanket to be tucked firmly under as additional lock to foot blanket.

10, To protect the head, grasp the long blanket at arrows 4 and 5 in Fig. 8. Tuck them in on each side of face.

11, In lifting this adaptation, care must be taken to grasp firmly the long blanket at the head, indicated by arrows 6 and 7 (vide Fig. 13).

414

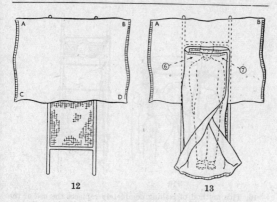

12, 13, To blanket a tall casualty.
14, 15, The blankets may be kept folded and ready for use.

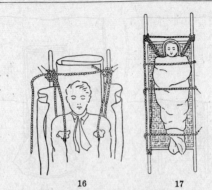

16   17

16, This method of lashing completely replaces the use of the
    chair-knot for casualties with injuries to the lower limbs.
17, Continue with normal cross-lashings.

SOME POISONS AND THEIR ANTIDOTES

A FTER accidental swallowing of any poisonous substances life can sometimes be saved and symptoms greatly minimized by giving a large quantity of water to drink. This dilutes and therefore weakens the poison, and delays absorption while other preparations for the evacuation of the stomach are being made.

Gastric lavage is carried out by means of a stomach pump, but this is contraindicated when strong mineral acids have been taken, as evidenced by staining of the lips and buccal mucous membrane. In the case of corrosive acids, *e.g.*, carbolic acid, a soft rubber tube gently inserted does no harm. A dilute solution of bicarbonate of soda or sulphate of magnesia may be used. Since the latter is a useful antidote in many poisons, some of it may be left in the stomach.

Emetics are substances which produce vomiting, but should not be used in strong corrosive or acid poisons.

Examples of Emetics :—

Sulphate of zinc, 30 grs. to half a pint of water.
Sulphate of copper, 30 grs. to half a pint of water.
Mustard, ℥ii to half a pint of water.
Warm water, copious draughts.
Salt, ℥ss to 1 pint of water.
Apomorphine, gr. $\frac{1}{10}$, injected hypodermically.

Demulcents are substances which soothe the mucous membrane of the gastro-intestinal tract, and include :

Milk.
Barley-water.
Albumen water.
Olive oil.

Stimulants are necessary in many types of poisoning. The following may be given :—

> Alcohol, *e.g.*, brandy or whisky.
> Black coffee (strong).
> Strong tea.
> Sal volatile.
> Smelling salts.
> Oxygen.

Shock and Collapse (for symptoms see pp. 90 and 314).—Treatment consists of :

1. The application of warmth by means of well-covered hot-water bottles and extra blankets.

2. The introduction of warm saline into the body.

3. The administration of suitable stimulants.

Some General Principles in the Treatment of Poisons :—

1. Send for the doctor.

2. Give the antidote (see p. 23). **(N.B.**—*If the stomach is to be washed out, or emetics given, this should be done first.*)

3. Treat for shock and for any other symptoms.

4. Keep any receptacle, such as cup, bottle, etc., which has contained the poison.

5. Keep for inspection any fæces, urine, vomit, or sputum.

6. Be guarded in what is said to relatives or friends of the patient.

7. Make a mental note of anything which may be said by the patient.

N.B.—*The last four points may be of the greatest assistance in a Court of Law.*

SOME COMMON POISONS

Poison.	Lavage or Emetic.	Antidote.	Other Treatment.
Aconite . .	Lavage or emetic	Tr. digitalis or liq. atropinæ, ℳii	Keep flat with head low. Stimulants. Treat for shock. Unceasing artificial respiration.
Alcohol . .	Lavage or emetic	..	Strychnine, gr. $\frac{1}{20}$. Cold douche, etc. Leave coffee in stomach after lavage.
Ammonia .	None	Weak acetic acid or vinegar	Olive oil and demulcents. Treat shock. Morphine. (Tracheotomy may be necessary.)
Antimony (*Tartar emetic*)	Not usually required	Tannin	Alcohol. Strong tea or coffee. Warmth. Treat shock. Keep prone. Give demulcents.
Arsenic . .	Lavage or emetic	Dialysed iron, ℥i every two hours for some hours	Large dose of castor oil to clear out intestines. Demulcent drinks.
Belladonna and Atropine	Lavage or emetic	Tannin or tea, morphine, gr. $\frac{1}{4}$	Free stimulation. Artificial respiration.
Camphor .	Lavage or emetic	..	Stimulants. Alternate hot and cold douches. Oils.

419

SOME COMMON POISONS

Poison.	Lavage or Emetic.	Antidote.	Other Treatment.
Carbolic, Lysol, etc.	Lavage with very soft tube	Mag. sulph.	Albumen water, oil, milk. Treat shock.
Caustic Potash Caustic Soda	} Neither {	Dilute vinegar or lemon juice	Treat shock. Oil and butter. Demulcents.
Chloral Hydrate	Lavage or emetic	Strychnine, gr. $\frac{1}{10}$, or atropine, gr. $\frac{1}{50}$	Stimulants. Artificial respiration. External warmth. Rouse patient.
Cocaine . .	Lavage or emetic	Strychnine, gr. $\frac{1}{10}$	Stimulants. Artificial respiration. External warmth. Rouse patient.
Corrosive Sublimate	*See Mercury.*		
Digitalis . .	Emetic and lavage (*zinc sulphate, gr. $\frac{1}{2}$*)	Opium and tannin	Keep in horizontal position. Free stimulation. Alcohol.
Fungi . .	Emetic or lavage	Atropine or morphine	Free stimulation and friction.
Hydrochloric Acid (*Spirits of salt*)	Same as for Sulphuric Acid.		
Hydrocyanic Acid (*Prussic acid*)	Lavage or rapid emetic	Ammonia inhalation. Ferri-sulph.	Alternate hot and cold douches. Artificial respiration. Treat for shock.
Iodine . .	Emetic or lavage (*used continuously*)	Starch in water	Demulcent drinks. Bread, arrowroot, flour.
Laudanum (*Opium*)	*See Morphine.*		
Lead Salts .	Lavage or emetic	Sulphate of zinc	Demulcents. Epsom salts. White of egg.

Poison.	Lavage or Emetic.	Antidote.	Other Treatment.
Mercury . .	Emetic or lavage	..	Demulcents. Treat for shock. White of egg.
Morphine .	Lavage with pot. permanganate or emetic (*apomorphine*, gr. ⅛)	Pot. permanganate. Atropine	Stimulation. Prevent sleep. Artificial respiration if necessary.
Nitric Acid .	Neither	Alkalis	Demulcents. Magnesia, lime water, or albumen water.
Nux Vomica .	*See* **Strychnine.**		
Opium . .	*See* **Morphine.**		
Oxalic Acid .	Lavage or emetics	Lime water and chalk	Castor oil. Free stimulation. Demulcents. Treat shock.
Phosphorus .	Lavage or emetics. ($CuSO_4$)	Permanganate of potash, gr. 5, in 1 oz. of water. Also $CuSO_4$, gr. 5	Avoid oils but give French oil of turpentine. Purgatives. Demulcents.
Ptomaines .	Lavage with Condy's fluid	..	Purgation and colonic lavage. Salines. Strychnine. Treat for shock.
Silver Nitrate (*Lunar caustic*)	Lavage and emetics	Large doses of common salt	White of egg, milk, and water.
Soda, Caustic .	*See* **Caustic Soda.**		
Strychnine .	Lavage before spasms appear. Emetic (*apomorphine*, gr. ⅛)	Tannin or charcoal. Chloral. pot. bromide	Chloroform inhalation. Morphine. Artificial respiration.

421

Poison.	Lavage or Emetic.	Antidote.	Other Treatment.
Sulphuric Acid (*Oil of vitriol*)	Neither	Dilute alkalis, *e.g.*, lime, soap, chalk, magnesia, etc.	Wall plaster in warm water. Oils. Demulcents.
Tobacco . .	Emetics	Tannin	Free stimulation. Strychnine. Recumbent position.
Turpentine .	Emetics	Mag. sulph.	Albumen water or milk.
Veronal . .	Lavage	Strychnine	Artificial respiration. Keep warm.
Zinc Chloride .	Cautious lavage, emetic (*apomorphine, gr. ½*)	..	Tannin. Egg albumen. Oils. Give demulcents freely.

METHOD OF WORKING OUT DOSAGE, ETC.

1. To find how much diluent to add in order to weaken a solution.

   EXAMPLE.—*Prepare 1 pint of carbolic lotion 1/80 from stock lotion of strength 1/20.*

   1/20 solution will contain 1 oz. of carbolic acid in 20 oz. of solution.

   ∴ 20 oz. of this solution diluted to 80 oz. will produce 1/80 solution.

   ∴ $\frac{20}{80}$ oz. of this solution dilute to 1 oz. will produce 1/80 solution.

   ∴ $\frac{20 \times 20}{80}$ oz. of this solution diluted to 20 oz. will produce 1 pint of 1/80 solution.

   $$\frac{20 \times 20}{80} = 5 \text{ oz.}$$

   ANSWER.—5 fl. oz. of stock solution is diluted to 1 pint.

2. *N.B.*—1 fl. oz. of water weighs 437·5 gr.

   1 fl. oz. of 1 % solution will contain 4·375 gr.

   A. To make up a solution of a certain percentage.

   EXAMPLE.—*Prepare 5 fl. oz. of a 4 % solution.*

   Multiply together 4·375, the percentage and the number of fluid ounces required.

   $$4 \cdot 375 \times 4 \times 5 = 87 \cdot 5 \text{ gr.}$$

   ANSWER.—Dissolve 87·5 gr. of substance in water and adjust the volume to 5 fl. oz.

   B. To make up a percentage solution of volume in volume, *e.g.*, pure lysol, the following method will be found useful:—

   EXAMPLE.—*Prepare 15 fl. oz. of a 5 % solution of lysol.*

   100 fl. oz. will contain 5 fl. oz.

   1 ,, ,, ,, $\frac{5}{100}$,,

   15 ,, ,, ,, $\frac{15 \times 5}{100} = \frac{3}{4}$ oz. = 6 fl. drachms.

   Dilute 6 fl. drachms of lysol to 15 fl. oz. with water.

3. *A.* To give a weaker hypodermic dose from stronger stock tablets.

EXAMPLE.—*Give morphia $\frac{1}{8}$ gr. from tablets $\frac{1}{4}$ gr.*

Dissolve the tablet in water, say 20 minims, then multiply the stock by the dilution, and divide by the required dose. Thus:

Stock tablets = morphia, $\frac{1}{4}$ gr.
Required dose = ,, $\frac{1}{8}$ gr.
Diluent = 20 minims.
$\therefore\ 4 \times 20 = 80 \div 8 = 10.$

ANSWER.—Each 10 minims contains morphia $\frac{1}{8}$ gr.

B. To give a stronger hypodermic dose when only weaker tablets are available.

EXAMPLE.—*Give morphia $\frac{1}{6}$ gr. from stock tablets $\frac{1}{8}$ gr.*

Take two tablets $\frac{1}{8}$ gr. $= \frac{1}{4}$ gr. Then dissolve these two in, say, 30 minims of water. Then follow the rule as before.

$4 \times 30 = 120 \div 6 = 20.$

ANSWER.—20 minims contains $\frac{1}{6}$ gr.

4. To estimate the amount of a drug in each dose of a prescription.

EXAMPLE.—*How much nux vomica is contained in each dose of the following prescription:—*

℞	Ext. cas. sag. liq. . . .	ʒiv
	Tinct. belladonna . . .	ʒii
	Tinct. nux vomica . . .	ʒii
	Sp. am. arom. . . .	ʒiv
	Sp. chlor.	ʒii
	Aq.	ad ℥vi

Sig. ℥ss. T.D.S.

Number of doses = 12.
Amount of nux vomica = 120 minims
$\therefore\ 120 \div 12 = 10$,,

ANSWER.—10 minims in each dose.

5. Young's rule for estimating the dose for a child under twelve years of age (at twelve years half the adult dose is given).

Divide the age by the age + 12 and multiply by the adult dose.

A. EXAMPLE.—*If the adult dose of strychnine is 1/60 gr., what proportion should a child four years old receive ?*

> The age of the child = four years.
> Adult dose   = 1/60 gr.

$$\therefore \quad \frac{4}{4+12} = \frac{4}{16} = \frac{1}{4} \times \frac{1}{60} = \frac{1}{240}.$$

The child should therefore receive 1/240 gr.

B. Dissolve the tablet, 1/60 gr., in a suitable amount of water, say 32 minims. Then follow Young's rule again.

$$\frac{4}{4+12} = \frac{4}{16} = \frac{1}{4} \times \frac{32}{1} = 8 \text{ minims.}$$

ANSWER.—To give 1/240 gr., 8 minims of solution are necessary.

AVERAGE NORMAL PHYSIOLOGICAL STANDARDS
Blood

Red blood cells . . .	5,000,000 per cub. mm.
White blood cells . .	6,000 to 10,000 per cub. mm.
Hæmoglobin . . .	100 %.
Colour index . . .	1.
Platelets	200,000 to 400,000 per cub. mm.
Reticulocytes . . .	Less than 1 %.
Average diameter of B.B.C.'s	7·1 to 7·5 μ (microns).
White cells . . .	Proportions of different cells.
Neutrophil polymorphs	50-70 %.
Lymphocytes .	20-40 %.
Monocytes . .	2-8 %.
Eosinophil polymorphs	1-4 %.
Basophil polymorphs	0·5-1 %.
Bleeding time . .	2-3 minutes.
Coagulation time .	2-8
Sugar	80-110 mg. per 100 c.c.
Non-protein nitrogen .	25-40 ,, ,,
Urea	20-35 ,, ,,
Urea nitrogen . .	10-15 ,, ,,
Uric acid . . .	2-4 ,, ,,
Creatinine . . .	1-2 ,, ,,
Creatine . . .	3-7 ,, ,,
Calcium . . .	9-11 ,, ,,
Inorganic phosphorus .	2·5-4·5 ,, ,,
Cholesterol . . .	140-180 ,, ,,
Chlorides . . .	450-520 ,, ,,
Total fat . . .	600-700 ,, ,,
Bilirubin . . .	Less than 0·5 Van den Bergh units.

426

Cerebro-spinal Fluid

Character	Clear ; colourless ; no coagulum.
Pressure	100-200 mm. of water.
Specific gravity . .	1,006-1,008.
Globulin (Pandy test) .	Nil.
Total protein . .	15-40 mg. per 100 c.c.
Sugar	50-60 ,, ,,
Non-protein nitrogen .	20-40 ,, ,,
Chlorides	720-750 ,, ,,
Cells	0-5 (lymphocytes).
Colloidal gold reaction .	Negative.

Urine

Reaction (fresh specimen) .	Acid.
Specific gravity . .	1,015-1,020.
Albumin, sugar, and acetone	Nil. to qualitative tests.
Urea	2 gm. per 100 c.c.
Volume passed per 24 hours	About 1,500 c.c.

URINE TESTING

T HE Collection of a Sample of Urine for Testing.

When possible a twenty-four hours' specimen should be taken. It is convenient to start the collection at 8 A.M., when the patient first voids urine. This is discarded, but all urine passed afterwards is kept until 8 A.M. the following morning. The urine is contained in a clean, closed receptacle. If it is likely to decompose, a preservative must be added, e.g., chloroform or toluol. The collection is stirred with a glass rod before taking a specimen from it.

Points to Observe about the Urine.

1. *Quantity Passed.*—Normally this averages 40 to 50 oz., but may vary according to (a) the degree of activity of the skin; (b) climate; (c) severe exertion; (d) nervousness and hysteria; (e) disease. An increased secretion is observed in renal tuberculosis, diabetes mellitus and insipidus, chronic interstitial nephritis. A decreased output of urine is present in feverish states, acute nephritis, acute diarrhœa. (f) Drugs, e.g., potassium citrate, caffeine, digitalis.

2. *Colour.*—Normally urine has an amber colour due to several pigments, chief of which are urochrome and urobilinogen. The colour may be altered by (a) the presence of bile, which gives it a greenish-orange colour; (b) blood, which gives a reddish or smoky colour; (c) drugs, e.g., carbolic acid gives a greenish hue, santonin causes an orange colour, etc.; (d) pus causes a white appearance. (e) In polyuria the urine is often pale and watery-looking.

3. *Odour.*—Normally urine has a characteristic smell. In certain conditions this may be altered, e.g., a diabetic urine loaded with sugar often has a sweetish odour, due to the presence of acetone. In cystitis the urine has a fishy smell. Drugs also affect the odour, e.g., turpentine gives a smell of violets.

4. *Sediment.*—A pinkish deposit is due to an excess of urates, whereas a whitish sediment is caused by phosphates.

5. *The Reaction.*—Normally this is distinctly acid, and is determined by testing the urine with litmus paper. Blue litmus turns red in the presence of an acid. Conversely, red litmus turns blue when in contact with an alkali.

6. *Specific Gravity.*—In normal urine this varies from 1015 to 1025. As a rule, the greater the quantity of urine passed the lower is the specific gravity. Febrile states in which there is a diminished output of urine show a higher specific gravity of the latter. The specific gravity is taken with a urinometer, which should float free in the fluid without touching the sides of the test-glass, and must be read off at eye-level. The urine should be cold before the specific gravity is taken.

Test for Chlorides.

A test-tube is half-filled with urine, and to this is added a drop or two of nitric acid, which holds the phosphates in solution. Then a 3 per cent. solution of silver nitrate is added to the specimen, drop by drop, till about six drops have passed. This forms a white, curdy precipitate at once. The test should be compared with a known normal specimen of urine. Diminished chlorides are found in chronic nephritis, early stages of pneumonia, malignant disease, and in gastritis. Chlorides are increased in a diet rich in salt, in rickets, and hepatic cirrhosis.

Test for Urates.

The presence of urates in urine is insignificant unless they are excessive. Urates can be dispersed by boiling the urine.

Test for Albumen.

Albumen in urine consists of a mixture of serum albumen and serum globulin.

1. The specimen of urine must be fresh.
2. The specimen must also be clear. To ensure this the safest way is to filter it through special filter paper. (Blotting-paper makes a good substitute.)
3. The urine must be acid.
4. The specimen must be cold.

There are many tests for albumen, but the most usual are the three given as follows :—

(a) *The Acetic Acid Test.*—Heat the top inch or so of a test-tube filled three parts full of urine over a spirit lamp. A cloudiness will form, which may be due to phosphate or albumen. Add 2 or 3 drops of acetic acid, and if the cloud disappears it is

429

due to phosphates, but if it becomes intensified albumen is present.

(b) *Heller's Cold Test.*—Take about ½ in. of concentrated nitric acid in a test-tube, and with a pipette carefully overlay it with the urine. An opaque line appears at the junction of the fluids. This may take a few minutes to develop.

(c) *Salicyl-Sulphonic Acid Test.*—(i) If necessary filter the urine through a double layer of filter (or blotting) paper to get it as clear as possible. Reserve a portion as a control. To about 2 ml. in a test-tube add 5 drops of the reagent. Mix and compare with the control. If there is no increase in cloudiness, albumen is absent. If there is an increase, confirm by doing the boiling test. (ii) Boiling test. Take about 10 ml. of the cleared urine in a test-tube. If necessary make it definitely acid to litmus by the addition of diluted acetic acid. Divide into two portions. Boil one portion and compare with the control. An increase in turbidity or a flocculent precipitate indicates the presence of albumen or, possibly, earthy phosphates. To the hot fluids add 2 drops of strong acetic acid. Any remaining turbidity is due to albumen.

Esbach's Quantitative Estimation of Albumen.

Apparatus required :

(a) An Esbach's albuminometer. This is a large test-tube marked with a scale for reading off the precipitate in grammes per litre. Above this is the letter U, and about 2 in. higher is the letter R.

(b) Esbach's reagent. Consists of :

Picric acid	.	. 10 gm.
Citric acid	.	. 20 „
Water	.	. 1 litre.

The following points should be noted before carrying out the test :—

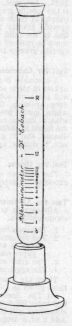

1. The urine must be acid.
2. Its specific gravity must be 1010 or below. If above this the urine must be diluted with an equal quantity of water, the final result being multiplied by 2.
3. The urine should be cold.
4. Keep the specimen in a room with a constant temperature.

Technique.—Pour some of the urine into the Esbach's tube up to the letter **U**. Then add reagent up to the letter **R**. Cork, and then gently invert the tube two or three times, taking care not to form bubbles. The tube is now set aside in an upright position and the precipitate allowed to settle for twenty-four hours. It is then read off on the scale as grammes per litre. If it is desired in grains per ounce the number of grammes is multiplied by ·4, *e.g.*, if the precipitate reaches the figure 4 it means that there is present 4 gms. of dried albumen to 1 litre of water. To bring this to grains per ounce $4 \times ·4 = 1·6$ gr. per ounce.

Test for Blood.

Take 1 in. of urine in a test-tube and add 1 or 2 drops of tincture of guaiacum. Carefully overlay this with $\frac{1}{2}$ in. of ozonic ether. Hold the tube in the hand to warm it for a few minutes. Blood is indicated by the appearance of a blue line at the junction of the fluids. The benzidine test has replaced the guaiacum test. Into a perfectly clean, dry test-tube place a small amount ("spatula end") of the solid benzidine. Add about 3 c.c. of glacial acetic acid. Agitate for a minute. To the solution, which should contain some undissolved benzidine, add an equal volume of 10 % hydrogen peroxide. Mix and pour over half into another perfectly clean tube. To one portion add 1 c.c. of the urine. The fluid rapidly acquires a deep blue tint if hæmoglobin or any of its derivatives is present. If the untreated fluid also develops a blue tint the test should be repeated, the control being treated with 1 c.c. of normal urine and the colours compared. By following this procedure the test is very conclusive.

Test for Bile.

There are several methods of testing for bile in the urine.
1. *Cole's Test.*—To about 1·5 c.c. of urine add 10 % barium chloride until no further precipitation is obtained. Mix and transfer to a centrifuge tube. Spin for three minutes. Pour away the supernatant fluid. Invert the tube and allow the fluid to drain

off as completely as possible. To the sediment add 3 c.c. of rectified alcohol (95 to 98 %) with a glass rod. Transfer the mixture to a dry test-tube and heat to boiling-point. Add a drop of 2 % potassium chlorate and boil again for at least half a minute. Allow the tube to stand until the precipitate of barium sulphate has settled. The supernatant alcohol layer is green or blue-green if bile pigments are present.

2. *Gmelin's Test.*—Overlay 1 in. of concentrated nitric acid with about 3 in. of the suspected urine. Bile is present when there is a play of colours at the junction of the fluids. This test can also be carried out by pouring some urine on to blotting or filter paper and then placing a drop of concentrated nitric acid on the moist paper. From the spreading edge of the drop of acid will develop a ring of various colours in which green predominates and forms the outer band.

3. *Iodine Test.*—Take an inch of the suspected urine in a test-tube and carefully overlay it with dilute tincture of iodine. A bright green ring will appear at the junction of the fluids if bile is present.

4. *Hay's Test for Bile Acids.*—Place 5 c.c. of urine in a test-tube. Sprinkle a small amount of flowers of sulphur on the surface of the urine. They fall to the bottom of the tube if bile salts are present, owing to the lower surface tension allowing the particles to get wet and then sink.

Test for Sugar.

Fehling's Qualitative Test.—Two stock solutions are used for this test :

Solution 1.

Copper sulphate	34·64 gm.
Conc. H_2SO_4 . . .	1 drop.
Distilled water . .	to 500 c.c.

Solution 2.

Sodium potassium tartrate . .	173 gm.
Sodium hydrate . . .	125 ,,
Distilled water . .	to 500 c.c.

Boil 3 c.c. of the reagent in one tube and the same volume of the suspected urine in another. The two hot solutions are mixed and allowed to stand. A brickish-red or orange precipitate indicates the presence of a significant amount of sugar (glucose). *N.B.*—Boiling of the mixture may lead to the formation of a greenish-yellow precipitate even with urines which do not contain an abnormal amount of sugar.

Quantitative Tests for Sugar.

Benedict's Method.—Dissolve 173 gr. sodium citrate and 90 gr. anhydrous sodium carbonate in about 600 c.c. of water. Filter and make up to 850 c.c. Dissolve 17·3 gr. crystalline copper sulphate in 100 c.c. distilled water and make up to 150 c.c. Slowly pour the copper sulphate into the alkaline citrate with constant stirring. The solution does not deteriorate, even on long standing.

Test.—To 5 c.c. of the reagent add 8 drops of the urine. Boil and maintain boiling for at least one and a half minutes. Allow the tube to cool in the rack for five minutes. Or boil the mixture and immerse the tube in a can of boiling water for three minutes and allow to cool in the rack. If glucose is present the whole body of the solution will be filled with a precipitate which may be red, yellow, or green in colour, depending on the amount of sugar. The test is positive with about 0·08 % of glucose. Since small amounts of glucose are always present in urine no significance should be attached to a faintly positive result.

A *Carwardines Saccharometer* can also be used to estimate the quality of sugar.

Test for Diacetic Acid.

Half fill a test-tube with freshly voided urine. Then add, drop by drop, some ferric chloride solution, which will cause a deposit of iron phosphate to form. Now filter the mixture and add a few more drops of ferric chloride. If diacetic acid is present a port-wine colour develops. The specimen is now divided into two, one being used as a control. One-half is boiled, when the colour will quickly disappear if it is due to diacetic acid.

Gerhardt's test with picric acid is still sometimes used, but is generally now replaced by the more reliable Rothera's test.

Test for Acetone.

Rothera's Test.—Into a test-tube place 2 in. of urine. Into another tube place 1 in. of powdered ammonium sulphate and a pinch of powdered sodium nitroprusside. Shake well for

433

about half a minute. Add 2 or 3 c.c. of strong ammonia. Mix and allow to stand undisturbed. A characteristic permanganate colour that may only develop above the layer of undissolved crystals indicates the presence of diacetic acid or acetone. The test cannot be regarded as negative until the mixture fails to show the purple coloration after standing for ten minutes.

Test for Pus.

Half fill a test-tube with the suspected urine and add some liquor potassæ. Then slowly pour the urine from one test-tube into another, and repeat this two or three times. The mixture will become thick and ropy if pus is present.

The presence of small amounts of pus is best detected by microscopic examination of the centrifuged deposit.

THE EXAMINATION OF FÆCES

THE microscopical and chemical examination of the fæces is principally the concern of the pathological laboratory, but much useful information may be gained by attention to the following points :—

1. *Quantity.*—The average adult stool weighs about 3 to 6 oz. The amount increases with the amount of vegetable matter in the diet.

2. *Form and Consistency.*—(a) Normally, soft and formed ; (b) hard, nodular, or scybalous in constipation ; (c) fluid or mushy in diarrhœa ; (d) flattened or ribbon-like in rectal obstruction or spastic colitis ; (f) frothy in fermentative conditions ; (g) greasy in jaundice, etc.

3. *Odour.*—This varies much with disease and dietary differences. It is most marked on a meat diet, and almost absent on a milk diet. Variations, such as sour, pungent, putrid, etc., occur in different diseases.

4. *Colour.*—Often important, influenced by diet, drugs, and disease.

  (a) Light brown to dark brown : normal.
  (b) Black : altered blood, charcoal, iron or bismuth medicines. Note that the benzidine test for "occult blood" is quite simple and sometimes gives valuable information in cancer of the stomach or duodenum.
  (c) Red : unaltered blood, beetroot.
  (d) Clay or putty coloured : bile deficiency in obstructive jaundice.
  (e) Very pale and greasy : undigested fats, jaundice.
  (f) Yellow : milk diet, rhubarb, santonin, senna.
  (g) Greenish : excess green vegetables, especially spinach, calomel.

5. *Mucus.*—Always important, and should be reported. Normally none seen. May occur (a) as superficial gelatinous streaks or blobs ; (b) mixed with the stool, and only apparent on making a thin paste with water ; (c) mixed with blood, as in dysentery ; (d) composing almost the entire stool, sometimes as firm bands or cords.

6. *Parasites.*—Various intestinal worms may be found. The

435

larger examples, such as tapeworms and round worms, are usually obvious, but the smaller forms, such as thread worms and whip worms, should be searched for by converting the whole stool into a thin paste with water and then sifting this slowly and carefully through a double layer of butter muslin or a fine wire sieve spread tautly over a bowl or basin.

7. *Reaction.*—The normal reaction is neutral or slightly alkaline. An acid reaction usually indicates some fermentation in the gut or an excess of vegetables in the diet. The stools of infants are usually acid.

BLOOD EXAMINATIONS

THE various chemical, serological, and cytological examinations on the blood are in the domain of the pathologist. Whenever blood is to be collected from a vein the following points should be observed :—

1. The syringe and needle should be not only sterile but either dry or washed out with sterile normal saline solution. In particular the syringe should contain no trace of alcohol or ether, and preferably no distilled water.

2. The blood withdrawn is put into test-tubes which are sterile and either (*a*) plain dry or (*b*) oxalated (*i.e.*, contain a small quantity of sodium or potassium oxalate powder).

(*a*) Plain tubes are required for : Wassermann reaction, Widal and other agglutination reactions, v.d. Bergh reaction, blood calcium.

(*b*) Oxalated tubes are required for : Blood sugar, blood urea, non-protein nitrogen (N.P.N.), etc.

3. Immediately the blood has been expelled from the syringe, this and the needle should be washed out with normal saline or *cold* water. In this way "jamming" of the piston is avoided.

DIETARY TABLES

These Tables were prepared by Miss A. F. Gent, late Sister-Tutor, Westminster Hospital, London, who has kindly given permission for their use.

SINCE diet plays such an important part in the maintenance of health and in the treatment of disease, the modern nurse must understand food values and their significance during illness and convalescence. An adequate general diet must contain the following food substances :—

1. Organic { Protein.
   Carbohydrate.
   Fat.

2. Inorganic { Water.
   Salts.

3. Accessory food factors or vitamins.

FOOD.	SOURCE.	FUNCTION.	ELIMINATION.
Protein . (Nitrogenous)	Lean meat. Fish. Eggs. Milk. Cheese. Certain fruits and vegetables.	Repair of body wear and tear, *i.e.*, it is concerned with the process of anabolism.	Is incompletely oxidized, and is not stored in the body but eliminated as waste matter in the form of urea, uric acid, and creatinin.
Carbohydrate .	Starches and sugars obtained chiefly from plants.	Produces and maintains body heat and energy.	Excess is converted into fat, and stored and used as such.

437

Food.	Source.	Function.	Elimination.
Fat	All animals and vegetable oils and fats.	Produces and maintains body heat and energy. Needs sufficient sugar for its complete oxidation.	Oxidized into $CO_2 + H_2O$, which is eliminated in the excretions. Fat can be stored when in excess and drawn upon when required.
Salts	Organic salts are derived from vegetable acids. Inorganic salts from the food generally.	Maintain the alkalinity of the blood, and aid growth, repair, and influence the action of heart and respiration.	
Vitamin	All animal and vegetable foods.	*See* **Vitamin** in "Dictionary."	
Water	Forms an important constituent of all foods, fruits, and vegetables. 2½ pints of drinking water should also be taken daily.	Essential to life.	In breath, skin, and kidneys.

CALORIFIC VALUE OF FOOD

THE amount of heat food can yield on complete combustion in the body is expressed in terms of calories (*q.v.*). It is known that—

> 1 gm. of protein yields 4·1 calories.
> „ carbohydrate yields 4·1 calories.
> „ fat yields 9·3 calories.

When the chemical composition of food is known, it is easy to estimate its calorific value. A well-balanced diet contains the three food substances in the correct proportions. Complete oxidation then occurs with a minimum of waste. Also—

1. A continued excess of protein throws too much work on the liver and kidneys.
2. Excess carbohydrate leads to digestive disorders, and results in faulty metabolism.
3. Fat requires sufficient carbohydrate for its complete combustion. Incomplete oxidation of fat results in acidosis (*q.v.*).

An average man, doing average work, needs 3,400 calories per day.

An average woman, doing average work, needs 2,500 calories per day.

An average child of ten needs 2,100 calories per day.

An average child of six needs 1,500 calories per day.

N.B.—Actual requirements are influenced by work, weight, build, season, and climate.

CALORIFIC VALUE OF COMMON ARTICLES OF DIET

Milk	100 gm. (3½ oz.)	yield	63⅗	calories.
Bread	„	„	„	296	„
Egg	„	„	„	142	„
Beef	„	„	„	172	„
Fish	„	„	„	65	„
Cheese	„	„	„	417	„
Bacon	„	„	„	490	„
Tomatoes	„	„	„	84	„
Pears	„	„	„	28	„

439

DIET IN DISEASE

DISEASE.	DIET.
Fever	Give 1. Minimum of fat—butter, milk, cream, and eggs. 2. Maximum of carbohydrate—sugar, starchy food, cereals, bread, potatoes, glucose, etc. 3. Bland fluids *ad lib.*—plain water, barley water, imperial drink, fruit juice, and water. Keep the bowels well open.
Rickets	Give a well-balanced diet with a sufficiency of protein and fat containing vitamins A and D. In addition, give— 1. Cod-liver oil ʒi t.d.s. ; or 2. Irradiated ergosterol. 3. Fruit juice, *e.g.*, oranges and limes.
Scurvy	Discontinue proprietary foods or sterilized and condensed milk for infant feeding, and give— 1. Fresh cows' milk. 2. Vitamin C in the form of orange juice, grape-fruit juice, or tomato juice, 1-2 tablespoons diluted with water and sweetened with sugar. 3. Potato cream. The flowery part of potato added to milk and creamed, and 6-8 teaspoonfuls given daily. 4. For adults, an abundance of fresh fruits and vegetables.
Heart Disease	Avoid heavy, indigestible meals and give— 1. Nourishing fluids, especially egg flip, milk, whey, and beef-tea. 2. Solid meals are given in small quantity, but frequently. 3. When œdema is present, fluids are restricted and salt is forbidden, also alcohol and highly seasoned foods.

DISEASE.	DIET.

Phthisis . The diet should be generous and varied, and the tastes and appetite of the patient consulted. Fatigue must be avoided and an hour's complete rest before the mid-day and evening meal is essential. The diet includes eggs, milk, cream, plenty of butter, soups, poultry, meats, salads and vegetables, suet pudding, cakes, fruit, tea, and coffee. Cod-liver oil, or cod-liver oil and malt, are usually ordered.

Gastric Ulcer . A. *Lenhartz diet*, or a modification, is usually prescribed. It consists of hourly feeds for ten days of eggs beaten up with milk, to which a little sugar is added. First day, 1 egg with 8 oz. of milk. One egg and 4 oz. of milk is added daily until the patient is receiving 6 eggs and 2 pints of milk. On the third day sugar is added. On the seventh day a little raw minced meat is given, after which the diet is gradually extended until full diet is being taken with comfort.

B. *Hurst's diet* may be prescribed :—

7.30 A.M.	Milk, 8 oz.	
9 ,,	Arrowroot or Benger's, 7 oz.; rusk and butter; red currant or apple jelly.	
11 ,,	Junket or custard, 8 oz.	
1 P.M.	Potatoes, parsnip, cauliflower, 8 oz.; rusk and butter.	
3 ,,	Milk, 8 oz.	
5 ,,	Arrowroot or Benger's, 7 oz.; rusk and butter.	
7 ,,	Junket or custard, 8 oz.	
9 ,,	Milk, 8 oz.	

Pernicious Anæmia The following may be given :—

1. Red meat, such as liver, kidney, heart, and also brains. Calf-liver is the best. If liver is not well tolerated, liver extract or ventriculin may be given.

DISEASE.	DIET.

2. Fresh fruit and vegetables.
3. Sometimes dilute hydrochloric acid is prescribed for an hour after a meal, taken in sips.
4. Carbohydrates are given in moderation.
5. Fats are restricted.

Diarrhœa . At first all food is withheld, but plenty of fluid allowed, *e.g.*, water, barley water, albumen water, and lime water. A chalk mixture is prescribed by mouth, and a starch and opium enema to relieve pain and tenesmus. Semi-solids are gradually introduced and the diet gradually built up. The patient must be kept warm, and a little alcohol may be ordered in the form of brandy.

Constipation . May be due, among other things, to—

(a) Deficient intake of cellulose.
(b) Weak peristalsis.
(c) Insufficient fluid.

The following should be given :—

1. Brown bread, porridge, vegetables (especially cabbage, turnips, spinach, onions), fruit, *e.g.*, apples, oranges, figs, prunes, etc.
2. A glass of water every morning and night.
3. Exercise.

Nephritis The diet depends somewhat on the type of nephritis present. In acute nephritis, fluid, especially milk, is given at first. Then farinaceous foods are gradually introduced, and later, fish, chicken, and light protein foods. When œdema is marked, fluids and salt are reduced to a minimum. In chronic nephritis, the diet consists chiefly of starchy foods, milk puddings, bread, butter, fish, green vegetables, salad, and fruit. In chronic interstitial nephritis, in which

DISEASE.	DIET.

the blood-pressure is high and there is little or no œdema, a low protein diet is indicated—red meat is restricted, and meat of any kind restricted to once a day. Vegetables, potatoes and fruit, milk puddings, bread, butter, and jam are allowed. Purin bodies, condiments, extractives, and alcohol are strictly avoided. Weak tea and coffee can be given once per day. Imperial drink, lemonade, and barley water are helpful.

Hyperpiesia .
(High blood-pressure.)

The diet should be arranged on vegetarian lines. Extractive and purin bodies withheld, carbohydrates in moderation, as they tend to cause obesity. Liquids and solid food taken in moderation.

(*See " Dietetics for Nurses," by I. Stewart. Faber & Gwyer Ltd.*)

Diabetes Mellitus

A disorder of nutrition in which not only carbohydrates are concerned, but also fat and protein. The diet combined with insulin must be so regulated that the patient can live and work comfortably. The calorific requirements of the patient are calculated 30, 35, to 40 calories per kilogram of body weight, according to hard work, moderate work, or rest. Many methods of dieting the patient have been evolved, but Dr Lawrence's " Diet Scheme " is one of the most modern methods in use. Each line represents 190 calories, and the patient is told how many lines he requires, and can choose his own dietary. The first half of each line indicates the carbohydrate, and the second half the protein and fat. The food must be carefully weighed, and only the stated amount taken. The physician prescribes the amount of insulin required by the patient, and each injection should be followed in twenty minutes by a meal. The injections are given twice a day, before breakfast and supper.

THE "LINE-RATION" SCHEME

By R. D. Lawrence, M.D., F.R.C.P.

One black portion added to one red portion=one Line ration.

Black Half-Lines.

Carbohydrate Foods (containing sugar or starch).

Black Portions (10 *gm. C.*).	*Oz.*
* Flour, rice, sago, tapioca (raw) . . .	2/5
Oatmeal, biscuit or toast; macaroni or prunes (dry) . . .	½
Bread (all kinds) . .	⅔
Potato, peas, broad beans, banana . . .	2
Parsnips or prunes (stewed); grapes	3
Beetroot; apple or pear (raw); dried apricots or peaches (stewed); ripe plums . .	4
Orange (skinned), or ripe greengages . .	5
Onions, carrots; cherries, peaches or gooseberries (all ripe) . . .	6
Milk; stewing apples or pears . . .	7
† Strawberries or apricots (ripe) . . .	8
Turnips, leeks, Jerusalem artichokes .	10
† Grape-fruit (in skin); blackberries (stewed)	10
† Brussel sprouts; raspberries or loganberries (raw) . . .	12

Red Half-Lines.

Red Portions (*Protein and Fat*). 7½ *gm. P. and* 15 *gm. F.* (*or* 9 *gm. F.*).	
1 egg and fat ¼ oz.	(0) oz.
Bacon 1 oz. . .	(lean only)
Ham 1 oz. and fat ¼ oz.	(0) oz.
Kipper 1¼ oz. and fat ½ oz.	(¼) ,,
Herring 1 oz. and fat ½ oz.	(¼) ,,
Lean beef or mutton 1 oz. and fat ½ oz.	(¼) ,,
Lean lamb or veal 1 oz. and fat ½ oz.	(¼) ,,
Lean pork 1 oz. and fat ½ oz.	(¼) ,,
Chicken or duck 1 oz. and fat ½ oz.	(¼) ,,
Tongue (tinned or fresh) 1 oz. and fat ¼ oz.	(0) ,,
Liver 1 oz. and fat ½ oz.	(¼) ,,
Kidney or tripe 1¼ oz. and fat ½ oz.	(¼) ,,
Rabbit or hare ½ oz. and fat ½ oz.	(¼) ,,
Cheese ¾ oz. and fat ¼ oz.	(0) ,,
White fish; sweetbreads 1¼ oz. and fat ½ oz.	(¼) ,,

THE " LINE-RATION " SCHEME—*continued.*

Black Half-Lines.

Carbohydrate Foods (containing sugar or starch).

Black Portions (10 *gm.* C.)   *Oz.*

†Red currants ;   stewing greengages, damsons, plums or apricots   .   12

†Melon (raw) ;   endive (raw)   .   .   .   14

(† Half portions of these are usually enough.)

Negligible Starch Content in Average Helpings of—Asparagus, green artichokes, French beans, cabbage, cauliflower, celery, cranberries, cress, cucumber, black currants, egg plant, stewing gooseberries, greens, horse-radish, lemons, lettuce, marrow, mushrooms, radishes, rhubarb, salsify, scarlet runners, sea kale, spinach, tomato (raw or cooked).

Red Half-Lines.

Red Portions (*Protein and Fat*). 7½ *gm.* P. *and* 15 *gm.* F. (*or* 9 *gm.* F.).

Sardines 1 oz. and fat ¼ oz.   (0) oz.

Salmon 1 oz. and fat ½ oz.   (¼) ,,

Crab or lobster 1½ oz. and fat ½ oz.   (¼) ,,

Pheasant, grouse, partridge, ¾ oz. and fat ½ oz.   (¼) ,,

Fats are meat fats, suet, dripping, butter, margarine, olive oil ; thick cream in twice the amount stated for other fats.

* Articles starred to be taken only if specially allowed by physician.

Extras of no food value.—Tea, coffee, soda, water, bovril, oxo, etc., ordinary condiments and flavourings.

N.B.—This diet scheme can be obtained in a card form suitable for patient's use from Messrs H. K. Lewis & Co. Ltd., Gower Street, London.

INFANT FEEDING

To feed a normal baby from birth to six months :—

The Feed.—

Boiled cows' milk, 1 pint.
Water, ½ pint.
Brown Demerara sugar, three level tablespoons.

Amount.—Of this mixture give the following :—

When baby weighs		5 lbs., give			6 feeds of		2½ oz.	
,,	,,	6	,,	,,	6	,,	2½	,,
,,	,,	7	,,	,,	6	,,	3	,,
,,	,,	8	,,	,,	6	,,	3½	,,
,,	,,	9	,,	,,	6	,,	3¾	,,
,,	,,	10	,,	,,	5	,,	5	,,
,,	,,	11	,,	,,	5	,,	5½	,,
,,	,,	12	,,	,,	5	,,	6½	,,
,,	,,	13	,,	,,	5	,,	6½	,,
,,	,,	14	,,	,,	5	,,	7	,,
,,	,,	15	,,	,,	5	,,	7	,,

Quick Feeding.—See that the hole of the teat is a good size, so that the baby can get the feed in ten minutes easily.

Times.—

Six feeds : 6, 9, 12, 3, 6, and 10 P.M.
Five feeds : 6, 10, 2, 6, and 10 P.M.

Breaking Wind.—Hold baby up for 20 minutes after each feed, till wind is broken twice.

Fruit Juice.—Give orange or tomato juice, 2 or 3 teaspoonfuls, diluted with water and sweetened with sugar, daily.

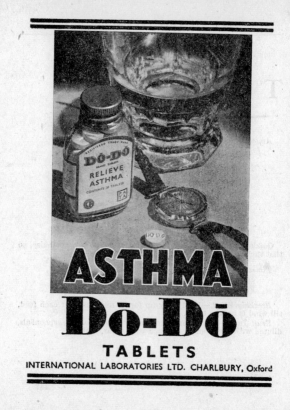

COMMENCEMENT OF MIXED FEEDING

Diet Sheet No. 1

For infants from six to nine months old.   (Weight, 15-18 lbs.)

6 A.M.	10 A.M.	2 P.M.	6 P.M.	10 P.M.
Milk (5 oz.). Water (2 oz.). Sugar (1 heaped teaspoonful), or breast-feed.	Milk (5 oz.). Water (2 oz.). Sugar (1 heaped teaspoonful). Robinson's patent groats, or Patentbarley, or Cream of rice (Groult's), or Allenbury's No. 3, or Glaxo Farex food. One heaped teaspoonful of any of the above, either in bottle or semi - solid from cup.	Bone and vegetable soup (2 tablespoons) mixed with milk (5 oz.). Sugar (1 heaped teaspoonful) or breast-feed.	Same as 10 A.M.	Same as 6 A.M.

Note.—Groats should not be given more than once a day. The juice of half an orange diluted with water and sweetened with sugar should be given daily, and all the milk should be well boiled.

If breast-fed, the cereal at 10 A.M. and 6 A.M. and the soup at 2 P.M. should be given from a cup or bottle made up with 1 oz. of water and 2 oz. of milk

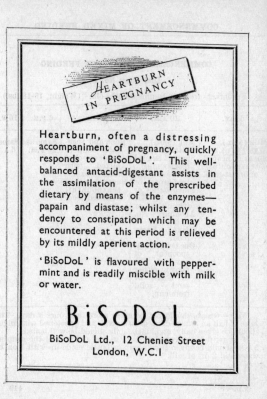

Diet Sheet No. 2.—Diet for children from nine months to one year. (Weight, 18-22 lbs.)

6 A.M.	8 A.M.	12.30 P.M.	4.30-5 P.M.	10 P.M.
Orange - juice or grape-juice (1 tablespoonful). 1 baked crust.	Porridge or groats from a cup given with a spoon (half a cup), or Baked crust and milk, or Half a Robb's biscuit with milk. Four mornings in the week, ½ egg. Two mornings, toast crumbs or crisp toast fried in bacon fat. Milk (8 oz.) to include that used above.	Bone and vegetable soup (4 tablespoonfuls). A little meat left on the bone and the soup thickened with potato and served with green vegetable (sieved). Cream of rice, tapioca, sago, or semolina (Groult's) (1 tablespoonful with sugar), or jelly or apple sauce. Milk (4 oz.) Water to drink.	Cream of rice, tapioca, sago, or semolina (Groult's), or Baked crust and milk or Robb's biscuit (half a cupful). Milk (8 oz.) to include that used above.	4 oz. of milk if necessary, but the child need not to be wakened for it.

Note.—As the child approaches its first birthday, the following may be added to the 12.30 meal : Brains or steamed or boiled fish or underdone scraped meat.

At the 4.30 meal, junket and stewed fruit or custard may take the place of the cereal foods given above.

Groult's cream of rice, sago, semolina, and tapioca will be found most suitable for children.

Diet Sheet No. 3.—Diet from one to two years

6 A.M.	8 A.M. Breakfast.	12.30 P.M. Dinner.	4.30-5 P.M. (6.15 P.M., see footnotes). Tea.
Juice of half an orange or a dessertspoonful of grape-juice.	Groats or porridge (1 tablespoonful), or Baked crust in milk, or Robb's biscuit in milk. Toast fried in bacon fat or small rasher of crisp bacon, or soft-boiled egg, with breadcrumbs, 2 per week only. Pounded, boiled, or steamed fish. Stewed apple or prunes (1 tablespoonful). Milk (boiled), 8 oz., including that given with groats or porridge.	Fish (boiled or steamed or Brains, tripe, scraped raw meat, or underdone meat, or Irish stew (1 level tablespoon of any of the above). Boiled, baked, or mashed potato (1 rounded tablespoonful). Sieved sprouts, cabbage, spinach, greens, cauliflower, or parsnip. Milk pudding (1 tablespoonful) or stewed apples, prunes, or junket or custard. 4 oz. of milk at the meal over pudding as junket. Water to drink.	Baked crust or Robb's biscuit and a small sponge cake, a little honey, seedless jam, or overripe banana (mashed), or Custard or junket. Milk (boiled), 8 oz., to include that used with above.

It ought not to be necessary to give anything after tea at 4.30-5 P.M. If the child requires a drink before being put to bed, a portion of the 8 oz. allowed for tea should be utilized.

N.B.—These three tables are used by Dr Donald Paterson, and supplied to out-patients at several London hospitals. They appear in Paterson and Forest-Smith's "Modern Methods of Feeding in Infancy and Childhood" (Constable & Co. Ltd.).

NOTES

NOTES

THE ELIMINATION OF PAIN

The administration of a safe sedative is often desirable in conjunction with the treatment of conditions which cause pain and distress.

'Anadin,' a well-balanced combination in the aspirin-phenacetin-caffeine group, can be relied upon for rapidity of action in the elimination of pain. It has no unpleasant after-effects and is unlikely to cause gastric disturbance. Moreover, 'Anadin' is not conducive to habit-formation and is, therefore, completely safe in the hands of the patient.

ANADIN Tablets